Mama might be better off dead

Phyllis and Herb
Goldberg,

To people who
understand and
have their own
stories to tell!

[signature]

LAURIE KAYE ABRAHAM

Mama might b

The University of Chicago Press ◆ *Chicago and London*

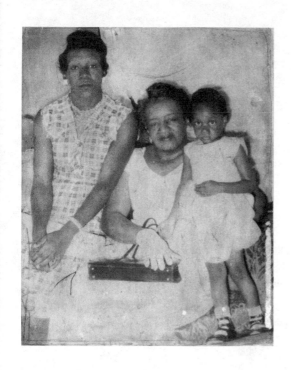

etter off dead

THE FAILURE OF HEALTH CARE IN URBAN AMERICA

LAURIE KAYE ABRAHAM, an award-winning investigative
journalist, has a master's degree in journalism from Northwestern University
and a master's degree in law from Yale University.

The University of Chicago Press, Chicago 60637
The University of Chicago Press, Ltd., London
© 1993 by The University of Chicago
All rights reserved. Published 1993
Printed in the United States of America

02 01 00 99 98 97 96 95 94 93   1 2 3 4 5
ISBN: 0-226-00138-5 (cloth)

Library of Congress Cataloging-in-Publication Data

Abraham, Laurie Kaye.
    Mama might be better off dead : the failure of health care in
urban America / Laurie Kaye Abraham.
        p.   cm.
    1. Urban poor—Medical care—United States—Case studies.
    2. Poor—Medical care—Illinois—Chicago—Case studies.
    3. Urban poor—Medical care—Government policy—United
States. I. Title.
    [DNLM: 1. Quality of Health Care—United States.
    2. Poverty—United States. W 84 AA1 A127m 1993]
    RA418.5.P6A26   1993
    362.1'0425—dc20
    DNLM/DLC
    for Library of Congress   93-15514
                                                                          CIP

Contents

Preface

This book followed the Banes family, Cora Jackson, and Tommy Markham from May 1989 to April 1990. I continued to gather material from their lives and research the book after that time, however, and so much of the data about the institutions or health care system is more current. This is indicated either in the text or the notes. Apart from the Epilogue, the only scenes involving the family that took place after spring 1990 are in chapter 8, chronicling doctors' appointments that I attended with Tommy Markham. The flashbacks to events which occurred before May 1989 are reconstructed from medical records and information the family provided. Scenes in which the family was not involved, such as those that took place in Mount Sinai Hospital's emergency room, happened anywhere between summer 1989 and fall 1991.

To protect their privacy, I changed the names of all family members, as well as other patients whose stories I told. The names of all doctors, nurses, and other health care professionals are real, except for Dr. Burton Stone, who is discussed in chapter 13. I interviewed all doctors, nurses, and health care "experts" quoted in this book, unless a footnote indicates otherwise.

Acknowledgments

J ackie and Robert Banes, the children—Latrice, DeMarest, and Brianna—Cora Jackson, and Tommy Markham made this book possible with their generosity of time and spirit. The longer I worked on the book, the more I came to respect this family, and care for them. Their willingness to share their lives, to let me into their home at all hours of day and night, sometimes astounded me. I always appreciated it. Jackie was the guiding light for the book, just as she is for her family. Her tough-mindedness, her humor, her indignation at injustice were alternately a joy and a challenge to me. I am forever grateful to Jackie and her family.

Many others deserve thanks for this book, and the best place to start is at the beginning. The publisher of the *Chicago Reporter*, Roy Larson, hired me in February 1989 to bring "people" into the investigative publication's health care reporting. We envisioned a series of stories on health care for the poor, though neither of us was sure what form it should take. But, Roy said, if the articles were successful, perhaps I might expand the series into a book. Roy's trust in me, his faith in both my writing and my ability to conceive and execute such a project, launched the book.

My editor and friend, Laura Green, made an equally important contribution. She moved to New York soon after I began the book, and in our effort to do the Baneses' story justice we spent long hours on the phone, and she spent many more hours carefully editing each chapter. Her skillful editing, her wonderful turns of phrase, and most of all her wisdom, permeate each page.

Deepest appreciation goes to the foundations and individuals whose financial support allowed me to write the book: the Community Renewal Society, which publishes the *Chicago Reporter*; the Joyce Foundation; the Robert Wood Johnson Foundation; the Retirement Research Foundation; the Woods Charitable Fund, Inc.; Richard J. Dennis, and Bernice Weissbourd. Thanks also go to Russell Hardin, who helped me find my way to the University of Chicago Press, and to senior editor John Tryneski, whose advice and reassurance kept me going once I got there.

This book is infused with the perceptions, sentiments, and facts and figures of countless people whom I interviewed—once, twice, and, in some cases, dozens of times. I thank them all. Nurses, doctors, social workers, and administrators at Mount Sinai Hospital and at Schwab Rehabilitation Center were enormously helpful. My gratitude to Benn Greenspan, chief executive of Mount Sinai, for his time and frankness at our breakfast meetings; to Dr. Karen O'Mara for guiding me through the emergency room; and to Sister Mary Ellen Meckley for showing me that the biggest inequities are found in the smallest places. I am especially grateful for the help and friendship of Diane Dubey. A former reporter herself, Diane knows what reporters want and how to get it. And I will not soon forget the honesty and compassion of the physician described in the book under the pseudonym of Burton Stone.

The staff at Lawndale Christian Health Center impressed me with their kindness and efficiency. I am particularly thankful for the inspiration and insight of the health center's founder, Dr. Arthur Jones.

For the chapters on dialysis and transplant, I am indebted to Patricia Barber, formerly of the University of Illinois Hospital's transplant program; Joan Shepard, executive director of the National Kidney Foundation of Chicago; Dr. Gordon Lang, president of Neomedica Dialysis Centers, Inc.; the staff at the Renal Network of Illinois, especially Cheryl Anderson; Dr. Raymond Pollak; and J. Michael Dennis.

At the Illinois Department of Public Aid, Dean Schott, Rose Dupont, Bill Opper, Fred Wood, and Diane Hayes were generous and patient. The same appreciation to Joy Getzenberg at the Chicago Department of Health; Jean Blaser, Illinois Department on Aging; Beth Yudkowsky, American Academy of Pediatrics; and the *Chicago Sun-Times* clip-library. For helping me wade through the Chicago Jewish Archives, thanks to Norma Spungen. Finally, when I needed a knowledgeable ear, I depended on Michael Gelder, Dr. Gordon Schiff, Dr. Terry Conway, Mary Gugenheim, and Dr. Quentin Young.

By writing this book, I realized how lucky I am to have so many gifted writers and editors for friends. Thanks to Todd Savage for his meticulous (and witty!) fact-checking, and to John Schrag, whose sensitive editing of the series helped shape the book. Apart from Laura Green, Glenn Coleman was the first person to read the book; his enthusiasm about it emboldened me to persevere. When Laura Green and I had become so close to the book that we worried we were losing our perspective, Lisa Chase stepped in. Before the second draft of the manuscript went to the press, Lisa copyedited every chapter, helping to trim the fat and smooth out what was left. Both Glenn and Lisa also gave me plenty of encouragement, sharing meals with me, comforting me when my confidence wavered, and just being there.

Steve Hetcher was also there—in my heart, as we were separated by a thousand miles while he was away at school. He, too, kept me from faltering, lending me courage, even a bit of his own bravado. In the beginning, he was the one who inspired me to think big, and he stayed with me until the end.

Finally, I want to thank my father, Harold Abraham, who has encouraged me to take risks since he coached my grade school softball teams, and most of all, my mother, Kaye Price, for always, always, believing that I could do it. Her passionate commitment to fairness and justice gave birth to this book.

Introduction

I n the fall of 1991, Harris Wofford, a relatively unknown Democrat
from Pennsylvania, won a seat in the U.S. Senate after making
sweeping health care reform the centerpiece of his campaign. The
victory surprised politicians, who had expected his opponent, Richard
Thornburgh, the U.S. Attorney General for the first three years of the
Bush administration, to coast into office. Wofford subsequently became
a symbol of Americans' dissatisfaction with the health care system and
desire for change. A January 1992 survey showed that the public
ranked health care as one of the top three issues the country's leaders
needed to address,[1] and ten months later, Bill Clinton took advantage
of that. Campaigning for president on a platform of change, he made
fixing the nation's ailing health care system one of his top priorities.
As of the spring of 1993, it was not clear what shape health care
reform would take under a Clinton administration, but the new president certainly had no shortage of proposals from which to choose. A
1992 article in the *Journal of the American Medical Association* summarized
just the "important" health care plans sitting on the nation's plate; there
were forty-one of them.[2]

The millions of uninsured Americans and the spiraling cost of health
care received progressively more attention through the last half of the
1980s. But what finally pushed health care reform to the top of the
national agenda, many believe, was the discontent of the middle class.
Middle-class families with sick children were being priced out of group
insurance, even plans offered by large companies; others were stuck in
dead-end jobs because "preexisting medical conditions" prevented
them from getting insurance from a new employer; and still others lost
medical coverage when they were laid off during the economic recession that began in mid-1990.

In some ways, this book has nothing to do with the insurance woes of the middle class; in others, it has everything to do with them. At the book's center are four generations of a black family who live in one of Chicago's poorest neighborhoods, called North Lawndale. The grandmother, Cora Jackson, was sixty-nine years old when I first met her in May 1989, and trying to cope with myriad chronic conditions, including high blood pressure and diabetes. She lived with her granddaughter, Jackie Banes, who cared for Mrs. Jackson as well as her own three children and her ailing husband, Robert. His kidneys failed when he was twenty-seven, and he then needed dialysis treatments three times a week to stay alive. Finally, there is Jackie's father and Mrs. Jackson's son, Tommy Markham, who was only forty-eight when he was disabled by a stroke caused by uncontrolled high blood pressure.

For the past three years, I have moved in and out of this family's life in an attempt to discover what health care policies crafted in Washington, D.C., or in the state capitol at Springfield, look like when they hit the street. This book provides a qualitative description that is now missing in our understanding of the much-studied problem of lack of access to care. As a reporter who has covered public health first for a socioeconomic medical newspaper and then for an investigative publication focused on race and poverty, I had written repeatedly about the big picture: high infant mortality rates, the surging uninsured population, the scourge of AIDS. Only by following a family for an extended period of time, however, was I able to get beyond the one-time tragedies and endless flow of health statistics that make the news and begin to understand the oft-repeated phrase "lack of access to care." It can be a slippery concept to grasp, perhaps because its meaning has been deadened by overuse but also because, for the poor, it manifests itself in more subtle ways than their being uninsured—ways that are inconceivable to most of us. I came to know Jackie Banes not as a helpless victim but as a resourceful woman who tried to work the health care nonsystem to the best of her ability. The lengths to which she went to get basic care for her family are one testament to the inadequacy of health care for the poor. The other is that her efforts so often failed.

Cradle-to-grave, this family has been largely left out of a health care system that is one of the best in the industrialized world for those who are affluent and well insured and embarrassingly bad for those who are not. Ten, even five years ago, those of us in the middle class might have dismissed the poor's struggle to get decent health care as something we would never come close to experiencing. No longer. Most everyone has a relative or friend who is uninsured and crossing her fingers, or who is overwhelmed by huge medical bills or insurance premiums. So far, their hardships may not have approached those the Banes family encountered when they tried to get medical care, but their experience carries a warning for us all: things will get worse, provided that private insurers continue the trend toward pushing all but the healthiest and wealthiest from their rolls, leaving the rest either uninsured or reliant on what are currently inadequate public programs.

But this book was not intended to persuade the middle class that some kind of health care reform is in their personal best interest. Just as doctors use CAT-scans and other instruments to uncover disease, this book exposes glaring inequities in health care access and quality that exist between the moneyed and the poor, inequities that existed long before the middle class began to feel the pinch. The place to start is with the uninsured. The poor are more likely to be uninsured than anybody else, and as Tommy Markham said: "You could be damn near dying, and the first thing they ask is 'Do you have *insurance?*'" Though his words succinctly express his indignation toward a system based on ability to pay, this book suggests that perhaps the *only* time the uninsured have a good chance of getting timely, quality care is when they are damn near death.

Robert Banes could not get reliable, steady medical coverage until his kidneys failed, and it took a stroke for Tommy Markham to get the same. Neither have held the kind of jobs that provide health insurance, and serious sickness or disability often are the only tickets to government health insurance for poor, single men under sixty-five.[3] During Jackie's first pregnancy, she was uninsured and delayed getting prenatal care for six months, when she went to one of the few places where the uninsured are certain to get care, if only after daylong waits: the emergency room of the city's overburdened, underfunded public institution, Cook County Hospital. Though no one would choose to have a baby at Cook County, where pregnant women are herded into narrow stalls like cattle and labor side by side separated by thin curtains, Jackie was lucky in some ways to have County to go to. Public hospitals in other cities, most notably Philadelphia, recently were forced to shut their doors when government support dried up.

Once Jackie gave birth to Robert's daughter Latrice, she and the little girl were covered by Medicaid—at least as long as Jackie stayed unemployed. Medicaid, the state and federal health care program for the poor, has never lived up to its promise to eliminate the country's two-tiered system of health care. First, Medicaid income restrictions are so tight that the program covers less than half of the poor, defined as those Americans who fall under the federal poverty level. Most of the working poor were and still are excluded from Medicaid and thus are uninsured, although some of their children are being progressively added to the program under reforms that began in the late 1980s. Those who manage to get Medicaid have struggled to find decent doctors. Medicaid pays physicians well below the rates of commercial insurers, and doctors perceive the poor as "difficult" patients, sometimes with reason. Poor patients' ailments are made worse by delays in getting care, and they show up at doctors' offices with more of what one physician called "sociomas," social problems that range from not having a ride to the doctor's office, to drug addiction, to homelessness, to the despair that accompanies miserable life circumstances. As for the physicians who do practice in poor neighborhoods, they may be there only because they are not good enough to work anywhere else. Poor families usually have no way of knowing whether local doctors are up to snuff, even when they have been disciplined by state medical regulators.

While Medicaid recipients are exceedingly vulnerable to the vagaries of state and federal budgets—benefits are cut when times are tight or whole categories of people are eliminated from the program—Medicare is an entitlement program that covers most Americans who are older than sixty-five and certain disabled people. Because Medicare is an entitlement, the federal government cannot cut people from the program willy-nilly. Payments to doctors and hospitals can be reduced, however, and they have been, though Medicare still pays much better than Medicaid, and its lower rates have not seriously curtailed the elderly's access to city doctors and hospitals. What bedevils the poor, as Cora Jackson could attest, are Medicare's gaps. It does not pay for medication, for transportation, for many basics that may sound wholly affordable to those with generous pensions or insurance to supplement Medicare. But such essentials strap the poor, who often end up going without.

The Banes family also faced a special set of hurdles because they are African American. The long wait Robert and other blacks face when they seek kidney transplants—almost twice that of whites—is a good example. While some of that is rooted in blacks' disproportionate poverty and even biological factors, subtle racism also came into play. Far too often health professionals tended to downplay the effect of race on their interactions with patients or the distribution of resources, and sorting out the influence of race from poverty was not always possible. But race had an undeniable effect in one particularly striking way. The history of hideous medical experimentation with black subjects, and its present day vestiges, made many blacks I interviewed suspicious of the medical system and sometimes compromised their access to care. More than a year after I met the family, I discovered that Tommy Markham had participated in a kind of medical research that today would be unthinkable. His experience helps to explain the persistence of AIDS conspiracy theories among blacks, something many whites perfunctorily disregard as paranoia.

While Medicaid and Medicare have failed poor patients, they also have failed to sustain the institutions that serve them. They, too, are a major part of the story of health care for the poor. The evolution of Mount Sinai Hospital Medical Center, which started the century treating poor Jewish immigrants and ended it treating poor blacks and Hispanics, provides ample evidence of the distortions in a system driven by the relative generosity of insurers. With Medicare and Medicaid paying at cost and below, hospitals have come to rely on a perverse system of cost-shifting: that is, covering the costs of uninsured, Medicaid, and Medicare patients by charging the privately insured higher and higher rates, which in turn increases the premiums employers and workers pay and contributes to the middle-class health care squeeze. It is a game of dominoes, but one that Mount Sinai and other hospitals that treat mostly poor patients cannot play. Only 6 percent of Mount Sinai's patients are covered by commercial insurance, leaving the hospital without shifting room. "It's hard to cost-shift 94 percent of your business to 6 percent," said Charles Weis, the institution's chief financial officer.[4]

Financial realities like these explain why Mount Sinai, which sits in the heart of North Lawndale, one of Chicago's sickest and poorest neighborhoods, spent much of the 1970s and part of the next decade trying to replace local patients with those from other parts of the city and the suburbs. It is not that Mount Sinai's leaders were particularly cold-hearted or greedy; rather, that is the way most hospitals did and continue to do business. Mount Sinai does not try to fight the inevitable anymore; more than perhaps any other hospital in the Chicago area, its leaders have chosen to devote the institution to serving its natural constituents, the poor. But only great ingenuity and commitment have allowed the hospital to survive, and it still continues to finish most years in the red. As one Chicago health care pundit put it, "I can't tell you Sinai won't go down in a year. Springfield [the state capital] could do it, a lot of things could do it." Hospitals in impoverished areas nationwide have fallen in great numbers, which sets up another game of dominoes, one in which the poor and their institutions are again the losers. The more hospitals that close, the greater the burden on those that remain and the higher the chances that they, too, will succumb. More is less for hospitals when more is more patients who cannot pay their way.

I observed the Baneses' interaction with dozens of doctors, nurses, and assorted health care workers during the course of researching this book. One discovery that at first surprised me, though in retrospect is completely understandable, was that the best of the lot had strong religious ties. Three of those people are discussed in some detail: Sister Mary Ellen Meckley, a home social worker and nun since her teens; Dr. Burton Stone (not his real name), an Orthodox Jewish internist who bases his practice at Mount Sinai; and Dr. Arthur Jones, an internist and urban Christian missionary who founded and runs a community health center for the poor near the Baneses' apartment. What set them apart was the compassion and respect they showed their patients. That is not as easy or common as it sounds. Benn Greenspan, president of Mount Sinai, described a hospital staff simmering with an anger that occasionally erupted. "What does it do to you when every day of your life you try to fulfill your professional responsibilities with less resources than you think you should have, with poorer [health] outcomes than you know you could get someplace else? You get angry, and you can take it out on your patients." Considering that the medical system is set up to reward doctors and other health care workers who care for not the sick but the sick and insured, I should have expected that those who did their jobs with uncommon skill and grace would have incentives other than the ordinary.

Dr. Stone, Dr. Jones, and Sister Mary Ellen worked in primary care, the front line of medicine designed to detect and treat illness before it becomes serious and costly. It is in this area that shortages are most dire in poor neighborhoods, as the crowds who seek basic care in Mount Sinai's emergency room attest. Once again, the medical reimbursement system takes much of the blame for discouraging physicians' interest in primary care, biased as it is toward acute, high-technology care.

During a meeting with Dr. Jones, I watched him read the results of electrocardiograms, tests that diagnose disorders of the heart. They were printed on strips of paper that Dr. Jones glanced at for a few seconds each. "See how long it takes me to read one of these," he said, disgusted. "And I get $8.65 for each of them [from Medicaid], versus $18.00 for a twenty to thirty minute office visit. It doesn't pay to sit and deal with people's emotional problems. It pays to do a procedure where all you have to do is walk in and walk out." The government has begun to try to correct some of the imbalances in Medicare payments, which may seep over into Medicaid, but the changes probably will not be big enough to lure many more doctors into primary care, especially in poor neighborhoods.

Yet Dr. Jones's half-hour sessions of explanation, the time for give-and-take between him and his patients, are as important to the poor as well-equipped hospitals and clinics. Lacking the education or confidence to push doctors and others for the information they needed, members of the Banes family often were in the dark about what was being done to them. And confusion sometimes turned to anger and alienation

The indifference to primary care reflected in the medical reimbursement system is mirrored by the devaluing of public health programs. Among other achievements, public health has benefited masses of Americans by controlling contagious disease and ensuring safe food and water, but the functions performed by local and state public health departments historically have been shortchanged, the legacy of which has tragic results for poor families. Despite a 1989 measles epidemic that killed nine Chicagoans, I found that the city Department of Health clinics, key providers of immunizations for poor children, were unorganized, understaffed, and unable to sustain a strong, consistent immunization campaign.

Medicaid, which is administered by the state's welfare department and sponsors its own program to promote immunizations and preventive care for children, was just as bad, if not worse. The chapter on preventive health care for children may have been the most sobering to write. If the public and private medical system has not found the will or the way to get basic preventive care to poor children—who, politicians insist, receive the highest priority—is it any wonder that poor women are dying in large numbers from cervical cancer, a preventable disease that can be detected by a simple pap smear?[5]

The Banes family was wonderfully generous with me. All they received in return for letting me snoop around their lives was a chance to share their troubles, perhaps, little else. My hope is that their story—and the stories of the hospitals and clinics that are barely surviving in poor neighborhoods—will be taken seriously by the leaders calling for change in America's health care system. Any reform plan that aspires to be both effective and just must pay careful attention to the day-to-day experiences of poor families. Anything less is not worth the effort.

1

"Where crowded humanity suffers and sickens":
The Banes family and their neighborhood

Robert Banes sat on the edge of his hospital bed, cradling his queasy stomach. A thin cotton gown hung on him like a sack. At five feet, eleven inches, Robert weighs only 137 pounds.

Robert's kidneys stopped functioning when he was twenty-seven. He received a transplant a year later, but his body rejected the new kidney after six years. Since then he has required dialysis treatments three times a week. Dialysis clears his body of the poisonous impurities that healthy people eliminate by urinating, but the treatments cannot completely restore his health, and Robert periodically spends a couple of days in the hospital. This time, he had been admitted to the University of Illinois Hospital because he had been urinating blood for a week, a problem that did not appear terribly serious to doctors but nonetheless had to be checked.

Feeling nauseated, Robert was not paying much attention to the game show that droned from his television. A nurse came in and stuck a thermometer in his mouth. Earlier in the day, Robert had undergone a cystoscopy, a procedure in which doctors put a miniaturized scope into his bladder to look for the source of his bleeding. He had not been told the results of the test, so he asked the nurse when his doctor would be stopping by. He also wanted to know how much longer he would have to stay in the hospital.

"You may have to go to surgery," the nurse said vaguely, flipping through his chart. A cloud passed briefly over Robert's face; the thought of surgery scared him, though he did not admit that to the nurse. Instead, he changed the subject.

"I guess I don't get dinner today," he said.

"You didn't get dinner?" she asked, surprised.

"I need some before I get sick."

"Don't do that," the nurse muttered as she walked out the door.

A minute later Robert hurried to the bathroom. "I was probably throwing up because I didn't have no food to push it down," he said, referring to the missed dinner. Robert returned to his bed and lay down, curling his knees into his stomach and pulling a blanket over his shivering body.

Four years before his kidneys failed, Robert was diagnosed with focal glomerulosclerosis, a progressive scarring of the kidneys that eventually destroys them. Focal glomerulosclerosis can be slowed though not cured, but Robert's disease went at its own destructive pace because he did not get medical treatment until his kidneys had reached the point of no return. None of Robert's low-paying, short-term jobs had provided health insurance, and he could not wriggle into any of the narrow categories of government-sponsored insurance, which are generally reserved for very poor mothers and children, the elderly, and the permanently disabled. In other words, Robert had not been poor-parent enough, old enough, or sick enough to get care.

The game show gave way to the news and a report about a "summer virus" that was infecting children. Robert frowned. He and his wife, Jackie, have two daughters and a son: eleven-year-old Latrice, four-year-old DeMarest, and one-year-old Brianna. "Don't tell me that," he sighed. That is Robert's typical response to bad news: he prefers to avoid it.

At the moment, however, Robert would not have minded a little bad news about his own condition. Since he had been admitted to the hospital on July 5, he had not been urinating as much blood, which frustrated him and Jackie. They felt he almost had to *prove* to doctors that he was sick.

Through his open door, Robert could see his wife arrive for an early evening visit. At five feet, ten inches, Jackie is only one inch shorter than her husband, but she weighs twenty pounds more than he does. When she smiles, her pretty, heart-shaped face gets full and round, captivating her baby daughter, who pokes at her cheeks and giggles, making Jackie giggle, too.

Jackie was not smiling that day, however. When she is in public, Jackie can look impassive, even defiant, though this vanishes when her curiosity gets the better of her. She walked slowly past the nursing station looking straight ahead, moving almost regally, her muscular thighs curving beneath her slacks. Next to her husband's brittle frame, Jackie stood like an oak.

She pulled up a chair next to the hospital bed, and Robert began to relay the sketchy medical update he had heard from the nurse. Jackie listened silently; then she responded in the way she sometimes does when she feels overwhelmed.

"I'm going away for a while," Jackie said coolly. "What are you all going to do without me?"

Robert did not reply. He knew, as she did, that she wasn't going anywhere; she was just letting off steam. Today had been her day to pay the bills, which she does in person since they are usually past due, and she had ridden the bus for hours in 90-degree heat.

Jackie told her husband to call home and tell Latrice to take some drumsticks out of the freezer for dinner. Jackie's invalid grandmother, with whom the family lives in one of Chicago's poorest neighborhoods, answered the phone, so Robert gave her the instructions instead. But a few minutes later Latrice called back because she was not sure her great-grandmother had heard the message correctly. In the way other children might memorize their parents' work numbers, Latrice had memorized the phone number for the university hospital, as well as for Mount Sinai Hospital Medical Center, where her great-grandmother frequently had been hospitalized. Jackie repeated the dinner instructions and hung up the phone. "I need the bed," she said.

She began to empty the stuffed grocery bag she had carried into the hospital. It contained two new T-shirts, underwear, and socks for Robert, a day-old piece of cake from Brianna's first birthday, which he had missed, a can of Sprite, and a bunch of grapes.

The couple watched part of another game show and talked about a report they had heard about a family found murdered mysteriously on the bottom of a lake. This story came from one of the tabloid news programs, whose bizarre stories the family regularly discusses. Then Jackie called home again to check on the children, who were home with her grandmother. The call was not reassuring: one of them had dropped cake on the rug, the other two had stepped in it, and DeMarest reportedly was taunting his great-grandmother.

"I need you to stay in here over the weekend so I can get things straightened out," Jackie wearily told her husband. When one or the other of her sick family members are hospitalized, Jackie sometimes considers it a chance to regroup, to get things together before she has to start taking care of everyone again.

Before Jackie left, she filled the plastic grocery bag she had emptied earlier. From Robert's belated dinner, she took a wedge of leftover chocolate cake home for DeMarest. She took packets of low-salt French dressing, salt, and sugar that Robert had squirreled away from his meal trays, as well as a roll of medical tape left by a nurse. Jackie carefully folded the foil Brianna's birthday cake had been wrapped in and stashed that in her bag, too.

Then she gave Robert $5.00 to pay for his hospital TV, which cost $3.25 a day. Robert slowly walked Jackie to the elevator, past a dimly lit room where the floor's patients congregated. One of the patients, a man about Robert's age, had earlier informed Robert that he was scheduled for a second transplant the next day. He told Robert that he had rejected his first transplanted kidney because he drank a case of beer in one evening—the kind of story that, true or not, flies back and forth among kidney transplant patients.

"This is my wife, Jackie," Robert said to a middle-aged woman sitting on the edge of the day room, closest to where the couple walked. "Nice to meet you," the woman said. Jackie smiled wanly, heading for the door.

The University of Illinois Hospital is part of what is known as the Illinois Medical Center, a 560-acre area just west of the Loop, Chicago's downtown. The center has the highest concentration of hospital beds in the United States, some 3,000 among its four institutions.[1] In addition to the University of Illinois, there is Cook County Hospital, one of the best-known, last remaining, and, as the ancient edifice continues to crumble, most notorious public hospitals in the country, and Rush-Presbyterian-St. Luke's Medical Center, an institution that caters to those who, unlike Robert and Jackie, are privately insured. The Veterans Administration West Side Medical Center is also located there.

The medical and technological might of the complex contrast dramatically with the area around it. Just past the research buildings and acres of parking lots lie some of the sickest, most medically underserved neighborhoods in the city. Medical wastelands abut abundance in American cities because health care is treated as a commodity available to those who can afford it, rather than a public good, like education. Though public schools invariably are better in prosperous suburbs than in poor city neighborhoods, every state at least provides every child with a school to attend, no matter what her family's income. The country has not even come that far with health care. Medicaid, the state and federal health insurance program intended for the poor, covers less than half of them, and much of the program is left to the states' discretion, so that a Southerner, for example, generally has to be poorer to receive Medicaid than a Northerner.

Even for those poor who manage to squeeze into Medicaid, the government's commitment to providing health care for them does not approach a commitment to equality. Just as education remains in practice separate and unequal, medical treatment for poor people with Medicaid or even Medicare (the government insurance for the elderly) is, in all but exceptional cases, conducted in a separate, second-rate environment.

The Banes family lives in the shadow of the Illinois Medical Center complex, twenty-five minutes southwest by way of the number 37 bus, which runs along Ogden Avenue. The street cuts diagonally across the city from the gentrified lakefront neighborhoods just north of the Loop to the bungalow enclaves of white ethnic suburbs that border Chicago on the southwest. Jackie and Robert live in between, on the West Side, the city's newest and poorest ghetto.

The streets were still lit by the late afternoon sun when Jackie climbed onto the bus for her trip home. Settling her bag on her lap, she fretted that doctors were going to release Robert before they figured out what was wrong with him. A person can only get so far with a "green card," she said, using the street name for the cards issued to families covered by Medicaid. "You need Palmer Courtland kind of money to get anywhere," she complained. Palmer Courtland is a self-made millionaire on "All My Children," a soap opera Jackie and Robert watch.

In addition to the hospitals and their services, programs in a clutch of other buildings near Ogden attempt to palliate what are often conditions born of poverty. There is the Illinois State Psychiatric Institute, the West Side Center for Disease Control, the Chicago Lighthouse for the Blind, and a bit further southwest, the Cook County Juvenile Court, which handles crimes by children, and those against them by their parents.

These buildings are strung along the Eisenhower Expressway, which zips from the booming Western suburbs into Chicago's downtown, whose dramatic growth in the past two decades has bypassed the West Side. Jackie rarely ventures into the Loop. From her perspective, the eight-lane highway is an escape route for the employees of the various hospitals and social service institutions, for people who do not carry poverty home with them in a plastic bag.

As Ogden turns more sharply to the west, it crosses into Jackie's neighborhood of North Lawndale, a name that carries the same ominous weight in Chicago as the South Bronx or Watts carry nationwide.[2] North Lawndale was the subject of a series in the *Chicago Tribune* in 1985 that examined the lives of the so-called underclass. Many people who work and live in North Lawndale were disturbed by what they thought was a distorted, overly negative picture of their neighborhood; the series' very name, "The American Millstone," is hated because it suggests a neighborhood that is no more than a burden to be cast off.

Jackie had never heard of the *Chicago Tribune* series; she reads the *Chicago Sun-Times*, whose pithy city coverage is preferred by poor Chicago blacks. Yet many of her observations of the neighborhood could have served as grist for the millstone.

"My auntie's building got burnt down," Jackie said matter-of-factly one day, pointing to an empty lot where her Aunt Nancy's apartment building used to stand. "Drug dealers moved in." The narrow lot is two lots away from the stone three-flat where Jackie grew up with her grandmother. The building has survived, though its balcony has disappeared and graffiti circles its porch columns. It is just a half-block away from where the family lives today. Since she was eight, Jackie has only once moved from this block, and that was a short three miles north to live with Robert at his mother's house. Her dreams of a better life are circumscribed by the neighborhood. She talks about getting out, but out means a strip of stone and brick three-flats about four blocks west. "I've always liked it up in that area," she said. "It looks like the middle-class people lives up in there, especially during the summer. All the trees are green and everyone has grass. And the buildings look well kept. You can just tell it's homeowners." Her assessment is accurate—the homes are better tended—but it is hardly out of the neighborhood. The buildings there may be relative castles, but the moat protecting them from the drugs and violence that pervade North Lawndale is narrow enough to step across.

As the bus hissed and groaned up Ogden, it passed Mount Sinai Hospital, which lives the same hand-to-mouth existence as the poor blacks and Hispanics it serves. More than the University of Illinois, Mount Sinai is the Baneses' hospital. It is where Jackie's grandmother,

Cora Jackson, had been repeatedly hospitalized because of complications from diabetes that eventually resulted in the amputation of her right leg. It's where Jackie's father was rushed after he suffered a stroke caused by high blood pressure. And on a happier note, it's where Jackie gave birth to Brianna a year ago.

At one time or another, the Baneses and Cora Jackson have sought (and not sought) health care in every way available to the poor. When uninsured—Robert, when his kidneys were deteriorating, and Jackie, when pregnant with Latrice—they delayed care, then went to Cook County Hospital. Later, when Jackie went on welfare, she and the children became eligible for Medicaid.

Meanwhile, some of Mrs. Jackson's medical bills were paid by Medicare, which covers the elderly and disabled, rich and poor alike. Robert also got Medicare but only after his kidneys stopped working. People with renal failure have special status under the program: they are the only group covered on the basis of their diagnosis and regardless of age or disability. Mrs. Jackson had been sporadically eligible for Medicaid, too, which she needed because Medicare does not pay for such important things as medications. Her Medicaid coverage had been fitful because she was enrolled in what is called the "spend-down" program. She qualified for Medicaid only during the months that her medical expenses were so high they forced her income to drop below a "medically needy" level set by the state. Notably, neither Mrs. Jackson, nor anyone else in the family, had ever been covered by private insurance.

Leaving Mount Sinai, the bus cut through Douglas Park, which spreads to the north and south of Ogden. Douglas and two other West Side parks were designed in 1870 as a system of "pleasure grounds" linked together by grand boulevards. Progressive reformers came to envision them as breathing spaces to provide respite from crowded tenements and other urban ills.[3] In its heyday from 1910 until 1930, when North Lawndale was populated by first- and second-generation Jews, bands gave free concerts on weekends, couples paddled rowboats on the lagoon just to the north of Ogden Avenue, and children swam in what was one of the city's first public swimming pools—which, with its baths, was considered as important for public hygiene as it was for recreation.

Except for the players and fans at soccer and baseball games, the park these days is barely dotted with people, a young Hispanic couple walking on a path on the south side of Ogden—the Hispanic side—or several dozen black children splashing in the lagoon to the north—the African-American side. Ogden is a dividing line between Hispanics and African Americans in North Lawndale, and the race line holds in the park as firmly as it does anywhere else in the neighborhood.

Though the park's glory has faded, it is the last piece of deliberately open land that Jackie passed on the Ogden bus. The rest of it consisted of a series of vacant lots, some of which run together for a block or more and which residents euphemistically call "prairies." As it was summer, some of the lots were covered with reedy grasses and weeds, frilly Queen Anne's lace, and deep brown stands of dock plant. Others were piled high with refuse—in one case, what looked like enough decaying furniture to fill an office. In another lot, a building had fallen in on itself, likely prey to the brick thieves who complete the destruction started when buildings are abandoned by landlords who can't afford their upkeep, then are stripped of sinks, stoves, and fixtures, and then finally picked apart, brick by brick. In still other lots, large fernlike weeds flourished, creating an urban jungle that suggests what a parish priest in a similar neighborhood in New Jersey called "panther beauty, beauty you don't want to mess with."[4]

As for the brick and stone two-flats, or old three-story apartment buildings still standing, it is often difficult to tell whether they are occupied or not. Rusty steel grates are locked across nearly every door, even those of the ubiquitous churches. Signs are hand painted and peeling, and since plywood is used to cover most street-level windows, even establishments that still do business have a boarded-up look.

Worse yet, dozens of storefronts have been reduced to gaping holes, outlined by shards of glass that form jagged frames for dark rooms of rubble. Only the foolhardy, or a drug addict desperate for a place to get high, would step inside.

The shrouded condition of the neighborhood unnerves Jackie. Even the local drugstore, whose windows are blocked with ugly, prehistoric stone, can seem foreboding. "You used to be able to see *in* the drugstore," Jackie complained. "Shoot, now you wonder if you get in somewhere, are you going to make it out safe?"

At one corner along the bus route, Jackie pointed to a currency exchange where several scraggly men clustered. "That's a hangout for IV-drug users," she observed with disgust, going on to tell about a nearby bar that peddled do-it-yourself packets for free-basing cocaine.

Jackie had noticed the drug paraphernalia when she once stopped at the bar to change a dollar bill. "When I saw that, I told the man I'd skip the change," Jackie said proudly, comparing herself to Father George Clements, a local African-American priest who mounted a boycott against stores that sold drug-related products.

Currency exchanges, storefront churches, auto parts shops, liquor stores and taverns, hot dog stands, and a beauty shop or two are the only businesses left on Ogden, which used to be one of the city's major commercial streets. The largest establishment in the neighborhood, Lawndale Oldsmobile, closed more than two decades ago. Its windowless, graffitied shell has been a fixture in North Lawndale since Jackie was a child. By the time she and her grandmother moved to Chicago from Tupelo, Mississippi, in the early 1960s, the neighborhood was already in rapid decline. The Eastern European Jews who had settled the area in the early part of the century had virtually vanished by the mid-1950s, replaced by black migrants from the South. Driven by the changing nature of their businesses as well as the deteriorating neighborhood, North Lawndale's major companies fled soon after: Sears Roebuck, International Harvester, and Western Electric either departed or reduced the size of their operations. Today, the bruised and battered buildings along Ogden give sad testimony to North Lawndale's knockout blow: the ravaging riots that followed Martin Luther King Jr.'s assassination in 1968. After that, most remaining middle-class blacks fled.

In 1960, Lawndale's population peaked at 125,000; by 1980, it had plummeted to 62,000; by the end of that decade, it fell to 47,000.[5] Statistics describing the economic status of the people who remain are discouraging: almost one of every two people is on welfare; three of every five potential workers are unemployed;[6] and three of every five families are headed by women,[7] whose earning power is, of course, significantly less than that of two-parent families.

Accompanying this kind of poverty is a shocking level of illness and disability that Jackie and her neighbors merely take for granted. Her husband's kidneys failed before he was thirty; her alcoholic father had a stroke because of uncontrolled high blood pressure at forty-eight; her Aunt Nancy, who helped her grandmother raise her, died from kidney failure complicated by cirrhosis when she was forty-three. Diabetes took her grandmother's leg, and blinded her great-aunt Eldora, who lives down the block.

Chicago's poor neighborhoods have always been its sickest. In 1890, a medical writer graphically described the conditions that were contributing to rampant disease among the city's immigrant industrial workers. "[Their] sole recourse usually is to the tenement where, heaped floor above floor, in a tainted atmosphere, or in low fetid hovels, amidst poverty, hunger and dirt, in foulness, want and crime, crowded humanity suffers, and sickens, and perishes; for the landlord here is also the airlord, the lord of sunlight; lord of all the primary conditions of life and living; and these are doled out for a price, failing which the wretched tenant is turned out to seek a habitation still more miserable."[8]

The diseases that killed in the nineteenth century lent themselves to such dramatic prose. They were the great epidemics, smallpox, cholera, and typhoid fever. Such bacteria-borne infectious diseases festered because of a water supply periodically tainted by sewage and were easily spread in the crowded living quarters of poor city neighborhoods. With the coming of better sanitation methods, which included reversing the flow of the Chicago River so that the city's sewage would be sent to southern Illinois and Missouri rather than into Lake Michigan, these epidemics were largely conquered, though other age-old communicable diseases such as tuberculosis, sexually transmitted diseases, and, recently, childhood measles, still disproportionately plague Chicago's poor.

One reason infectious diseases retain their foothold among the poor remains substandard housing, which is bad and getting worse in North Lawndale. A recent survey by an economic development group found that only 8 percent of the neighborhood's 8,937 buildings were in good to very good condition. The rest were abandoned, on the verge of collapse, or in need of repair.[9]

Dr. Arthur Jones has visited many of these decrepit buildings on house calls to patients too sick to make it into his clinic, which is located on Ogden almost directly behind Jackie's apartment. The clinic, Lawndale Christian Health Center, was founded by Dr. Jones and several other urban missionaries in 1984 and has succeeded, by most all accounts, at providing affordable and humane health care.

Dr. Jones told of one woman who was suffering a severe case of hives caused by an allergic reaction to her cat, yet repeatedly refused to get rid of the animal. "I really got kind of angry," Dr. Jones remembered, "and then she told me that if she got rid of the cat, there was nothing to protect her kids against rats." Another woman brought her two-year-old to the clinic with frostbite, so Dr. Jones dispatched his nurse practitioner to visit her home a block away from Jackie's. The nurse discovered icicles in the woman's apartment because the landlord had stopped providing heat. The stories go on, most involving landlords who cannot afford to keep up their buildings and tenants who cannot afford to leave them.

By these standards, the Baneses' apartment is in good shape. They have to contend with an occasional rat and wage a constant battle against roaches, but the landlord has kept the two-flat in decent repair; his sister lives on the first floor.

For the most part, the diseases that Jackie and her family live with are not characterized by sudden outbreaks but long, slow burns. As deadly infectious diseases have largely been eliminated or are easily cured—with the glaring exceptions of AIDS and now drug-resistant tuberculosis—chronic diseases have stepped into their wake, accounting for much of the death and disability among both rich and poor. The difference is that for affluent whites, diabetes, high blood pressure, heart disease, and the like are diseases of aging, while among poor blacks, they are more accurately called diseases of *middle*-aging.

In poor black neighborhoods on the West Side of Chicago, including North Lawndale, well over half of the population dies before the age of sixty-five, compared to a quarter of the residents of middle-class white Chicago neighborhoods.[10] Though they occur more often on the West Side, the three most common causes of premature mortality in the two areas would correspond—heart disease, diabetes, and high blood pressure—were it not for one fatal condition that increasingly is considered a major public health problem: homicide. It ranks sixth in the white neighborhoods but is the number two killer of West Siders under sixty-five.[11] Alcohol and drugs are the poisons that induce many of the West Side's deaths, whether from homicide or heart attack. Thirteen percent of fatalities in that part of the city are directly attributable to alcohol and drugs, four times the rate in white, middle-class neighborhoods.[12]

These statistics are not, of course, unique to Chicago. A study of premature mortality in Harlem showed that black men there were less likely to reach the age of sixty-five than men in Bangladesh.[13] "When sixty-seven people die in an earthquake in San Francisco, we call it a disaster and the President visits," said Dr. Harold Freeman, one of two Harlem Hospital Center physicians who conducted the study. "But here everyone is ignoring a chronic consistent disaster area, with many more people dying. And there is no question that things are getting worse."[14]

Though genetic differences still are occasionally cited in medical literature in order to explain disproportionate disease among blacks, nearly all health experts put most of the blame on poverty—and the lack of access to care and hardscrabble lifestyles that accompany it. The situation worsened during the mid-1980s when the gap in life expectancy between the two races began to widen for the first time in history. Blacks' life expectancy has been less than whites' for as long as health statistics have been gathered, though since the turn of the century both races have lived a little longer each year. But from 1985 to 1988, blacks' life expectancy declined each year while whites' continued to creep ahead.[15] In 1989, blacks regained some of the time they lost, when their life expectancy rose slightly, but only to the 1984 level of 69.7 years.[16]

The starkest contrast in longevity is between white and black men, largely because of spiraling rates of homicide and AIDS among minorities. DeMarest, who was born in 1985, can be expected to live for sixty-four years and ten months, whereas an average white boy born that year will live eight years longer.[17] Jackie knows her son's chances of living a long life are not good, but she does not spend much time brooding about the dangers that await him. For now, she keeps him close to home and hopes for the best.

When Jackie stepped down from the bus after visiting Robert at the hospital, it was late in the day; the sun was about level with her shoulders. As she waited to cross Ogden, she glanced back toward the city, where the 110-story Sears Tower was silhouetted against the blue sky. The tower had been a beacon to Jackie as a child. "That was one ambition me and my cousin used to have. We wanted to walk to the Sears Tower." They never made it past a local shopping strip.

Jackie proceeded across Ogden toward the back of her own stone and brick two-flat, which, fortunately, is about a half-block removed from the harsh four-lane street. Her second-floor back porch, where her children had been playing earlier, was now empty. They had gone inside, since they are under orders not to venture beyond the fifteen-square-feet of the porch. To help make sure they don't, Jackie locks a metal gate across the steps.

The day before Robert was hospitalized, the family had gathered on the porch to celebrate the Fourth of July. It was a normal holiday, normal at least for a family that resigns itself to sickness in the same way that other families resign themselves to being polite to an unwelcome guest.

Robert slumped in a chair, next to the grill, spatula propped up on his knee. His eyes were glassy and he looked more drained than usual. Suffering the side effects of whatever was causing him to urinate blood, he had not been eating well. The rest of the family welcomed the light breeze that cooled the porch, but Robert was shivering despite his long-sleeved sweatsuit.

While Robert listlessly tended the grill, Jackie tossed a salad in the kitchen, then mounded uncooked chicken, ribs, and hamburgers into a large aluminum roasting pan. She took the meat out to the porch for her husband to grill, but when she saw how tired he looked, she took over.

Jackie has not worked outside of her home since Latrice was little and does almost all of the cooking for the family. This pattern was established long ago, when Jackie was a young teenager living alone with her grandmother, whom she calls "Mom," or "Mama." By the time Mrs. Jackson got home from her job cooking and waitressing at a truck stop, she wanted no part of the kitchen, so Jackie began making dinner on week nights. "I became sort of like the Hazel in the family. Mom the hubby that go to work; I was the wife."

Jackie said she rather enjoyed being in charge at home, picking up after her grandmother, chiding her for tossing her bra and girdle over the shower-curtain rod when she came home from work. But Mrs. Jackson, who left for work at 5 A.M., was not moved by her granddaughter's requests to please, please put her clothes in her room. "I lay them where I take them off," Mrs. Jackson would tell Jackie. And that was the end of it.

Mrs. Jackson has never been one to waste words with her family, Jackie said, but as she has grown sicker, she has spoken less and less. The Fourth of July was no exception. While the rest of the family talked and listened to Latrice's portable radio on the back porch, Mrs.

CHAPTER ONE

Jackson sat quietly in her wheelchair in the front room, eating from a plate Jackie had fixed for her.

Mrs. Jackson's right leg was amputated in late April because of an infection. First, half of her foot had been removed in February, which doctors had hoped would obviate the need for further amputation. But after a month and a half of erratic outpatient care, Mrs. Jackson's condition worsened, and her leg had to be amputated, too. Like many diabetics, Mrs. Jackson suffers from peripheral vascular disease, a chronic illness that causes blood vessels to thicken and restricts the flow of blood so that infections cannot heal.

Though she wasn't saying much, Mrs. Jackson looked fresh and more alert than she had recently. Wearing a red-and-white gingham dress, she sat up almost erect in her wheelchair, and when Brianna scuttled into the room, she watched her quizzically. Mrs. Jackson had to wait for the family's life to parade before her since she refused Jackie's offers to push her to the back porch. Several notes from hospital social workers in Mrs. Jackson's medical chart said the elderly woman worried about being a burden to her granddaughter, and perhaps that was part of the reason she chose to stay inside.

Then, too, getting the wheelchair through the kitchen to the back porch is something of a production. Jackie has to move the kitchen table and chairs, and even then, Mrs. Jackson's wheelchair barely fits through the narrow hallway connecting the living room and kitchen. The five-room apartment does not easily accommodate three children and three adults, especially since Mrs. Jackson began to require extra equipment such as a portable commode, a walker, and, of course, a wheelchair.

Mrs. Jackson's world had shrunk to include her bedroom and the front room that adjoined it. Emblems of her life cluttered her dark wood dresser. There were a dozen or more brown pill bottles, two Bibles, gauze pads and antiseptic spray, an unopened pack of Red Man chewing tobacco (for a habit she had acquired in Mississippi), latex gloves, and a small photo album. A picture of Latrice in first grade was stuck in the dresser's mirror. A black patent leather handbag and two church hats, one a deep red knit with fur trim, the other decorated with large gold sequins, hung on its corner. The hats were getting dusty. Since Mrs. Jackson's leg was amputated, she had not been able to go to the First Baptist Church on Sundays, her favorite activity of the week. The situation was especially sad because she had not been

22

a woman who spent much time at home, according to Jackie. "As long as I know this lady, she's been the get-up-and-go type. She has really been stripped of all her worldly duties." Jackie remembers her grandmother as her conduit to the outside world; she often boasts about Mrs. Jackson's legendary knowledge of bus routes. "Mama used to show me this way, showed me that way; she got around." Though it is hard to imagine somebody being so stoic, Mrs. Jackson never complained about being homebound, Jackie said, or pined for fresh air and sunshine.

Back on the porch, it was relatively quiet, except when two fire trucks screamed out of the station behind the apartment. No trees or bushes grow on the small patch of dirt and weeds in the back yard the Baneses share with the tenant below, but a tree on the lot behind them provides some shield from the constant traffic on Ogden.

Robert perked up when his twenty-year-old half-sister Lativa and her boyfriend arrived. "See, he looks a lot better," Jackie said ruefully. "He gets tired of the same old faces."

The couple indeed brought a burst of vitality to the porch. Lativa was home on leave from the Army, and brought birthday presents for Brianna, whose first birthday was two days away, and for DeMarest, who would not turn five until after Lativa returned to her base in North Carolina.

After dinner, Jackie allowed Latrice and DeMarest to walk to a nearby liquor store to get snowcones, a favorite in the neighborhood. On sweltering summer days, adults and children drag folding chairs and coolers out to the curb and settle in. They pump red, blue, or green syrups into paper cones filled with scoops of chipped ice and sell them to passers by. Latrice cherishes the rituals of holidays, including the trip for snowcones, so she made sure she and her brother honored the Fourth with their choices, blue-raspberry and watermelon flavors for Latrice, blue-raspberry and strawberry for DeMarest.

Munching on their snowcones as they walked home, the two children passed a narrow general store that was closed for the holiday. Its owner, Jim Downing, a tough sixty-year-old with the hard body of someone thirty years younger, sells a little bit of everything. Hand-painted signs propped outside his establishment hawk pecans, extermination service (by Mr. Downing, who went to jail for several weeks for using dangerous, illegal chemicals), roach spray, and $39 burglar gates, one of which the Baneses bought and Mr. Downing mounted across their back door. Jackie does laundry in the two washing machines that are crammed into Mr. Downing's store, and Latrice comes here regularly to buy candy, or pick up soda or a gallon of milk for her mom. Mr. Downing tots up her charges on the back of a brown paper sack, testing Latrice's arithmetic as he goes. If the Baneses are running short of cash, he lets them run a tab.

Dessert and dinner finished, the family waited for darkness to fall, then went to the back yard to set off Roman candles and firecrackers that popped when Latrice or DeMarest flung them to the ground. During the night, Robert continued to urinate blood, and the next morning, he reported to the University of Illinois Hospital.

He went home after three days, on a Friday. Doctors told him to return the next Monday for surgery. The medical tests had revealed that the blood was coming from the stump of his rejected kidney, and they wanted to correct the problem. They called late that afternoon and told him they had changed their minds; they would wait to see if the bleeding cleared up on its own. It did.

2

The rigors of kidney dialysis for Robert Banes

Robert was thinking about frying some bacon for breakfast when the driver who takes him to the kidney dialysis center sounded his horn from the street. This was unusual because it was just a little after 5:30 A.M., and Robert is scheduled for a six o'clock pickup, Mondays, Wednesdays, and Fridays. Robert has known drivers to be late, sometimes by hours; he has known drivers not to show. They are rarely early.

Still sleepy, he dropped down on the couch to pull on his leather high-tops. A lamp glowed orange in one corner of the living room; otherwise, it was early-morning gray. Latrice slept next to him. Her long, brown legs stretched the length of the couch that does double-duty as her bed. She lay on top of a rust-colored throw that Jackie uses to cover the couch's thinning, stained upholstery. Jackie was already up, washing in the bathroom. Her grandmother lay still in her bed, she had not yet called for her breakfast or morning drink of water.

The living room is substantially longer than it is wide and is divided into two main sections. The back area, where Robert sat and Latrice slept, holds Jackie's furniture, the couch and a matching love seat she brought when she, Robert, and Latrice moved in with her grandmother in 1986. A dark wood hutch, built into the back wall, is filled with pictures of the family. Some of the photos are old and tattered, their frames tarnished, but none of that seems to matter much. The pictures look as if they have been there for a long time and will remain for a long time to come. A light-colored wood bookshelf next to the hutch is overflowing with knickknacks: ceramic figurines Jackie gave to her grandmother, mixed with animals made from shells (souvenirs of a craft project at a nursing home where Mrs. Jackson worked), mixed with a dozen basketball trophies that Robert won in high school and junior college.

Toward the front, outside Mrs. Jackson's bedroom door, sits a more formal-looking couch, upholstered in faded gold, that the old woman has owned since Jackie was a girl. DeMarest is an active little boy and has torn and poked through its plastic slipcover until it no longer provides much protection, but Jackie resists removing it. Her grandmother insisted on the plastic cover, and Jackie does not want her to think the family is defying her now that she cannot do anything about it. A low-slung credenza, about thirty years old, with a working radio and a broken turntable inside, is across the room from Mrs. Jackson's couch. Three color TVs are stacked together near it, although only one works.

Robert finished tying his shoes. Eyes half shut, he pushed aside a vinyl recliner the Baneses put in front of the door at night for extra security and descended the stairs that lead down to a small front porch. "Heh, Banes, I knew I'd get you today," called the driver, who has transported Robert before. Each weekday, private companies that contract with the Chicago Transit Authority take Robert and twenty-five hundred other disabled Cook County residents to medical appointments and wherever else they need to go. In the summer of 1989, there were five transportation companies working for the CTA (subsequently one of them was kicked out of the program for fraud, as another had been earlier in the year). Robert used SCR Transportation, which had the worst on-time record in the program. SCR arrived on time for about half of its rides; the rest of the time, drivers were anywhere from ten minutes to more than an hour late.[1]

Nonetheless, the ride was a blessing because the dialysis clinic is a good hour away on the bus or train. Robert would have to leave for the clinic in the dark, an unsettling proposition in a neighborhood imprisoned by nightfall. The Baneses rarely go out at night, and even at dusk, when Latrice wants to run down to her cousin's apartment less than a block away, Jackie watches her come and go from the front porch. Robert also appreciates the ride home after dialysis because sometimes he feels weak and shaky, not at all in the mood to be jostled on the bus.

As soon as Robert got into the car, he pulled a pack of cigarettes out of his jacket and lit one. "My wife doesn't know I smoke," he said. Robert tries to curry Jackie's favor with small gestures such as pretending not to smoke and buying her a box of candy when she gets mad. What Jackie wants most, though, is for him to stay away from cocaine, and that he has a harder time doing. He sometimes goes weeks, even a month or two, without using cocaine but then binges and spends every cent he can find on drugs. That leaves Jackie straining to meet her household budget, and it cannot be good for Robert's health. Robert refuses to discuss drugs with anyone but Jackie and then only if she pushes the issue.

The twenty-minute ride to Neomedica Dialysis Center, located in the most exclusive area of Chicago, had the feel of a boys' night out. The two men bantered about NBA stars they had met, gangsters the driver had chauffeured, and the high cost of dating.

"Give me some cash and I can go out, buy some drinks for the ladies," the driver boasted.

"So you can make things *happen*," Robert said with a vicarious thrill.

Robert wears a dialysis uniform of sorts: a navy and white nylon sweatsuit and a red Bulls cap. His arms are still sculpted from his basketball-playing days, but the muscles look as if they have been sanded down. All that's left are a few bulges covered by a thin layer of skin. He has lost twenty pounds in the six months since he began dialysis, a big enough drop that the clinic nutritionist said she plans to put him on a supplemental diet. On the warmest days, Robert gets cold, and when he sees a woman walk down the street in shorts and a sleeveless shirt, he often says, "I wish I had her blood." Like most dialysis patients, Robert is chronically anemic.

Neomedica's clerk calls patients back for dialysis two or three at a time, so Robert found a chair in the waiting room and turned to the *Sun-Times* sports pages. Other patients killed time with talk of the Bulls and high blood pressure pills, the Cubs and the restrictive diets patients are supposed to follow. Robert was one of the last patients left when he was summoned at 7:30. That is his regular dialysis time, but Robert gets to the clinic a little after six because he has found that the earlier the pickup, the more likely the transportation company is to be on time. When patients are late getting to Neomedica, they may wait hours to be dialyzed.

Upon hearing his name, Robert pitched his paper and walked to his recliner, past a score of patients tethered to blinking, beeping machines. Two thin plastic tubes, reddened by steady streams of blood, snaked from each of the patients' forearms. On their inner arms, dialysis patients have knots called fistulas, where doctors connect a vein and an artery to enable them to receive dialysis. The arterial tube feeds blood into the dialyzer, where a six-inch filter composed of dozens of tiny strawlike tubes draws out wastes the kidneys can no longer expel. The cleansed blood is then pumped back into patients' bodies. Without dialysis, Robert and the other patients would die within a few weeks.

Fourteen of the patients on Robert's morning shift at Neomedica are black, five are Hispanic, two are white, and one is Asian. The racial mix of the group nearly matches that of Chicago's dialysis population, though the center has fewer whites than the city as a whole.[2] Nation-wide, the incidence of kidney failure among blacks is four times that among whites.[3]

Much of that racial difference results from kidney failure caused by hypertension, a disease that usually can be controlled by medication. In other words, a significant portion of the kidney failure among blacks is largely preventable with regular care. For those who are poor, the reasons they do not receive care range from inadequate or nonexistent insurance, to a misunderstanding of the seriousness of the condition, to an inability to cope with anything other than immediate threats to their well-being. A sad mix of all three caused Jackie's father, Tommy Markham, to suffer another of the consequences of uncontrolled high blood pressure, a stroke, when he was only forty-eight.

Tommy gives only sketchy details about his youth, but he apparently had a contentious relationship with his parents, Mrs. Jackson and her first husband. He stayed behind in Mississippi when the couple moved north, to Gary, Indiana, though his young daughter, Jackie, went with them. Jackie's teenage mother had given her daughter to Mrs. Jackson to raise. After Tommy got into trouble for car theft, he moved to Chicago, where Mrs. Jackson had gone after she split from her husband. Tommy's run-ins with the law did not stop, however. The way Tommy tells it, he got fed up with a man who wrongly accused him of "going with his woman" and "beat the shit out of him." He was convicted of armed robbery and spent seven years in Illinois's Stateville Correctional Center during his twenties. (Tommy huffily denies the robbery: "I didn't rob the dude. I just beat him up. . . . He was laying there in the gangway, and peoples from the lounge ran out. They took the money off him.")

When Tommy was released in 1971, Mrs. Jackson continued to raise Jackie. He lived with his mother and ten-year-old Jackie for a few days, but Mrs. Jackson threw him out because of his "attitude," Jackie said, and he returned to the West Side's streets. He worked off and on as a bartender, butcher, and exterminator, all the while guzzling beer, whiskey, and cognac. Six feet, two inches tall, with muscle built in the prison gym and still evident today, Tommy was menacing to Jackie and, evidently, to a lot of other people. "Everybody would be scared of Tommy, Tommy, Tommy," Jackie chanted. So intimidated by her violent father was Jackie that she has fonder memories of him when he was imprisoned than when he came out. She and her grandmother took the Greyhound bus to visit him in Joliet once a year. "I remember my father giving me bottled pop and peanuts," she said. "It used to be a nice ritual for me. The prison had beautiful flower gardens and afterward we'd go shopping in Joliet."

Tommy's stroke did not come out of the blue. He knew he had high blood pressure, but he stopped taking antihypertensive medication because of its side effects—impotence, for one. His alcoholism and smoking also almost certainly contributed to the stroke. But high blood pressure does not cause any discomfort for most people, which is why doctors call it the "silent killer," and so Tommy, who generally does not look past the next day, paid no attention. "Nature will takes its course," he likes to say. And it did. The left side of his body is now paralyzed, and he spends most of his time in a wheelchair, though he can walk very slowly with the assistance of a brace and cane. As Tommy tells the Currency Exchange clerk with whom he flirts when he picks up his welfare check, "I can't run no more yards; the All-American Tom Cat done slowed down."

The casualties that high blood pressure inflicts on blacks are enormous; they suffer strokes at twice the rate of whites,[4] and there are sixty thousand excess deaths a year among blacks from hypertension-related diseases.[5] In Chicago, where the population of blacks and whites is roughly equal, there are more blacks with kidney failure caused by high blood pressure than whites with kidney failure *regardless of cause.*[6]

Hypertension does not account for all of the difference in black and white kidney-failure rates. Blacks with diabetes also lose kidneys more than whites.[7] But the main reasons that high blood pressure, diabetes, and even Robert's relatively rare focal glomerulosclerosis take a higher toll on blacks are probably similar: a third of blacks are poor, and for lack of money, or understanding, the poor easily can get shut out of medical care.

Robert was born thirty-five years ago at what was then called the Illinois Research and Educational Hospital, part of the University of Illinois medical school complex. He still goes there for care, as an outpatient in the transplant program.

As a boy, Robert moved between the West Side apartments of his young mother and his grandmother. Fearing he would get tangled up with a gang, they sent him to Panola, Alabama, when he was seventeen to live with relatives. Panola was so small, Robert says, that "by the time you raise your hand to wave to somebody, you're out of town."

His next stop was a Tennessee community college where he studied and played basketball until he dropped out in the spring of 1975. Not long after, Robert returned to Chicago and his mother's house, located several miles away from where Robert and Jackie live today. He met Jackie at a birthday party for his mother in 1977, the same year he received the first sign that his kidneys were failing. A job physical revealed protein in his urine—a warning that his kidneys were not functioning well. A renal biopsy later that year showed the focal glomerulosclerosis.

There is no cure for focal glomerulosclerosis—it progressively scars kidneys until they are destroyed—and doctors are baffled by the disease's cause. Steroids and chemotherapy are used to slow its progress, but they may or may not work. Robert received no treatment for this potentially fatal condition. He did not even see a doctor again until four years later, in April 1981, when he showed up at Cook County Hospital's emergency room. Robert had been unusually tired for several months and had trouble keeping his food down. When his ankles began to swell at Latrice's third birthday party, a friend drove him to the hospital. There, doctors discovered his kidneys were working at less than 5 percent of capacity.

The chairman of general medicine at Cook County Hospital, Dr. Terrence Conway, has seen hundreds of patients with advanced, untreated conditions similar to Robert's. His first experience at County came during the Vietnam War, when he was assigned to the hospital

as an orderly to fulfill conscientious objector requirements. After graduating from medical school in 1976, he worked at a federally funded
health clinic on the South Side, then as the medical director of another
such clinic in the Cabrini-Green housing project, and in 1988, he
returned to County. When Robert came there, he was near death, Dr.
Conway said. "His blood pressure was high, blood clotting was not
very good. His fluid was backing up, which could have caused heart
failure. He probably could have gone another three weeks without one
of his systems failing, but not much longer."

Why Robert waited until he was in such crisis to seek medical care
is not entirely clear. In the medical record, a Cook County social
worker wrote that Robert told her that he didn't have any money to
pay his hospital bill. None of his short-term, minimum-wage jobs provided medical insurance to pay for diagnostic kidney studies, or medications, or follow-up visits to the doctor, and he was not consistently
enrolled in Medicaid, which has very limited coverage for single adults,
anyhow.

Beyond Robert's inability to pay for care is the fact that he did not
seem to understand the gravity of his illness, or that medical care could
have extended the life of his kidneys. Cook County's medical history
for Robert says: ". . . a renal biopsy at Columbus Hospital showed focal
glomerulosclerosis, but Mr. Banes neglected to continue his follow-up."

This is what Robert recalls: "I was thinking there wasn't that much
wrong. I thought whatever it was might clear up on its own. They told
me I had something on my kidney, but nobody told me to come back."

Patricia Barber, a nurse and clinical transplant specialist at the University of Illinois, coached Robert through his first kidney transplant
in 1982. In January 1989, his body rejected the transplanted organ,
and Barber was preparing him to get onto the transplant waiting list
for a second time. "When patients come into Cook County with
chronic renal failure and say, 'Nobody ever told me this could happen,'
they're partly right. They've been told but not in a way that sticks,"
says Barber. "Robert was referred back for treatment, but being young
and feeling well, he did not have a lot of motivation to follow through."

Then, too, people who can barely afford food and shelter may not
think they have much to gain from spending scarce dollars for doctors'
visits. "For someone who is poor, health care is not the highest priority," Dr. Conway said, an observation offered repeatedly by doctors
and nurses who work with poor patients.

CHAPTER TWO

It's also possible that friends and family were not pushing Robert to go to the doctor, Dr. Conway continued. "People in Chicago's poorer neighborhoods are used to a lot of sick people around. When someone says 'Something's wrong with my kidneys,' the automatic response is not 'Well, what doctor are you going to?' When you live on the North Shore [the affluent suburbs north of Chicago], that's the first thing people ask you."

Dr. Conway also speculated that since Robert's disease is a chronic one, doctors may have told him that "there was nothing they could do," a phrase that can mean one thing to patients and another to doctors. "It sounds black-and-white, but it's not. We can't cure AIDS, but we don't say 'You're on your own. Don't come back.' We can do things to prolong life."

Doctors may face a particular challenge getting that message across to people as fatalistic as Robert and Jackie. Asked at least a half-dozen times to discuss her feelings about her family's unrelenting illness—did she think they were unusual or especially cursed?—Jackie got exasperated. "Look," she finally said, obviously hoping to close the subject, "I just say it *happens*."

The fantastic and horrid deaths that mark their daily lives feed such fatalism. Perhaps only the most stout-hearted—or delusional—could retain a sense of control over their destiny. One day, a thirtyish-looking man spotted Jackie in a car and ran up to the side window, puckering his lips in an exaggerated kiss. "I went to school with him," Jackie said, laughing at his foolishness. Then, without skipping a beat: "They found his brother dead right up under the house, this tall building right up on the corner. I heard rumors when I was in grammar school. The kids was playing and they kept saying they smelled something foul, like dead rats, and it was his brother's body down in the sewer."

Then there is the death of Robert's beloved mother. The official version of her story is that she went out drinking with friends after work on a Friday, returned home, and passed out in the garage with the car running. The unofficial version is considerably more vivid. "She was murdered," Jackie said once. Then she corrected herself. "Carbon monoxide, that's what's on the death certificate. But [Robert and his family] say there was scratches and blood. And I've heard that she was disrobed halfway. And I remember Robert getting her bra and there was blood stains on it, so we feel like, the family felt, there was foul play somewhere."

It would be easy to dismiss this as an example of devoted children unable to face the mundane but ultimately tragic circumstances of their mother's death. And that may be all it is. But in a neighborhood where the cliché "truth is stranger than fiction" takes on pointed meaning, who knows for sure?

There has been little rigorous study of how fatalism and other accompaniments of poverty influence communication between doctors and patients, but at least one investigator of the subject found that doctors spend more time discussing diagnoses and treatments with well-educated people, resulting in a "paradoxical situation whereby patients most in need of education receive the least."[8] At the same time, blacks report more often than whites that doctors do not adequately explain the seriousness of their illnesses or how medications work.[9] Robert, for one, is often confused by doctors, but he rarely if ever asks them for more information.

Several days before he was admitted to University of Illinois Hospital because of the blood in his urine, Robert had visited a urologist at the university's outpatient clinic. He had never seen the doctor before, but Barber, the transplant nurse, made him an appointment because of the unusual bleeding. At that appointment, the doctor told him he would have to be hospitalized. He also told Robert that before he could be admitted to the hospital he would need blood tests and an ultrasound study of his kidneys.

"When am I going to have to have surgery?" Robert asked, certain of that eventuality though the doctor had not mentioned it.

"That's only if the ultrasound shows us something like a cyst, like cancer on the kidneys," the doctor said flatly.

"Don't tell me that, please," Robert pleaded. The doctor smiled sympathetically and walked out of the examining room without explaining further.

Through the open door, Robert could see but not hear the doctor conferring with a nurse who was holding a small plastic cup of blood that seemed to be Robert's.

"Don't be whispering," he said to himself. "Tell me, too."

But when the doctor returned moments later, Robert did not ask him what he had been talking about. He lay back on the examining table and offered up his arm for his blood pressure to be taken. If Robert wondered what the chances were of his having cancer, he said nothing.

Robert says he is not angry that no one effectively explained to him that his kidneys were failing. Then again, Robert does not admit that much of anything disturbs him. "I look at dialysis like a setback. Why should you get down? It just makes you sicker."

It's understandable, perhaps admirable, that Robert does not want to dwell on his illness. But Robert is so matter-of-fact and publicly emotionless about how he got sick—and even the most devoted doctors and nurses are so used to situations like Robert's—that it is easy to be lulled into taking it all for granted. Whose fault is it that Robert did not have health insurance, and that at least thirty-five million Americans are without it today?[10] What about doctors' inability to communicate to patients in a way that makes them understand their illnesses—whose fault is that? Who is responsible for the many poor minorities who are so socially and economically isolated that they cannot take advantage of the medical system in the same way that many whites can?

No one is forced to take responsibility for these inequities. Medical ethicist Larry Churchill describes well the forces that allow the United States to remain the only industrialized country other than South Africa that does not provide at least basic health care to all of its citizens. "Access to health care is mostly contingent on having a way to pay for it, either out of one's own resources or with some form of insurance," he writes. "The essential point is that [this] allocation by price is a rationing scheme—one which we have easily accepted in health care as an extension of a basic economic philosophy, and one which largely absolves any particular person from responsibility for the results. Since no one actually decided to exclude the poor (as it is their lack of money that excludes them, not our actions) no one is responsible and no one is to blame."[11]

The morning the dialysis driver arrived early, Robert fell asleep within minutes after his blood began cycling through the dialysis machine at Neomedica. Before settling in for a nap, he covered himself with a blue bedspread he'd brought from home to ward off the chill he gets during dialysis. The elderly Hispanic woman who sat next to him had the opposite problem: she brought a small fan to cool her as she slept. Cigarette smoke curled over the backs of several of the recliners spread across the room. Some patients watched a TV that hung from the ceiling; others chatted quietly.

Dr. Gordon Lang, the medical director of Robert's facility, had begun making his rounds. With graying, curly hair, a strong-boned face, and stylish ruby-red glasses, he is quite handsome. He quickly scanned medical charts, exchanged a few words with patients, and was gone within a half-hour. Dr. Lang is also the president of Neomedica Dialysis Centers, Inc., and along with monitoring the medical care of the downtown clinic's patients, he has to oversee this expanding for-profit dialysis chain, which in 1989 included eight other Chicago-area dialysis units.

Dialysis is one of few areas of medical care dominated by for-profit providers, and it has been at the center of a nationwide debate about the costs and quality of proprietary medicine. Medicare pays dialysis units a fixed fee for each dialysis session—Neomedica currently gets $131 per treatment[12]—but exercises little control over how that money is spent. Officials at the Health Care Financing Administration, which administers Medicare, charge that, to preserve high profit margins, many centers compromise patients' care by reducing staff and shortening treatment times.[13] Such cost-cutting changes have been made at Neomedica, Dr. Lang freely admits, but he said they do not threaten patients' health. Neither, he said, do Neomedica's physician-owners earn excessive profits.

Dr. Lang founded Neomedica with another doctor when Medicare began to pay for dialysis in 1972 and today owns 14 percent[14] of the $6.7 million chain.[15] Public documents do not show how much Dr. Lang makes as the corporation's chief executive, but his job as a medical director of Robert's unit, which Dr. Lang estimated occupies him for three or four hours a week, pays well: $68,480 in 1989, according to Medicare cost reports.[16] Completely apart from what he makes for running Neomedica, he earns a monthly fee as the nephrologist for Robert and forty-five to fifty other dialysis patients.[17] For that work, Medicare pays doctors an average of $173 per patient per month, which would mean Dr. Lang earns roughly another $100,000 each year from Medicare.[18] Finally, a medical practice he maintains outside of the dialysis unit further enhanced his income. Dr. Lang will not say how much he currently makes a year, but according to the Internal

Revenue Service, his taxable income in 1985 was $362,964.[19] (That figure comes from a suit Dr. Lang filed against the IRS to block the agency's attempt to recover $160,000 for alleged improper deductions he took on a ski resort condominium in Utah.)

Dr. Lang's manner with the dialysis patients at Neomedica's downtown unit was brisk and efficient if not cursory, but for Robert, at least, he is "the man." Though Robert and the other patients regularly grumble about every aspect of dialysis, little of their anger seems directed at Dr. Lang. The technicians and nurses take the brunt of it, even though it is Dr. Lang who has ultimate responsibility for the way the unit is run.

Robert's chair sat back-to-back with that of a pencil-thin Puerto Rican girl who had shimmied into the unit in stretch pants, an oversized T-shirt, and powder blue heels. Before he dozed off, Robert had predicted that she would start "hollering" from cramps that some dialysis patients suffer as excess fluid is rapidly drained from their bodies. Sure enough, she began whimpering softly, then louder. Her cries were like a sharp pinch, awakening one to a reality that can easily be lost among the banter of the patients who swap stories like old friends at a weekly poker game: dialysis is a painful process for men and women (and boys and girls) who are dying by inches. Once on dialysis, the average person lives for five years suffering from the cramps and chills of the procedure, the fatigue of chronic anemia, and the nausea that accompanies kidney failure.

Many of the young people who require dialysis live longer than that, but Robert remembers those who did not. On the way home from dialysis that morning, Robert talked about an eighteen-year-old girl whose chatter about her senior prom had accompanied him through his first spring on dialysis. She never made it to the dance. "She had a heart attack right on the operating table," Robert said, shaking his head.

That Medicare pays for dialysis for the 150,000 Americans who need it is unusual because the federal health insurance program primarily covers medical expenses of the elderly and disabled. Kidney failure is the only disease that makes people of all ages eligible for Medicare, through what is known as the End-Stage Renal Disease program. But Medicare pays for only 80 percent of dialysis. At least part of the remaining 20 percent comes from one of three different sources: Medicaid, the government program for the poor; private insurance; or in

Illinois, a special program sponsored by the state Department of Public Health that picks up patients who would otherwise fall between the cracks, those not poor enough to qualify for Medicaid but too poor to afford private insurance. This state program covers only hemophiliacs and dialysis patients, who are able to attract extra state dollars for one of the same reasons Congress voted to extend Medicare coverage to renal patients in 1972: death from kidney failure (as well as hemophilia) is both swift and certain.[20] There is no net to catch borderline poverty-level people who need medical treatment for chronic diseases such as cancer, whose progress is slower but just as fatal if left untreated.

Robert and thirteen other patients in his dialysis group are impoverished enough to be eligible for Medicaid. Six more are covered by private health insurance, and two qualify for the state public health program. National estimates put half of the dialysis population below the poverty line.[21]

Like Robert, Adelle is one of those who are poor. She has been on dialysis for twenty years, since she was thirty-one. Her kidneys failed, she figures, because of a series of kidney infections she suffered as a young woman in San Antonio. She never saw a doctor. She and her husband, Mexican immigrants, worked the kind of low-skill jobs that usually do not offer insurance, and she had little money for medical care. "I would have had to pay out of my own pocket," she said in a calm, unflinching way, sounding as if, presented with the same circumstances today, she would make the same choice.

Despite her failing health, she said she enjoys life. She walks in shopping malls for exercise and dances for short spells when she gets the chance. "I get all out of breath, so I wait until the middle of the record to start." She also takes pleasure from indulging in several of dialysis patients' forbidden foods: a small piece of avocado, a half cup of pinto beans once a week, and an occasional Snicker's bar.

Three years ago, Adelle's situation improved for what may sound like an unlikely reason: her husband of thirty-three years, whom she still cares for, moved out. "Once we separated I qualified for everything," she said. Before that, she was only eligible for the Illinois Department of Public Health program, which, though it covers the portion of dialysis treatments leftover by Medicare, does not pay for anything else. On her own, Adelle became eligible for monthly Supplemental Security Income (SSI) payments of $368 a month for elderly and disabled people who have no other means of support. Eligibility for SSI automatically made her eligible for Medicaid, which pays for the $50 to $100 worth of medication she needs each month. Her husband's job as a shipping clerk had disqualified her from receiving either of these benefits.

Though her husband still faithfully picks her up from dialysis—"He likes to take me home because sometimes I don't feel so good"—Adelle said they have no plans to live together any time soon.

A social worker for another dialysis center in Chicago said she sometimes advises patients to separate from their spouses, if only on paper. "I'm not proud of it, but my first responsibility is to the patients," she said. "[Being single] makes it so much easier. They won't feel like they're taking food out of their children's mouths to buy medication." So maybe Adelle's husband left, and maybe he didn't. It's hard to tell sometimes.

Adelle had given up hope of ever working, but Robert still felt capable of holding down a job. Soon after he was discharged from the University of Illinois Hospital, he found work as a nighttime security guard for $4.50 an hour. The job made his dialysis schedule particularly grueling.

Wearing a blue baseball cap with SECURITY printed across it, Robert emerged from the marble lobby of a downtown office building at five o'clock one Friday morning in mid-July. That gave him an hour or so to kill before dialysis. At 3 A.M., Robert had eaten a salami sandwich Jackie had made for him, so he was not hungry, and he felt awake, so he did not want a cup of coffee. With nothing to do but wait, he took the bus to Neomedica and sat outside, watching for a technician to unlock the door.

Robert said he felt okay that morning, but he seemed wistful. He reminisced about the pleasures that life afforded before he became sick, like drinking icy beers after an afternoon of basketball in the hot Alabama sun. "The beer was so cold it felt like glass cutting my throat; it hurt but it felt good. That was in the good old days, when I didn't have no kidney problems, wasn't nobody calling me 'Daddy.'"

After dialysis that morning, Robert went home to bed. He worked from 8 P.M. to 4 A.M. the same night, and continued that shift for six straight days, during which he was dialyzed three times.

"Back to work?" asked Dr. Lang as he passed Robert on his rounds the next Friday.

"Yeah, but I'm sitting most of the time," Robert responded. Dr. Lang was on to the next patient and did not seem to hear.

A hand-lettered sign pinned to the bulletin board in Neomedica's waiting room said: "Do not let dialysis discourage you from WORKING. Continue to develop your skills and strive for who you want to be. There are many agencies willing to help you seek employment."

Something about the sign, perhaps the bright orange kindergarten-capital letters in which WORKING was printed, was condescending. Its cheery simplicity rang hollow to anyone who knows how rare jobs are among dialysis patients. Not only do the poor get sicker, but the sick get poorer.

Only one-third of all patients who dialyze at a clinic return to work once their treatments begin.[22] The Illinois Department of Rehabilitation Services has had little success with the few dialysis patients it has tried to help.[23] DORS is better equipped to handle disabilities such as deafness and blindness than it is kidney failure, which is more like an illness. Rehabilitation agencies' responsibility for dialysis patients is a holdover from an earlier era. Before Medicare started paying for dialysis, the machines were in short supply and so the treatments were reserved for people who had the potential to be "contributing members of society," to return to work. Thus, dialysis often fell under the jurisdiction of state vocational training programs.

Today the high unemployment rate in the dialysis population comes from a number of factors. First, dialysis itself is easily a part-time job. Counting travel, waiting, and treatment time, the process can eat up six hours a day, three times a week. In addition, almost all dialysis patients are anemic. An eight-hour day can leave them exhausted.[24] Robert knows that all too well. Asked how he is feeling, he invariably responds, "Tired."

Potential employers are wary of limitations like these, fearing that dialysis patients will miss too many days of work. They also avoid hiring dialysis patients because of the possibility that they will drive up health insurance costs.

Even for the patients who feel up to it, fear of losing their federal benefits keeps them from seeking work. "I'd like to work part-time, but they say if you work at all, your Social Security will get cut off," said Anne, a forty-six-year-old dialysis patient on Robert's shift. Before Anne went on dialysis sixteen years ago, she worked at a factory, but she was not rushing into anything these days. Dialysis was work enough, she said. Indeed, she often dressed for it as she might a secretarial job, in a plaid skirt topped with a tomato-red blouse, for example, with matching red earrings and purse. The only sign of Anne's illness was her swollen legs; people with kidney failure do not rid their bodies of fluids the way normal people do.

Though social workers who work in dialysis units say some patients use Social Security as an excuse, their trepidation about working is not unfounded. The Social Security Administration gives people with disabilities a nine-month work-trial period during which they may keep all their wages. At the end of that time, if they are earning a "substantial" income—usually about $300 a month—their disability payments are cut off. (They do not, however, lose their health insurance coverage under Medicare.)

"Nine months is a reasonable time if your disability is one that peaks and then levels off, like losing your legs," says Rosa Mizzoni, who has been a social worker in dialysis units for more than a decade. "But dialysis doesn't peak. It peaks and valleys, peaks and valleys for all of someone's life."

Soon after he went back to work, Robert learned he was losing $278 a month in disability benefits. Ironically, it was not because of the new job, but one he had held the year before. He had never reported it and had not intended to. "When you need the money, who needs to report it?" he said. But because the Internal Revenue Service shares its records with Social Security, the agency eventually found out.

A thirteen-year veteran employee of Social Security said almost no one on disability reports it when they return to work. "They say, 'I'll get what I can get and worry about the future when it comes.' I can't blame them."

If Robert keeps his security guard job for a year, he will earn less than $10,000, about $5,000 under the annual federal poverty level for a family of five in 1989. The Baneses "get over," as Jackie says, with the help of $619 her grandmother receives in Social Security retirement benefits each month. "I need her as much as she needs me right now," Jackie says.

Jackie used to receive $386 a month in welfare payments from Aid to Families with Dependent Children (AFDC), but the Illinois Department of Public Aid realized that Robert's disability payments were not being counted as part of the family's income. So the agency budgeted part of Robert's check for family expenses and reduced Jackie's grant accordingly. As a result, she began to receive only $90, even though, of course, Robert's disability checks were subsequently eliminated.

There is one exception to the pattern of unemployment among dialysis patients: those who learn home dialysis in Chicago are twice as likely to return to work as those who are treated at a clinic.[25] Home dialysis patients may work more because they are healthier to start with; people with many complications need the medically supervised dialysis that clinics provide. The at-home procedure also makes working easier by increasing patients' independence and control over their schedules.

But most inner-city residents—who tend to be poorer and less educated than their suburban counterparts—attend clinics, according to the executive director of the National Kidney Foundation of Chicago, Joan Shepard.[26] Some physicians may not offer the home procedure to the poor, assuming they cannot handle it. For example, Dr. Lang said many of his inner-city patients do not have the partners who are necessary to help with home dialysis. Ironically, Neomedica's records at this time said Robert was separated from his wife. He tells that story to anyone who he believes might have the authority to somehow interfere with his disability checks, or Jackie's payments from Public Aid, or the Social Security retirement payments Mrs. Jackson receives.

Yet poverty creates real barriers to home dialysis. People on what is called continuous home peritoneal dialysis must remove wastes three times daily via a catheter surgically implanted in their abdomens. "If there are six people sharing a bathroom, you may not have the sterile environment you need," Shepard said. In addition, people with little education often are leery of taking charge of their own medical care. Doctors would have a tough time persuading Robert and Jackie to bring dialysis home with three children and a bedridden grandmother. "Let the experts handle it," Jackie says.

At dialysis units, social workers are charged with helping patients get back to work. In general, they do not provide the aggressive vocational rehabilitation, or in many cases, vocational *initiation*, poor minority patients might need. Many did not work regularly even before their kidneys failed; 22 percent of working-age black men in Chicago are unemployed,[27] a percentage that is almost certainly higher in places like North Lawndale. Before Robert lost his kidneys, he worked in a hospital kitchen, a car wash, a United Postal Service office; nothing lasted more than a couple of months.

The most social workers usually do is give patients employment referrals, but, as the department of rehabilitation's experience suggests, few outside programs are designed to meet the needs of dialysis patients, who are more likely than people with other disabilities to be routinely sick and tired.

The social worker at Neomedica's downtown unit, Mark Strobel, spent thirty-four hours a week tending to the needs of about 110 dialysis patients, an average caseload for Chicago dialysis units.[28] Though his caseload may not be too far from the norm, social workers in the field say it is nearly impossible to provide intensive job assistance, never mind emotional support, for that many people. That may be especially true since a good part of Strobel's time seemed to be spent trying to enhance not the lives of patients but Neomedica's bottom line.

IMPORTANT NOTICE: PLEASE READ! said a hand-out Strobel gave to Robert and the other patients that summer. "Dear Patients: Due to changes in the Medicare program, it is very important for you to bring any of [sic] all letters from Medicare to me to read over; especially letters requesting you to produce employment status. Failure to comply with Medicare can cause one to lose Medicare coverage and thus be billed for any of [sic] all medical expenses."

Though the letter seemed to warn that patients who lost Medicare would be forced to pay for their dialysis treatments, Neomedica's accounts managers were well aware that the chances of the company recovering from patients were slim. Most simply could not afford it, no matter how many "payment due" notices they received, so to help make sure Neomedica would be paid, the business managers used Strobel to urge patients to comply with Medicare rules.[29]

Strobel's preoccupation with other matters may not have made much difference to Neomedica's regulars since most did not seem to trust him enough to seek his help anyway. Hardly an effusive man, the kind who relied too much on exclamation points to express enthusiasm, Strobel almost seemed to squirm in patients' presence, and he did not stay around long enough to feel at ease. He left the job in July after less than a year, leaving behind a notice on the bulletin board. "I enjoyed my stay at Neomedica, and I will miss you all!" it read. "Good luck and God be with you!"

After he left, social workers from Neomedica's other units had to cover the downtown branch for a time. By early 1991, only six social workers covered all eleven of Neomedica's units (two new locations opened in 1990), which gave them caseloads of 150 to 180 patients each, the highest in Illinois.[30]

The tragic absurdities of a health care system governed by patients' ability to pay are underscored by comparing social work at Neomedica to social work at a dialysis unit in Highland Park, one of the wealthy suburbs north of the city. The dialysis unit is part of Highland Park Hospital, a modern brick and glass structure that is located just past a rolling green golf course and country club where the pool shimmers aquamarine on a clear summer day.

There, through large picture windows, patients take in views of the woods that envelop the hospital. They sip soda from the well-stocked refrigerator, soothe upset stomachs with crackers and soup from the unit's kitchen, and sit on recliners covered with fresh linen, changed between each dialysis session. Each nurse and technician is responsible for two patients, as opposed to four and sometimes more at Neomedica. As at most dialysis units, Medicare is the primary insurance of nearly all of Highland Park's patients; their secondary coverage is what allows them to luxuriate. Only two are covered by Medicaid, the rest by private insurers whose reimbursements are much more generous.[31]

One social worker spends sixteen hours a week at Highland Park serving fifty patients, which makes her caseload 25 to 50 percent smaller than that of Neomedica's social workers. That is to be expected. But after the director of Highland Park's unit offered these numbers, she laughed. All of the patients who want to work do so, she said. "One woman has Picassos hanging in her house. It would be a joke to ask her to work." There really is not much for the social worker to do, she continued, except to make arrangements for patients to receive dialysis when they travel to Europe or Hawaii.

3

Gaps in government insurance
for Mrs. Jackson

Jackie climbed up onto a trunk at the head of her grandmother's bed. She put her right foot on the bed frame, inches from Mrs. Jackson's ear, and her left on the wheelchair that was wedged between the bed and the dresser. Legs spread, her head almost touching the ceiling, she stood there for a second, towering over her grandmother and the crowded bedroom. Jackie crouched down and grabbed her grandmother underneath her arms. She pulled. Mrs. Jackson jerked back a few inches. Jackie yanked again. Mrs. Jackson drooped in Jackie's arms, where Jackie wanted her. Still supporting her grandmother, Jackie carefully stepped down from the wheelchair, then the mattress, and gave one last pull, this time to the left. Mrs. Jackson plopped into the waiting wheelchair.

"We push and pull each other all day," Jackie said later, "and we don't get anywhere."

After Mrs. Jackson came home from Schwab Rehabilitation Center, where she spent three weeks in May after her leg was amputated, Jackie assumed responsibility for all of her care. A home occupational therapist had tried to teach Jackie how to move her grandmother with a canvas belt, but Jackie thought her own technique was better because the room was so cramped. It was also dingy and musty-smelling; a bare bulb on the ceiling provided the only light. And despite Jackie's efforts to eliminate roaches, an occasional one found its way into Mrs. Jackson's room, crawling on the wall next to her bed, or creeping across her sheets. "Home contains architectural barriers to successful rehabilitation, poor, cluttered environment," Rose Murry, a nurse from Mount Sinai's home health agency, had written in Mrs. Jackson's file.

Feeling the watchful eyes of Rose and several other health professionals who came to her home to check on Mrs. Jackson, Jackie often tried to give the apartment a quick cleaning before they arrived. But in some ways her efforts were in vain; she could dump the children's toys in a cardboard box in the living room, or wipe off surfaces, but the smudged walls and water-warped coffee table were beyond help. So was the shag carpet, the casualty of the children's sticky candy, too much spilled pop, too much wear. Only under Mrs. Jackson's couch, which had not been moved for years, were its gold and white hues still recognizable.

Since Rose (Jackie called nurses by their first names) was expected later that morning, Jackie decided to change her grandmother's night-gown. She pulled the pink nylon one Mrs. Jackson was wearing over her head and replaced it with an identical blue-green gown. The whole time, Mrs. Jackson looked straight ahead, her eyes blank, her mouth set in a frown. The elderly woman had raised Jackie, and their recent shift in roles made Jackie uneasy. When Mrs. Jackson first became incontinent, she would stare silently at Jackie when she cleaned her up. "Close your eyes Mama," Jackie told her grandmother. "Don't look at me when I'm doing this."

Jackie handed her grandmother her glasses from the dresser, and Mrs. Jackson carefully put them on. In old pictures Mrs. Jackson has a slight double chin and a thick neck; she looks healthy, if overweight. These days, the largish pale pink glasses rest on distinct cheekbones, with hollows underneath, and her neck is thin, the wrinkled skin pale and delicate.

Jackie wheeled her grandmother into the living room, where Robert slouched on the couch, his eyes closed. He had come home from dialysis a short while ago and felt tired. The treatments wear him out, but even when he is feeling well, he does not help Jackie care for her grandmother. DeMarest and Brianna were chasing each other, weaving around Mrs. Jackson's wheelchair. Two years older, DeMarest had the advantage and playfully grabbed at his little sister's shirt. "Tell him not to hit you or we'll get on him," Mrs. Jackson said gruffly to Brianna, who stared at her uncomprehendingly before going on with her game. Too young to understand, Brianna did not appreciate Mrs. Jackson's attempt to side with her against DeMarest.

Rose rang the doorbell shortly after Mrs. Jackson was settled in her chair. The nurse was stopping by to check the stump of Mrs. Jackson's amputated leg, which had not yet healed completely, as well as to monitor her diabetes, high blood pressure, and heart disease. She also needed to check her darkening left toe and her bedsores, one on her buttocks and another one developing on her left heel.

Rose quickly went to work. She put a thermometer in Mrs. Jackson's mouth. While she waited for her temperature to register, she wrapped a blood pressure cuff around her arm. Mrs. Jackson kept her eyes lowered.

Next, Rose crouched down in front of the wheelchair to inspect Mrs. Jackson's foot. "I don't like the color of that toe," she said. But the toe was still warm to the touch and had a pulse, which meant gangrene had not set in.

"You're going to have everything cut off," Jackie said bluntly, perhaps trying to shock her grandmother into conversing with the nurse. Jackie wanted her grandmother to speak for herself; she worried that she might leave something out that could prove important.

Rose cut Mrs. Jackson's disposable stretchy slipper up the center to ease the pressure on her toe. Mrs. Jackson had been asking Jackie to cut her toenails, but Jackie refused on instructions from doctors. Any mishaps could cause wounds that might not heal because of the poor circulation diabetics develop in their extremities. Jackie thought her grandmother was beginning to resent her for refusing to perform this seemingly simple task, so she asked Rose what she should do.

"Jackie shouldn't be cutting your toenails so don't get mad at her when she says 'No,'" Rose counseled.

"Thank you, ma'am," Mrs. Jackson responded curtly.

Jackie asked Rose whether Medicare or Medicaid would pay for the adult diapers her grandmother needed. Rose said she didn't think either would.

"I'll see you Monday. We'll look at your foot, your stump, and your behind," Rose said to Mrs. Jackson as she left.

Mrs. Jackson nodded.

Nurses, physical therapists, and other health professionals who visit sick people in their homes have become more important because of changes in federal health care financing for the elderly over the past decade. Congress liberalized coverage of home health care services under Medicare in 1980. The change eliminated a hundred-day annual limit on home health visits, as well as a requirement that patients be hospitalized for at least three days before qualifying for home care. A more well-known change that increased the use of home health services was Medicare's introduction of DRGs, or diagnosis-related groups, in 1983. In an attempt to control costs, Medicare began to pay hospitals predetermined rates for patients, depending on their diagnoses. Since hospitals receive a set amount for patients regardless of the cost of care, they have an incentive to discharge patients as soon as possible. The result is that patients who might have spent a few extra days in the hospital recuperating are now discharged "sicker and quicker" and need care from a home nurse. It also means that families are left with the responsibility of caring for more seriously ill relatives, a burden that falls heaviest on poor families like Jackie's, who have few resources to draw upon.

Despite the growth in Medicare reimbursement for home health services—a 24 percent annual rate of increase from 1974 to 1986[1]— expenditures still are mostly for acute, hospital-based care. The $2.5 billion Medicare spent on home care in 1989 accounted for only 2.7 percent of the agency's total expenditures.[2]

Mrs. Jackson and Jackie were expecting another visitor from Mount Sinai's home health agency that day, Sister Mary Ellen Meckley, a social worker who visits homebound patients to assess whether they are receiving the community services available to them. Sister Mary Ellen had not set a firm appointment but was expected sometime that afternoon, so Jackie decided to start on her grandmother's hair. She had just finished loosening her tiny braids, which had grown frizzy, when the buzzer rang again.

Sister Mary Ellen bustled into the living room. "How are you?" she asked Mrs. Jackson cheerfully. The lines around Sister Mary Ellen's eyes crinkled as she smiled; she looked genuinely pleased to see Mrs. Jackson again. The last time she had been out to the house Mrs. Jackson still had her leg; only her foot had been removed.

"All right," Mrs. Jackson said in a low voice that did not attempt to match Sister Mary Ellen's enthusiasm.

Surprise flashed almost imperceptibly across Sister Mary Ellen's face—the last time she had seen Mrs. Jackson she had seemed much more lively—but she did not dwell on the old woman's low spirits. She plunked down on the worn couch and asked Jackie what she needed. Dressed in a crisp white blouse and navy skirt, the colors Mount Sinai home workers are required to wear to signal their benign intentions, she exuded a warm efficiency.

Jackie told Sister Mary Ellen that Rose, the nurse, had informed her that neither Medicare nor Medicaid would pay for adult diapers, which cost $45 for a box of forty-eight. "No, no," Sister Mary Ellen corrected her, explaining that Rose was new on the job. "It's Medicare that doesn't cover diapers. Medicaid covers them. It's crazy."

"Thank you," Jackie said, putting a lilting emphasis on "thank" in the way that she does when another person confirms her beliefs.

Medicare pays for Mrs. Jackson's home health services and virtually all of her hospital costs, after she pays a $560 annual hospital deductible. For a $31.90 monthly premium, it also pays for 80 percent of her doctors' bills. The $7,428 annual income she receives from Social Security puts her about $1,400 over the federally defined poverty level,[3] and so she does not qualify for a program Congress created in 1988 to exempt the poor elderly from Medicare's deductibles and copayments.

Ironically, even if Mrs. Jackson were poor enough, chances are she would still be paying those expenses out-of-pocket. A study conducted by a senior citizens' advocacy group concluded that about half of the four million poor elderly thought to be eligible for the extra benefit were not receiving it. That is because it is up to the elderly to apply for the program, and the agency that administers Medicare, the Health Care Financing Administration (HCFA), said it could not afford to identify and contact everyone who might be eligible.

Critics say the government could find many potential recipients by using its own computers. "If this benefit were for the four million richest Americans, I'd bet that the White House would make sure they got every penny of it," charged Ronald Pollack, executive director of the Families United for Senior Action Foundation, whose report suggested that HCFA was not informing people to save money.[4]

Deductibles and copayments aside, Medicare does not cover many things that Mrs. Jackson and other chronically ill people need, such as medications, transportation to doctors' appointments, and, as was the issue this day, adult diapers. According to HCFA rules, Medicare covers only services or supplies that are "medically necessary." And adult diapers are not, according to an official at HCFA's regional office in Chicago. "They are bought without a prescription; they are more of a convenience," she said. Many devices or supplies that can prevent disease and disability from worsening are not covered by Medicare because its reimbursement criteria emphasize curing acute conditions rather than maintaining health or improving daily functioning—a policy that may be penny-wise but pound-foolish. Adult diapers, for instance, can prevent bedsores, as well as allow people to get out of their homes. Another example of shortsightedness, criticized in a report by the Institute of Medicine, a health policy group based in Washington, D.C., was Medicare's denial of coverage for grab bars in bathrooms. They are considered convenience items, although bathroom falls are a leading cause of hip fractures and other often devastating injuries among the elderly.[5]

The convoluted logic used to justify coverage of certain items as opposed to others can sound preposterous to lay people like Jackie. When another Medicare official was asked why, if Medicare doesn't cover diapers, it covers home catheters also used for incontinence, she replied, "We would consider the diapers and Chux [absorbent pads for Mrs. Jackson's bed] more as comfort items, whereas a tube or catheter would be considered a medical type of supply."

Though Medicare covers both rich and poor, the poor, of course, are much more vulnerable to its shortcomings. Elderly people more affluent than Mrs. Jackson do not have to worry about coming up with $45 for a box of diapers. They also often retire with supplementary health insurance provided by their employers, or buy "Medigap" insurance, special policies that pay for some of the care Medicare doesn't cover. Even if Mrs. Jackson could afford Medigap insurance, her "pre-existing" medical conditions probably would preclude her getting such commercial coverage, which she has never had in her life. The closest Mrs. Jackson came to a Medigap insurer—in the months she qualified—was Medicaid.

Since Medicaid covered the adult diapers, Sister Mary Ellen offered to call a medical supply company to order them. Jackie appreciated her help because the day before she had pored over the Yellow Pages trying to figure out which companies would bill one of the government insurers for the diapers rather than require cash up front.

Jackie's pleasure was fleeting. The suburban medical supply company, Peiser's Medical Supplies and Services, refused to fill the order for the diapers. The clerk said she had no proof Peiser's would be reimbursed by Medicaid. When she punched Mrs. Jackson's name into the computer, "spend-down not met" had popped onto the screen. Mrs. Jackson's $619 monthly income is too high for her to qualify outright for Medicaid. Her spend-down is akin to a deductible, a set amount of money she must spend every month on medical needs before Medicaid kicks in.

Jackie set down her jar of hairstyling grease and grabbed a piece of paper sitting on the hutch. It was a letter she had received from the Illinois Department of Public Aid, which administers Medicaid. It said her grandmother's spend-down had been met nine days earlier, starting the first of the month.

Sister Mary Ellen picked up the phone again, this time to call Jackie's local Public Aid office. Sitting on the couch, she rested the mouthpiece under her chin as the phone rang and rang. Sister Mary Ellen's first trying encounter with the spend-down program had come days after it began in 1981, she told Jackie. "I got this call from this nurse saying her patient's blood pressure was way high, and the woman was going crazy because she could not get a green card to buy her meds."

Sister Mary Ellen guessed that Mrs. Jackson's spend-down problem stemmed from a delay at IDPA in entering her eligibility into the computer. But she could only guess because no one answered the phone.

"They're not supposed to go on break until 3:15," Sister Mary Ellen sighed.

As Jackie wove her grandmother's hair into tiny new braids, Brianna walked tentatively toward the wheelchair. Mrs. Jackson's face softened. She put out her hand. Brianna ran off.

"I can't believe you're so quiet," Sister Mary Ellen said to Mrs. Jackson, who was still sitting in her wheelchair.

"Yup," she responded. Mrs. Jackson met Sister Mary Ellen's eyes for a moment, then looked away, toward a homemade wind chime that hung near the front door. Crafted from a plastic soda bottle, "Cora" written across its base, it had been a gift from a resident in a nursing home where Mrs. Jackson had worked as an aide.

"How was your stay at Schwab?" Sister Mary Ellen pressed.

"It was all right." Mrs. Jackson's mouth barely moved.

Sister Mary Ellen set down the receiver. "I guess the caseworker got an early break."

To get Medicaid without a spend-down in 1989, single elderly and disabled people could not bring in more than $292 a month—what is known as the medically needy level in Illinois.[6] On paper, Mrs. Jackson received $686 from Social Security each month, but she actually got only $619 because Medicare's $31.90 monthly premium was taken from her check as was a deduction for an overpayment she erroneously received in years past. The Department of Public Aid based its calculations on what she was entitled to, however, not what she got, so Mrs.

Jackson had to put at least $394 ($686 − $292) toward medical expenses each month in order to get a green card.

She was one of nearly twenty-six thousand aged, blind, and disabled Illinois residents who participated in the spend-down program.[7] They have less than $2,000 in assets, another requirement for the program, but their incomes are too high to qualify for Medicaid without a spend-down. That does not mean that twenty-six thousand people actually are covered by Medicaid at any one time. It just means that they could get green cards if they met their spend-downs; the Department of Public Aid says it has no statistics on the number of people who do so regularly.

The program was designed with good intentions: to provide some relief for people with medical costs that dwarfed their incomes. But its strict income limits, as well as its cumbersome rules, have made it a headache for people who are chronically ill. Its inherent erratic nature runs counter to a basic tenet of good primary health care: detect small problems quickly and treat them regularly so they do not balloon into serious illnesses that are more debilitating, and far more costly.

It was Jackie's responsibility to gather medical bills or receipts month by month and take them to the local Public Aid office, a chore she understandably did not enjoy, especially since she felt like she was dumping the bills into a vacuum. The Public Aid caseworker told her she need not make an appointment to drop off her grandmother's receipts; she should simply leave them at the front desk. "It might be two days later until [the caseworker] comes to pick them up," Jackie complained. "How am I supposed to know?"

Two days can make a big difference. People become eligible for a green card on the day of the month that their medical bills and receipts show they have met their spend-down. If Mrs. Jackson meets her spend-down on the twentieth of the month, she qualifies that day for the rest of the month. So ten days after she becomes eligible, her coverage expires. As Jackie says, "By the time I get the card, it's time to do it again."

Jackie also was bitter because for years her grandmother had received a Medicaid green card without having to pay a spend-down first. "When she didn't need the green card, she got it like clockwork." Jackie suspected that as her grandmother got sicker, and the pile of medical bills grew, Public Aid had resorted to the spend-down to cut costs. It was reasonable to question the agency's motives: her grandmother's income had not changed since 1985, so why only now was she being informed of a $394 spend-down?

The answer is that the Department of Public Aid had made a mistake. Records at Mrs. Jackson's Public Aid office show that a spend-down amount had been calculated for her in 1985 when her income increased, but somehow it had never been picked up on the computer. As a result, she had received a medical card every month without a spend-down.[8]

That Mrs. Jackson slipped through the system did not surprise the staff at the local Public Aid office on Ogden Avenue, a short walk from Jackie's apartment. Until the late 1980s, the two or three spend-down workers there handled an astronomical 1,500 cases each, despite the complexity of their job compared to others at the agency: the constant flow of medical bills, the hand calculations required, the inquiries from hospitals and doctors' offices. In addition, during the early 1980s, spend-down procedures regularly changed in response to a flood of lawsuits that forced Public Aid to administer the medical program more fairly. Jackie would find it hard to fathom, but before the lawsuits were settled, the spend-down program was even more unpredictable and confusing. Since its inception, Medicaid has been tied to welfare, and messes like this one persuade public health experts that an agency with the primary mission of putting people on welfare rolls (or taking them off) is not equipped to run health care programs.[9]

Jackie's hypothesis about the reason her grandmother now had to pay a spend-down was partially correct. Though there was no conspiracy to deny Mrs. Jackson coverage, her increased flow of medical bills probably jogged Public Aid to review her case. In that review, the department discovered its own mistake. Sister Mary Ellen weighed this kind of factor when she advised one of her clients who was receiving a green card without a spend-down *not* to use it for covered medical transportation. She knew the old woman's income was way too high for a green card without strings attached, and Sister Mary Ellen worried that if she started using it too much, Public Aid would be alerted to the mistake and put her on spend-down. "I told her to keep calling her nephew for a ride," Sister Mary Ellen said. "She needed to keep the card for medication."

Mrs. Jackson did not know this, but she could have received a green card without having to spend half of her income first if she and her second husband had not worked enough to receive Social Security. There are two primary tracks to provide income and medical care to elderly and disabled people. Mrs. Jackson was on the first track: she received Social Security and was covered by Medicare.[10] The second track is for disabled people who either worked very little over the course of their lives, or worked at jobs where contributions are not made to the Social Security System (cleaning women, for instance, often fall into this latter category). They receive very low Supplemental Security Income payments—$368 a month in Illinois in 1989—and are covered by Medicaid. The dialysis patient Adelle received SSI and Medicaid, and so did Mrs. Jackson's son, Tommy, after he was disabled by the stroke.

The hitch was that although Mrs. Jackson was on the first track and received the more generous Social Security pension, as well as Medicare, she still needed Medicaid as backup insurance for medications, adult diapers, transportation, and the like. To get it, she had to spend down her income to the state's medically needy level. In Illinois, again, the medically needy level was $292 in 1989, or 58 percent of the federal poverty level. Meanwhile, SSI recipients are allowed to keep their full $368 a month *and* get Medicaid green cards.

Tom Grippando works for United Charities as a legal aid attorney who helps poor Chicagoans like the Baneses get fair treatment from the Department of Public Aid. He was particularly incensed about what he calls the spend-down program's discriminatory treatment of workers (remember, many SSI recipients never worked). "SSI recipients are $76 ahead of people who had the misfortune of working for a living," said Grippando. He argues that the Department of Public Aid should disregard the first $368 of all elderly people's incomes so that workers are not cheated. But that seems unlikely. A Public Aid official conceded the system was "harsh and unjust," but he said his agency cannot change its rules unless federal law is amended.

If this all sounds incredibly confusing, that's because it is. Because the United States does not provide a basic level of health care to all its citizens, the country is left with a patchwork of state and federal programs among which inconsistencies are inevitable. People are divided into groups and subgroups, and then divided again. Administrative costs consume up to a quarter of America's health care spending (public and private), whereas they add up to no more than 11 percent in Canada.[11] That country guarantees health care to all its citizens and does not fritter away dollars determining who should get care and, more to the point, who should not.

If Mrs. Jackson were feeling better, she probably would scoff at the spend-down inequity for Social Security recipients, but she would not bother fighting it. Instead she would find a way around it. Mrs. Jackson was an "old pro" at working the system, Jackie said, taking her pay in untraceable cash and using a variety of other methods that serve as unofficial tax deductions for the working poor. Sometimes her grandmother went by the book; sometimes she did not.

In the living room hutch, a snapshot of Mrs. Jackson in a tarnished gold frame hints at what she was like in her prime. She is pictured with a favorite cousin, B.J. His arm is slung over her shoulder, and she leans into him. Her short hair is swept back from her broad, fleshy face, and she is wearing a pale blue dress. It has a high scoop neck but is fitted and does not hide her figure. B.J. is smiling broadly, almost laughing, his teeth flashing. Mrs. Jackson, too, looks like she gets the joke, but her burgundy-shaded lips are pressed together in a smile that is more cryptic, a bit flirtatious, perhaps. Cora Jackson looked like a woman who played her cards close to the vest.

"The truck drivers loved her," Jackie said of her grandmother, who for some years worked as a cook and waitress at a nearby truck stop and bar. "They'd slip dollar bills into her apron pockets." Jackie knows this because during high school she also worked at the truck stop, making beds for the drivers who rented rooms on the second floor of the establishment. Over the holidays, she and her grandmother put wrapped "Christmas boxes" by the cash register so they could pick up extra tips.

"I thought we had tall bucks," Jackie said, remembering the "silver" that her grandmother would lay out on top of the console television when she came home. She worked there twelve hours a day, from 5 A.M. to 5 P.M., Jackie said. Before and after that job, she worked as a health aide in nursing homes and in private homes.

At work, Mrs. Jackson used another name, Cora Stone, with another Social Security number, which Jackie guessed her grandmother obtained when she first moved to Chicago in the early 1960s. Sometimes she paid taxes under this name, and sometimes she didn't have to worry about taxes because her jobs paid cash, such as the job at the truck stop. This way, she was able to collect about $200 a month in

Social Security disability benefits that she was awarded in 1971 on the basis of high blood pressure and arthritis (conditions that plagued her before diabetes became a serious problem). Cora Jackson knew that her money would have been threatened had Social Security known she was working.

Jackie said her grandmother also enhanced her income illegally when her boyfriend died. Percy Jackson had been living with Jackie and her grandmother for about a year when a police officer knocked on the door one day in 1975 and informed them that Mr. Jackson had been badly burned trying to stamp out a fire at his factory job. Jackie remembers that her grandmother had been cooking a dinner of fried liver, rice, and rolls. "With Mr. Jackson there, she would actually set the table, put out bowls with silverware," Jackie said. "He was good to Mama. He was a railroad man and worked around the steel mills; he had plenty of money."

After about a month in the burn unit of Cook County Hospital, Mr. Jackson died. At that point, according to Jackie, Mrs. Jackson, who had used her first husband's name, decided she "needed to get hold of the cash this man had coming." After all, there was no one else to claim it; Mr. Jackson had never been married to Cora or anyone else. Shortly thereafter, a marriage certificate arrived in the mail, sent by one of Mrs. Jackson's sisters who lived in Cleveland, Ohio. Cora and Percy had never been to Cleveland, but Social Security accepted the evidently bogus marriage certificate, and Cora took the last name Jackson.

When she turned sixty-five in 1985, she began to receive widow's benefits from Social Security (Mr. Jackson's retirement income). That's when her official income jumped from $250 a month in disability payments to more than $600.

Jackie said she told her grandmother she was going to get caught one of these days and get shipped off to jail. But Mrs. Jackson never seemed too worried. "I'll cross that bridge when I come to it," she told Jackie.

From a middle-class point of view, Mrs. Jackson's finagling yielded very little extra income. If she had not worked and only collected disability, she and her granddaughter would have been forced to live on $200 a month. She was entitled to the disability payments: the Social Security Administration had investigated her case and declared her disabled because of her arthritis and high blood pressure. But as

Robert knows, that entitlement ends if disabled people manage to work and earn more than about $300 a month. Then disability payments are cut off, on the assumption that if people can work at all they are not, by definition, disabled.

Mrs. Jackson's solution was to work under an assumed name, earning another $500 a month and enabling her and Jackie to live more comfortably, though their annual income always hovered around the poverty level. When Mrs. Jackson decided to retire at sixty-five, she relied on her deceased "husband's" Social Security retirement payments to replace her lost income.

Equally important, if not more important than the $200 extra a month Mrs. Jackson received after she was declared disabled, was the medical insurance to which she was entitled. Two years after people begin receiving Social Security Disability payments, they are eligible for Medicare, as well as for secondary insurance from Medicaid, providing their incomes are low enough.

If Mrs. Jackson had not sought disability, she would not have had health insurance until she turned sixty-five and became eligible for Medicare. None of her minimum-wage jobs provided insurance. As a working-age single adult she could not have received Medicaid because she did not fall into any of the right groups. There are a series of gates the poor must pass through to receive Medicaid, the first being "categorical eligibility." The categories of people covered were, and for the most part still are: single parents (grandparents raising their grandchildren usually don't count), children of single parents, and the aged, blind, or disabled.[12] Rules like these, as well as a second gate that shuts out all but the poorest of poor (though it is inching open for young children and pregnant women because of recent Medicaid reforms), explain why only 36 percent of people under sixty-five with incomes below the federal poverty level were covered by Medicaid in 1989. The proportion was somewhat higher for poor children; 46 percent of them were covered.[13]

By waitressing, cooking, and caretaking on the sly, Mrs. Jackson avoided becoming one of the uninsured whom numerous studies have shown to have worse health indicators than any other group. They see doctors the least often, are sicker when they do, and even when hospitalized, they receive fewer medical procedures than others.[14]

Yet even with Medicare and sporadic Medicaid coverage, Mrs. Jackson's access to medical care was far below the standard most middle-class Americans expect. Although it is impossible to know exactly what would have happened had Mrs. Jackson told the whole truth and become one of the working uninsured, it's not hard to imagine that she would have skimped on her high blood pressure medication to make ends meet, or foregone a doctor's appointment to have her hypertension monitored. Her health could have deteriorated much earlier than it did, and she might not have been around to finish raising Jackie.

A few days after Sister Mary Ellen's visit, Jackie stood at the door of her grandmother's bedroom as Rose, the home nurse, began another checkup. Mrs. Jackson looked almost lost in her double bed, lying flat on her back in the middle of the pink sheets. Rose suggested that Jackie get a hospital bed with a crank so that Mrs. Jackson could sit up more easily. Jackie was using a large throw pillow to prop her grandmother up, but it often slipped out of place. Jackie knew that Medicare would pay monthly rental for the bed, but she was not sure she wanted one. She wanted to keep her grandmother's large mattress and cherry wood headboard, but she had no place other than the bedroom to store them.

Jackie helped Rose dress her grandmother's bedsores, then left the nurse to finish the job while she folded her children's laundry into small squares in the living room. Her grandmother's Medicaid spend-down still had not been officially approved, which was a problem as she was due for a doctor's appointment later in the week.

The Baneses have little choice but to hire a special medical van, called a medicar, to take Mrs. Jackson to doctors' appointments at Mount Sinai's outpatient department. Even if they had a car, Jackie and Robert probably could not maneuver Mrs. Jackson from their second-floor apartment to the street. It takes two attendants to lift her onto a stretcher and carry her downstairs to the medicar. (For that reason, Mrs. Jackson was not eligible for the Chicago Transit Authority program that Robert used; recipients must be able to get "curbside" under their own steam.)

Medicaid covers medicars, but without the spend-down approval, Jackie faced the prospect of coming up with $70 for the round trip to Mount Sinai, about a mile away. Medicare, of course, pays for 80 percent of Mrs. Jackson's doctors' bills, but it does not pay to get her to their offices. Again, Medicare covers only "medically necessary" transportation; nonemergency trips to the doctor's office do not count.

"I'm ready to go back to the work world so bad, but I got to find me something midnights," Jackie lamented as she tried to figure out how she was going to come up with the money to get her grandmother to the doctor. Jackie had not worked regularly outside her home since her children were born, but she often talked about going back. She had been a clerk at JC Penney's, at Montgomery Ward's, and at the offices of an automobile importer. She also was an office cleaning lady, the job she seemed to remember most fondly. "I worked in the VIP area, where you had the glass tables, the carpeted floors, the little bars," she said, smiling at the memory. She and her co-workers occasionally stole a nip from the bar; other times they were invited to take home leftover food and drink from a party or meeting.

Though Jackie sometimes sounded like she would embark on a job search the next day, she was ambivalent about working, partly because she did not trust Robert to watch the children. "I have gotten home and Brianna would be standing up in the window, and Robert would be on the couch asleep. I told him I didn't enjoy seeing my baby up there walking in the window."

Rose emerged from Mrs. Jackson's bedroom carrying her small black bag. "Do you want to test Mom's sugar?" Jackie asked, sitting next to her pile of laundry. Rose said she wanted to see Jackie do it, since part of her job is teaching Jackie to care for her grandmother on her own. Jackie didn't budge from the couch. She had learned to change her grandmother's bandages using sterile procedures, and to monitor her blood sugar and other vital signs, but she obviously was not in the mood to practice her skills. Rose got the message, suggesting that they wait until next time to check Mrs. Jackson's diabetes. Jackie wasn't off the hook yet, however.

"Can I see what she's been eating?" Rose asked.

Jackie got up and went to the kitchen, returning with a plate that contained Mrs. Jackson's mostly uneaten breakfast: a biscuit, rice, and two strips of bacon. "I saw bacon on her plate, which she shouldn't be having," Rose chided.

"I'm buying low-salt bacon," Jackie protested weakly, "and boiling it to get rid of the salt."

Rose did not look convinced. "I'll see you in a couple days," she said as she headed for the door.

"OK, then," Jackie said with finality. She followed Rose out onto the second-floor landing and watched her walk down the stairs, watched until she could see her no more. Then Jackie returned to the apartment, and firmly shut the door.

Though Rose obviously got on Jackie's nerves sometimes, she was much more comfortable with her and the other nurses than she was with the doctors her grandmother saw at the hospital. She had actually liked another home nurse, Michelle, who went on maternity leave and was replaced by Rose. If Jackie had recently changed her grandmother's bandages, Michelle would not bother to do it herself. "Michelle would skip it because she had confidence in me. If I come in here and tell her I done did it, she'd say, 'OK, I'll go on.'"

While Jackie talked more freely with the nurses than doctors, she did not hesitate to hold back certain information if she thought they would not approve. Some days, when Rose or Michelle told her that Mrs. Jackson's blood pressure was good, Jackie skipped her medication for the rest of the day. She thought she could not afford to do otherwise. A month's worth of medication to control Mrs. Jackson's high blood pressure, diabetes, and other problems costs at least $75. Medicaid usually would pick up the tab, but Mrs. Jackson's coverage was too unpredictable for Jackie to depend on it, so she rationed. She also counted on Mrs. Jackson's frequent stays in the hospital to keep drug costs down. When her grandmother received medicine from the hospital, she did not have to use the pills in brown bottles on top of her dresser.

Jackie thought that so far she had been a pretty fair judge of how much medication her grandmother needed. One time, she took Mrs. Jackson to the doctor after she had gone three days without high blood pressure pills. "Wow, keep doing what you're doing," Jackie said the doctor told her. "Her pressure is good."

4

Fitful primary care fails Mrs. Jackson

A few days after Rose's visit, Mrs. Jackson saw her internist at Mount Sinai, Dr. Boris Gurevich.

"Can you feel this?" asked Dr. Gurevich. He was examining Mrs. Jackson's remaining leg, poking the top of her blackening left toe with his index finger. Mrs. Jackson did not reply immediately.

"No . . .," she began.

". . . or does it feel like it's dead?"

Dr. Gurevich, Jackie, and her grandmother were squeezed tightly into a small medical suite at Mount Sinai, where on Thursday mornings, between about 8:30 and 10, the physician sees patients from the West Side.

Jackie watched the exchange between Dr. Gurevich and her grandmother carefully. After prodding at her dark toe, he looked at the sore on Mrs. Jackson's heel. He did not ask about her diabetes, or check the deepening, half-dollar-size bedsore on her buttocks, which Jackie brought to his attention.

"Bring her back in two weeks," he said.

"Why can't we admit her today before it gets worse?" Jackie demanded. "We have to pay for the medicar, and we may not be able to come back."

Dr. Gurevich did not respond to Jackie's plea. Instead, he picked up the phone and rang Mrs. Jackson's podiatrist, Dr. Robert I. Steinberg. Then he called Mount Sinai's admitting office.

Irregular primary care had been a problem for Mrs. Jackson from the start, when diabetic gangrene was first diagnosed in her right foot in February. That infection, of course, had led to the amputation of her right leg, and Jackie feared that events were about to repeat themselves. Diabetics who lose one leg have a 50–50 chance of losing the other.[1]

Back in the waiting room, Mrs. Jackson leaned forward to take the pressure off her bedsore. The only time she got out of the house was to go to the doctor, and she was dressed for the occasion in a mauve housecoat with china-blue roses and a navy turban. Jackie wore a fuchsia blouse and matching slacks. At home, she wears cotton house dresses and tennis shoes with the backs crushed down into makeshift slippers, but she would never leave the house like that. "I have two appearances, my inside appearance and my outside appearance," Jackie says. "My family tells me they like the way I look when I'm walking out the door."

Mrs. Jackson's lips were pressed tightly together. She began to moan softly every minute or so. "I wish they'd hurry up," she said in the first sentence she had spoken all morning. "My poor back is hurting me." Though Jackie had told her that it confuses doctors, Mrs. Jackson prefers to call her buttocks her back.

A half hour passed before the admitting clerk arrived. The wait was not overly long, but Jackie had become increasingly agitated as she watched her grandmother grimace in pain. "This ain't no hotel," Jackie said finally.

Worried about her grandmother's foot and not wanting to miss the appointment, Jackie had been stewing all week about how to scrape together the money to get her grandmother back and forth to see Dr. Gurevich. Finally, the day before the appointment, Public Aid's computer registered that she had met her spend-down. With Mrs. Jackson's name in the computer, the medicar companies would transport her to Mount Sinai without requiring cash up front, as they trusted that Public Aid would pay the bill. Otherwise, Mrs. Jackson probably would have missed the appointment because Jackie could not spare seventy dollars for the two-mile roundtrip ride to Mount Sinai. For that reason, Mrs. Jackson had missed an appointment earlier in the week with the podiatrist, Dr. Steinberg.

Jackie had inquired about scheduling all of her grandmother's doctors' appointments on the same day, but that did not fit the physicians' schedules. Neither Dr. Steinberg nor Dr. Gurevich have offices at Mount Sinai; they only see outpatients there for a couple of hours each week. Dr. Steinberg's office is in Oak Park, a suburb on the western border of Chicago, fairly close to the Baneses' home in North Lawndale. But seeing Dr. Gurevich at his office was out of the question. He is based far from the hospital in a Russian-Jewish enclave on the northwest side of Chicago, a trip of at least a half-hour each way by car. Dr. Gurevich bases his practice there because many of his patients are Russian-Jewish immigrants, as he is; the physician came to the United States in 1978.

As an attending physician at Mount Sinai, Dr. Gurevich gets additional patients when he is on call in the hospital's emergency room one day a month. Patients who are admitted to the hospital through the emergency room on that day but who do not have a doctor may be referred to him. These patients are almost always blacks and Hispanics from the neighborhood. He picks up a few additional West Side patients through referrals from other physicians, which is how he came to be Mrs. Jackson's doctor.

Dr. Steinberg had been the first doctor at Mount Sinai to examine Mrs. Jackson, when she visited him at his Monday-morning clinic four months before in February. "We put her in the hospital right away," Dr. Steinberg said, remembering her gangrenous foot. "Her big toe and part of her foot were as black as coffee." As a podiatrist, Dr. Steinberg does not have the training to treat Mrs. Jackson's significant medical problems—diabetes, high blood pressure, and peripheral vascular disease—so he asked Dr. Gurevich to accept her as a patient.

Some of the most fundamental deficiencies in Mrs. Jackson's care can only be found by going back to this time, to the events that led to the amputation of her right leg in April, and even further back, to the years when she lacked the basic care necessary to prevent the crippling complications of diabetes. There, little support can be found for the notion that Medicare assures the same quality and quantity of care to the middle-class and poor elderly. The episodic, uncoordinated nature of Mrs. Jackson's treatment conspired against her health, until, as Jackie would say, "It look like Mama going to have to get just about everything cut off."

For people who believe in bad signs, and Jackie and her family do—Robert tells of being alerted to his mother's death by a howling cat—Mrs. Jackson's first attempt to have her diabetic gangrene treated in February was ominous.

The big toe on her right foot was infected and had become progressively painful and dark over the course of several weeks. "It was very foul," Jackie said. "But her being Miss Doctor, she thought it was a bad bruise." Mrs. Jackson's diabetes was not severe enough to require insulin injections, but she had known she was diabetic and had taken medication for the condition for some years. Despite that, she evidently did not know that foot problems often accompany diabetes. Even if she had, she may not have realized that without prompt treatment infections can quickly turn gangrenous and require amputation.

She was not putting off the doctor's appointment for lack of insurance. Then as now, Mrs. Jackson was covered by Medicare, which paid for her visit when she finally decided to seek help from Dr. Hector Marino, a general practitioner whom the family had visited for all manner of problems since Jackie was a girl.

Dr. Marino had been prescribing medication in a not too successful effort to control Mrs. Jackson's diabetes for about a decade. When he saw her foot one Friday in February, he decided to refer her to another doctor. Jackie said he told her grandmother to visit a podiatrist but did not recommend anyone in particular, so Jackie planned to take her to one the next Monday. But by Saturday, her grandmother was in such pain that Jackie called 911 for a Chicago Fire Department ambulance. She spoke to a dispatcher. "I was telling them my grandmother's toe was messed up and she needed to get to the hospital. They said they was no cab service for somebody who got a hurt toe."

She called again on Sunday and embellished her story, making her grandmother's condition sound more serious, and the dispatcher agreed to send out an ambulance. Mrs. Jackson was lying in bed when the paramedic arrived. He asked her some questions about her health, took her blood pressure, then pulled out a penlight and illuminated her toe. He switched it off.

"The hospital isn't going to do anything but wrap it up and send her home," Jackie said he told her.

"You bring her back then," Jackie responded.

"We don't do that," he said, and left.

Later, Jackie would hone the skill of making her grandmother's illness "sound a little more impossible than it is." In November, months after the above incident, when the old woman was vomiting and refusing to eat, Jackie again called the fire department, which does not require payment up front. "My grandmother had a fall," Jackie lied, "and her stomach is paining her." The fall did the trick; the paramedics promptly arrived to take Mrs. Jackson to Mount Sinai, where she was sick enough to be admitted.

But back in February, Jackie was still a novice at working the system. So the Monday morning after the paramedics refused to transport her grandmother, she called a couple of foot doctors whose offices were relatively close to the house but none could see her grandmother that day. This was not a simple task: although the Yellow Pages has a one-page display advertisement of podiatrists according to neighborhood, no poor neighborhoods are included. The individual listings are ten pages long and in small type; Jackie went through, skimming the addresses after each doctor's name. With the morning wearing on, she decided to call Mount Sinai directly, where Mrs. Jackson's sister Eldora went for her diabetes. Here her luck changed, at least for a moment.

Fortunately, it was a Monday, because Mount Sinai's podiatry clinic is only held once a week, for three hours on Monday mornings. Dr. Steinberg was working the clinic and agreed to see Mrs. Jackson right away. He told Jackie to get her grandmother to the hospital's outpatient Kling building by 12:30 P.M.

Jackie returned to the Yellow Pages. Since she didn't think her grandmother could make it on the bus, she called several private ambulance services. The first two quoted prices of $100 to take her grandmother one way to Mount Sinai. Finally, a smaller outfit said they would carry her for $35.

Dr. Steinberg hospitalized Mrs. Jackson immediately. Over a two-week stay, most of her right foot was amputated and surgeons inserted a synthetic blood vessel in her thigh to route blood around her own obstructed vessel. They hoped to increase circulation to the remainder of her foot so that any leftover infection could be cleared away. Mrs. Jackson went home in early March, under the care of a home nurse who was to visit once a day for the first week and twice a week for eight weeks thereafter.

From here on, Mrs. Jackson would be cared for through Mount Sinai's outpatient department. Dr. Marino did not follow her at Mount Sinai, though he had when she was admitted to Saint Anthony Hospital in 1987 after suffering a stroke, from which she recovered almost completely. Jackie did not push for Dr. Marino to come to Mount Sinai because she had the impression from doctors there that he should have immediately hospitalized her grandmother when he saw her gangrenous foot. For his part, Dr. Marino said that for convenience's sake he prefers to restrict his practice to one Chicago hospital, Saint Anthony.

Both hospitals border Douglas Park, Saint Anthony to the south, and Mount Sinai to the east. The Catholic institution traditionally has been the hospital of choice for South Lawndale residents, most of them Hispanic. Mount Sinai, on the other hand, has drawn more of its patients from the all-black North Lawndale. These boundaries do not hold tight because of doctors' practice patterns and other factors. Were it not for Jackie, for example, Mrs. Jackson easily could have ended up at Saint Anthony several times, despite her connections at Mount Sinai. Fire department rules say ambulances must take people to the closest hospital, and paramedics sometimes decide that, from Jackie's apartment, located on the border between North and South Lawndale, Saint Anthony is closer. "I would beg for them to take her to Mount Sinai, and they'd look at each other and say, 'OK,'" Jackie said. Doctors who practice in Chicago's inner city say that because of paramedics' rules, it is not unusual to be assigned to a case only to discover several weeks later that the patient recently had been hospitalized at a different institution. Because the patient was too sick or docile to relay the information, the new doctors had to start from scratch—which wastes time and money and sometimes delays proper treatment.

With Jackie as her advocate, that did not happen to Mrs. Jackson. Nonetheless, two decades worth of Mrs. Jackson's medical history were never transferred from Dr. Marino to Mount Sinai, as would be routine for middle-class patients. Her new physicians may have assumed that, like many other poor blacks, she did not have any regular source of primary care, or that the information from a "storefront doctor" would not have been reliable. Another reason may be that since Dr. Gurevich and Dr. Steinberg saw Mrs. Jackson at the hospital instead of at their offices, a secretary was not available to track down her medical history.

Generally considered less desirable than private doctors' offices because of the lack of continuity, hospital outpatient departments are used much more commonly by poor minorities than others. Before Medicaid and Medicare were introduced in the 1960s, there was a substantial difference in the number of annual doctors' visits for rich and poor, black and white. That gap has narrowed because of the two government insurance programs[2] (though many health experts contend that minorities and the poor still are not getting enough primary care, that they should in fact be visiting doctors *more* often because national surveys continually show they are the sickest Americans).[3] What has not changed is that race and class still determine the setting in which people get care, and, not surprisingly, separate is not equal.

In 1989, 20 percent of blacks, compared to 12 percent of whites, reported in an annual federal health survey that their last contact with a physician had been at a hospital outpatient department. The gap between rich and poor was similar: 18 percent of survey respondents from families with incomes lower than $14,000 reported a hospital outpatient department as their last physician contact, compared to 11 percent of people with incomes higher than $50,000.[4]

The National Health Interview Survey data do not distinguish between visits to hospital clinics and emergency rooms. The latter, of course, get more public attention. Other research that factored out emergency room visits shows that the poor still rely on hospital outpatient care more than others. A pioneering study of hospital discharge data in New York City found that while elderly New Yorkers in the poorest areas use emergency rooms one and one-half times more than their counterparts in affluent areas, they visit hospital outpatient departments four times as often.[5]

There is no obvious reason for hospital outpatient departments to offer poorer primary care than private doctors' offices. And, in fact, the clinical quality of the care in hospitals may be no different, and even better. The problems at hospitals are more subtle. Typically, patients see medical residents who spend only a few months in one clinic before rotating to the next. "People who go to outpatient departments don't have a physician who is really in charge. There seems to be a sense that there is some institutional responsibility for the patient, but that's really kind of hollow," explained Melvin I. Krasner, senior director of research for the United Hospital Fund of New York, which conducted the hospital discharge study. "The poorer patients need even more than the middle-class patient in terms of continuity and management, but they get less."

Mrs. Jackson's situation was somewhat different since Dr. Gurevich, an attending physician rather than an intern or resident, became her physician, but the continuity and coordination problems remained. Dr. Gurevich's home base on the other side of town meant that he spent only a few hours each week seeing outpatients at Mount Sinai. When he was there, Jackie often could not afford a medicar to take her grandmother to see him. In sum, nobody was aggressively steering Mrs. Jackson's care.

The problems of getting Mrs. Jackson to the doctor were especially acute after she went home in March with a partially amputated right foot. During that delicate time, she had to be followed carefully if she were to have any chance of keeping the remainder of her foot and her leg.

Mrs. Jackson had appointments with Dr. Steinberg on Mondays and Dr. Gurevich on Thursdays. Jackie never took her grandmother to both because she was unaware that she could get her to them for anything less than a $70 roundtrip. "I didn't know that ASC [a medicar company] and them take Medicaid," Jackie said later. "I had to hear that from the nurse. I thought they were cash-only people." To her chagrin, about the same time she made that discovery, she realized her grandmother had been put on the spend-down program, which meant she was not eligible for Medicaid every month.

So four days after Mrs. Jackson was discharged from the hospital following the amputation of her foot, Jackie paid $70 to get her grand-mother to and from an appointment with Dr. Steinberg. She skipped Dr. Gurevich's Thursday morning appointment three days later, decid-ing to wait until the next week. She figured she would alternate; Steinberg one week, Gurevich the next. It was not a bad strategy given the circumstances, but a strategy nobody would willingly choose.

The following week, on a Thursday morning in late March, the medicar was a little late, so Jackie called the outpatient suite at Mount Sinai to let Dr. Gurevich know she was on her way. She was assured that the physician would still be around, but when Jackie hurriedly pushed her grandmother in her wheelchair into the clinic at about 9:30, he had gone.

"I was so mad," Jackie said. "I rolled her right over to the emergency room. I told them they had to see her."

Mount Sinai cannot locate the medical records from this encounter. All that is left to document it is a large red emergency room logbook. It shows that Mrs. Jackson was brought to the emergency room at 9:39 A.M. suffering from "leg edema," a swollen right leg, and was sent home eight long hours later at 5:40 P.M.

There are also laboratory tests from that day, evidently ordered by the emergency room staff. They show that Mrs. Jackson was beginning to have a dangerous reaction to Coumadin, a drug she was taking to keep her blood from coagulating and thus allow it to flow to her leg and what was left of her foot.[6] The drug was prescribed in an attempt to prevent further amputation, but while Coumadin can be beneficial, it has a very narrow therapeutic margin. It's easy for a patient to overdose on it and bleed uncontrollably.

A test called a prothrombin time (PT) measures patients' coagulation levels. A normal level is about 11, but Dr. Gurevich did not want Mrs. Jackson's level to be normal; he wanted to prevent her from developing blood clots, which were more likely to form in her sluggish circulatory system. To do the job, her Coumadin level needed to be one and one-half to two times the normal reading. Accordingly, the ideal level for Mrs. Jackson would have been between 16 and 22. That day in the emergency room, however, Mrs. Jackson's PT level registered 35— more than three times the normal level—so high that her coagulation level needed to be monitored closely in the next few days, lest she begin to bleed to death. Yet, according to medical records, no such monitoring took place. How that happened shows how a primary care system made from fraying cloth can rip apart, leaving patients exposed to dangerous illness, even death.

Mrs. Jackson supposedly stopped taking Coumadin the day after her emergency room visit, on doctor's orders. The next week, however, she missed her appointments with both Dr. Gurevich and Dr. Steinberg because Jackie did not have the money to get her there and did not understand the gravity of the situation. The problem could have been solved had the home health nurse drawn Mrs. Jackson's blood for a PT test during that week, but presumably because of inadequate communication between Dr. Gurevich, the emergency room staff, and the nurse, that never happened. Judging from the nurse's notes, she did not seem to be aware that Mrs. Jackson was regularly missing doctors' appointments where her coagulation level might have been measured.[7]

The inevitable happened. On a Saturday morning, after two missed doctors' appointments, a private ambulance took Mrs. Jackson to the emergency room. Her nose had bled all night. The diagnosis: "Coumadin toxicity." Her PT level was 40, higher than it had been the last time she visited the emergency room, suggesting that somehow Mrs. Jackson had mistakenly continued to take Coumadin.

Medicare paid for this ambulance trip because it resulted in a hospitalization and was thus deemed "medically necessary." The federal health insurer would not have paid to get Mrs. Jackson to the doctor earlier in the week, when her high Coumadin level might have been detected and brought under control. Not only would an earlier visit have been better for Mrs. Jackson's health, but it could have saved the government several thousand dollars for the week-long hospital stay needed to treat the Coumadin poisoning. But even such minimal "prevention" does not comport with Medicare policy, which again, summarily defines nonemergency trips to the doctor's office as medically unnecessary.

Dr. Gurevich visited Mrs. Jackson the day after she was admitted to the hospital. "Patient supposed to see me as out-patient ten days ago, but she missed the appointment," his notes say. "Was [warned] about the Coumadin risk."

The hospital record also included a note from Dr. B. S. Iyer, the surgeon who had inserted a synthetic blood vessel into Mrs. Jackson's thigh during her first hospital stay. Evidently, Dr. Iyer had examined her in the emergency room the day she missed her appointment with Dr. Gurevich. As a surgeon, he would not be the physician responsible for monitoring her Coumadin level, but he, too, noted in the hospital record that she had not followed doctor's orders. "I had seen this patient in ER 10–12 days ago. She was to come back and see me in 1 week, which she never did," Dr. Iyer wrote.

Without the emergency-room medical record, it is impossible to know what arrangements the ER staff made for Mrs. Jackson's follow-up care. Dr. Iyer speculated that she was discharged from the overburdened emergency room before the equally overburdened hospital lab processed the tests showing her high PT level. "That's always a problem at Mount Sinai," he said, "It can take eight to ten hours to get labs."

The chief of emergency medicine, Dr. Karen O'Mara, conceded that Mrs. Jackson may have been discharged before her lab results came back. (Because of the constant delays, Dr. O'Mara had checked into setting up a satellite lab for the ER, but the $50,000 start-up cost was beyond Mount Sinai's shoestring budget.) Even so, normal emergency-room procedure would have been to contact Mrs. Jackson's doctor with the results once they were completed so that someone could order a PT test. Whatever the exact chronology of events, Dr. O'Mara said it was evident that there was a communication breakdown somewhere along the line. Perhaps Dr. Gurevich was not informed of the lab results, or he received them but neglected to order the nurse to perform a PT test. Dr. Gurevich declined to be interviewed.

It is not unusual for physicians to have only cursory involvement with home health patients at Mount Sinai and elsewhere. Nurses typically draw up care-plans and physicians sign them. One reason for some doctors' lack of attentiveness is that Medicare and other insurers do not reimburse them for supervising home patients. In a 1987 home care survey, 44 percent of physicians said the paperwork required too much time; 39 percent said home cases increased their potential for malpractice suits; and 73 percent griped about not being paid for the work. "At this time, I see home care as charity work that physicians are doing," said the founder of the American Academy of Home Care Physicians, Dr. Paul Hankwitz.[8]

After a week in the hospital, Mrs. Jackson was stable enough to go home. But not for long. A week later she was back in the emergency room. "Robert was on the dialysis machine," Jackie remembered. "Mama got up and made it to the first of the carpet at her bedroom door, and fell over belly down." Jackie went downstairs and asked the neighbor to help move her grandmother. "We drug her from the bedroom to the reclining chair. She wasn't conversating. She was just getting sicker and sicker, like an infection was taking over her body."

It was during this hospitalization that Mrs. Jackson's right leg was amputated up to the thigh. The infection in her partially amputated foot had not healed and was beginning to spread. Doctors had no choice but to amputate.

No one knows the exact cause of noninsulin-dependent diabetes, the kind that afflicts Mrs. Jackson, her sister Eldora, who was blinded by the disease, and more than 90 percent of all diabetics. It seems to be triggered by obesity and runs in families, which suggests a genetic link.[9]

Some studies have shown that the disease, which prevents the body from using glucose properly, is more common among poor, less-educated Americans, but when researchers control for obesity and age, the importance of socioeconomic factors diminishes.[10]

While poverty and the fragmented primary care system that accompanies it may not explain why blacks get diabetes more often, it may explain why they suffer such serious complications. The amputation rate among blacks is twice as high as among whites; diabetes-related kidney failure is three times as frequent; and black women are three times as likely to be blinded by the condition.[11]

Another provocative finding of the United Hospital Fund's study was that, despite many similarities in the reasons that rich and poor elderly are hospitalized, diabetes and other chronic diseases stand out as exceptions. In poor areas, diabetes ranks as the sixth most common reason for admission, whereas it barely makes the top twenty in neighborhoods where less than 10 percent of the population is poor. The report concluded that although Medicare puts rich and poor elderly on more equal footing than younger people who do not have the benefit of government-sponsored insurance, disparities in access and "ability to make the dietary and lifestyle changes necessary to manage the disease" persist.[12]

Dr. Paula Butler, an endocrinologist who runs a clinic for diabetics at Mount Sinai, pointed to one simple example of the access gap. Since Medicare does not cover medications, poor diabetics with erratic secondary insurance, or none at all, may not be able to afford the drugs and equipment necessary to control their disease. "The medicines are expensive, the home blood-sugar tests are expensive," she said.

Mount Sinai dietician Janine Ricketts-Byrne told of diabetics who have spent several days subsisting on bread and sugary Kool-Aid when food banks were empty or closed for the weekend. "The diabetic diet does not involve lobster, but it costs money," she said.

The real fight against Mrs. Jackson's encroaching peripheral vascular disease should have begun in the years before she showed up at Mount Sinai with a gangrenous foot. But, once again, having insurance is not a guarantee of good care for the poor; the skills and training of many doctors who practice in their neighborhoods may be substandard. Mrs. Jackson saw Dr. Marino regularly, but he said he had trouble bringing her blood sugar under control. When her blood sugar levels became increasingly high, he said he urged her to replace the oral diabetes medication she was taking with more potent insulin, but she refused because she did not want to give herself injections. Mrs. Jackson considered her high blood pressure—the probable cause of her 1987 stroke—to be her most serious problem. And it was, until, as the years passed, her blood sugar levels began to rise, too.

A general practitioner whose patients range from old women to pregnant girls to adolescent boys, Dr. Marino was a trusted family doctor for Mrs. Jackson and the Baneses. He saw Jackie when she was a little girl, and he delivered DeMarest. Mrs. Jackson first began to visit Dr. Marino in the early 1970s when his office was located in the heart of North Lawndale on Madison Street. When that office burned down a decade later, Dr. Marino moved a few miles west to a small storefront on the border of Chicago and suburban Oak Park, and Mrs. Jackson followed him. These facts paint a picture of a Norman Rockwellian doctor of the kind that health planners say are in desperately short supply in the inner city: a family practitioner who over two decades provided basic primary care for three generations of poor people.

What Mrs. Jackson and her family had no way of knowing was that Dr. Marino had failed a peer review by the Department of Public Aid's Medical Quality Review Committee. The five-doctor panel investigated fifteen cases beginning in 1988 and concluded that Dr. Marino had overprescribed narcotics, prescribed antibiotics without documenting a need for them, failed to order appropriate laboratory studies, and had not consistently provided proper checkups for children.[13] In one case, a forty-six-year-old alcoholic died from kidney and liver failure twenty-three days after his last visit with Dr. Marino, yet nowhere in the physician's records was "there any indication of an illness of this severity," the reviewers wrote. "Even an abbreviated physical exam would have found the jaundice, ascites [a swollen abdomen often associated with alcoholic liver failure] and peripheral edema [swollen extremities that may be caused by cirrhosis or renal failure]."

The peer review team recommended that Dr. Marino revise his practices in accordance with their findings and take ten hours of Continuing Medical Education in pediatrics. He was put on "continuous monitoring status," which meant his performance would be reviewed after nine months. To put Dr. Marino's case into perspective, the physicians' panel found such serious quality-of-care deficiencies with only sixty-seven of twenty-one thousand doctors who accepted Medicaid during 1991. Twenty-three of those physicians were terminated from the Medicaid program altogether; one was suspended; and forty-three (including Dr. Marino) were put on "continuous monitoring status."[14]

Dr. Marino has what is considered a large Medicaid practice; he treated more than one thousand Medicaid recipients in both 1989 and 1990, earning $65,217 the first year and $80,976 the second.[15] Practices consisting mostly of Medicaid patients—often called "Medicaid mills"—are worrisome because they have been associated with short visits and inadequate preventive care. A dramatic example of the segregation of Medicaid patients was reported by former University of Illinois political scientist James Fossett and public health researcher Janet Perloff. They found that in 1986 fewer than two dozen obstetrician/gynecologists cared for more than one-third of all Medicaid patients in Cook County and St. Clair County, also a poor, urban area in Illinois.[16]

Another charge against Medicaid mills is that they do not provide steady, reliable care, partly because the doctors who run them may not be allowed to work in hospitals. Hospital privileges are usually reserved for doctors who have had residency training and who are certified by a medical specialty board, which, although not a prerequisite to practice medicine, is an easily quantifiable measure of competence. But doctors who establish solo practices in poor neighborhoods often lack one or both of these credentials, a common reason being that they earned their medical degrees in foreign countries and did not pursue further training here.

Dr. Marino, for one, graduated from medical school in the Philippines in 1972 and started but did not finish a residency at a Chicago hospital. Although he is not certified by a medical specialty board, he does have privileges at Saint Anthony and a suburban hospital. Nevertheless, Mrs. Jackson's care still lacked continuity. Dr. Marino said he referred her to a specialist, but he did not remember who it was, and he did not note the doctor's name in his chart. He even wavered on what kind of specialist he would have chosen for her, a vascular surgeon, perhaps, but he was not sure. Mrs. Jackson, of course, told Jackie she was supposed to see a podiatrist. Such vague referrals are a problem in a medical system where specialists hesitate to take patients who have not been referred by another doctor. The problem is worse in poor neighborhoods where medical specialists are scarce.

Mrs. Jackson could have received something closer to state-of-the-art diabetic care at Mount Sinai's outpatient department, which adds another complicating piece to the puzzle of health care in ghettos. The revolving door for medical residents may interfere with continuity at outpatient departments, but young physicians' knowledge of current diagnostic techniques and treatments is often significantly better than that of doctors who practice in the city's poor neighborhoods.

The diabetic outpatient clinic may offer the best of both worlds. It is regularly staffed by two full-time physicians who supervise residents but also have close contact with patients. Held two mornings a week, the clinic is run more like a traditional office-based practice than is usual for hospital-based primary care.

Patients make appointments and generally visit their doctors every two months. The clinic tries to get all of its diabetics to use home test kits, so that when they detect a significant fluctuation in their blood-sugar levels, they can call the clinic for an appointment or a medication adjustment. This helps to prevent the wild swings in blood-sugar levels that doctors believe contribute to the development of kidney failure, blindness, and peripheral vascular disease. Patients also get another bonus that a general practitioner like Dr. Marino could not afford to provide: a diabetic health educator.

Clinic director Dr. Butler said the health educator was invaluable. "He spends a lot of time talking to people about what they should be doing, with their diets and everything else. We really badger them a lot, though at some point, you tell them it's in their hands." Perhaps the health educator could have taught Mrs. Jackson to take proper care of her feet before it was too late. Jackie said her grandmother's feet had been tender for years. "She'd grab people by the collar who stepped on her feet on the bus."

The amputation of Mrs. Jackson's right leg the last week of April had not, of course, put an end to her medical worries. She seemed destined to spend the summer going in and out of the hospital.

The day that Mrs. Jackson was admitted to Mount Sinai by a seemingly reluctant Dr. Gurevich, Jackie escorted her to a room on the sixth floor. The room had a nice view of Douglas Park, though it was a dreary, unseasonably cold summer day. As two nurses started to prepare Mrs. Jackson's bed—she needed a special mattress for her bed sores—Jackie took the elevator back downstairs for a cup of coffee and doughnut in the hospital cafeteria.

She was pleased that she had persuaded Dr. Gurevich to admit her grandmother, as opposed to simply having her foot examined again at her next appointment. "In two weeks [the infection] would have done gone through her whole foot," Jackie said. "I know what they would have told me. It's gotten so bad, we're going to have to . . ." Jackie made a chopping motion with her hand.

Upstairs, as Mrs. Jackson was getting settled in, a middle-aged woman who occupied the bed next to her's was getting ready to leave. A curtain separated their beds, but Mrs. Jackson could hear the woman on the phone, flirting with a male friend who evidently was coming to pick her up. She was wearing a hot-pink sun dress, which inspired a few whistles of admiration from the nurses.

"Push that curtain back so I can see you," Mrs. Jackson said after listening for a while. The woman complied and took a turn in her dress. Mrs. Jackson nodded approvingly. "You're going out, and I'm coming in," she said with resignation. The woman smiled sympathetically, gathering her things.

"You be good," Mrs. Jackson said as the woman headed for the door.

"I'll pray for you," the woman responded. And she was gone.

The rest of the afternoon Mrs. Jackson was rarely alone; a series of medical professionals came by to check her in.

First was senior resident Dr. Mark Angel. "We're going to do the best we can," he said.

"I know that," Mrs. Jackson responded.

"But I can't promise anything spectacular," Dr. Angel continued, inspecting Mrs. Jackson's left toe. "We may have to amputate again."

"Oh, I hope not."

The next visitor was a dietician. She surveyed the lunch tray in front of Mrs. Jackson. Her meal consisted of tea, apple and cranberry juices, raspberry Italian ice, and chicken broth.

"Are you ready for solid foods?" the dietician asked.

"I don't know," Mrs. Jackson said tersely. Her tone said, "I'm the patient; you're the dietician. You tell me what to eat."

After the dietician came a technician pushing an electrocardiogram machine. "Going to do an EKG on you, Mrs. Jackson," she said, as she helped Mrs. Jackson slip out of her hospital gown.

"Uh-huh."

"You've had a lot of these."

"Uh-huh."

The technician attached tiny electrodes to Mrs. Jackson's chest, stomach, and thighs, then connected them to the portable recording machine via a cable. The whole process took a few minutes.

A nurse arrived to take her medical history.

"How tall are you?"

Mrs. Jackson did not answer right away. She had been asked that earlier and had not answered, but this time she looked as if she were mulling it over. She was about to say something when the nurse jumped in. "You look about my height."

"Okay," Mrs. Jackson responded.

The nurse asked about her bowel movements, and Mrs. Jackson said they were "doing well," though she had told a doctor earlier that she had not had one for a week. Taking Mrs. Jackson's medical history without Jackie around was an arduous task, rife with imprecision.

The most painful moment of the afternoon came during a visit from medical resident Dr. Kyu-Jang Oh.

"Can we start your IV?" Dr. Oh asked.

"Hmmmm," Mrs. Jackson replied. She had learned by now that in hospitals, questions and statements are the same thing.

With Dr. Oh was a medical student, Nancy Church. He was teaching her how to insert intravenous tubes.

Dr. Oh told Mrs. Jackson to close her fist as he and Church bent over her forearm in search of a vein. They probed with the needle. Mrs. Jackson's eyes squeezed shut and she raised her free fist to the sky.

No luck. Dr. Oh left for another needle.

"Sorry about this. Sorry we have to stick you again," Church consoled.

The second time, Church grabbed Mrs. Jackson's free hand in a gesture of support. She held it in her own plastic-gloved one until the needle took. The ritual of Mrs. Jackson's fourth hospital stay in five months had begun.

5

Mrs. Jackson's melancholy

Outsiders who entered the Baneses' apartment that summer seemed to be disturbing the still, stale air. That was especially true for home physical therapist Talha Ahmed Shamsi, who paid Mrs. Jackson a visit shortly before Dr. Gurevich rehospitalized her at Mount Sinai.

Right away, Shamsi crouched down in front of Mrs. Jackson's wheelchair, trying to make eye contact with her. It was late afternoon, and Mrs. Jackson had been waiting up for him, dressed in her pink nightgown and powder-blue robe. Usually she would be back in her room by this time, but Jackie had pulled her grandmother out of bed in the morning to receive the nurse's ministrations and had left her sitting in the same spot in the middle of the living room. Mrs. Jackson did not seem to mind. Bed or chair, her unceasing frown and clipped conversation suggested that things looked grim from wherever she sat or lay. For the past couple of hours, she had faced the front door, never reaching down to adjust the position of her wheelchair, to turn it toward the images that flickered across the television, perhaps, or to roll it closer to the hutch filled with the family pictures that were so dear to her.

Shamsi began peppering Mrs. Jackson with questions, trying to determine her level of functioning. A native Pakistani, his accented voice rang out against the low hum of the television and Mrs. Jackson's infrequent mumbled responses. Like Sister Mary Ellen, he seemed to hope that if he spoke loudly enough his energy might somehow seep into her tired bones.

"Can I see the prosthesis?" Shamsi asked, looking up from Mrs. Jackson and toward Jackie, who was watching the exchange from the couch.

Jackie explained that her grandmother had never received an artificial leg because she had been too ill to respond to physical therapy while she was at Schwab Rehabilitation Center.

"On my referral, it says prosthesis training and stump care," Shamsi pressed Mrs. Jackson. "Were you doing any exercises at the hospital?"

Jackie did not wait for her grandmother not to respond. "No, she couldn't get any of them," she said, at which point Shamsi began to address all of his questions to Jackie.

"Was she totally independent before the amputation?"

"Once they took her toes off, that slowed her up."

Shamsi continued discussing the possibility of an artificial leg, which was frustrating to Jackie. All she wanted was for him to lighten the burden of caring for her grandmother; walking seemed out of the question. "She can't even get out of her wheelchair," Jackie protested. "She can't slide onto the commode."

Instead of directly responding to Jackie, Shamsi began an evaluation of Mrs. Jackson's strength. He told her to straighten her knee. "Straighten your knee, come on, straighten it, straighten it, straighten it," he commanded. "Bend your elbow. Come on, bend it hard. Bend your elbow." He picked up Mrs. Jackson's forearm and pushed it toward her, showing her what he wanted.

He helped her to stand. "Take your weight on your leg. Go on. Straighten. We won't let you fall. Straighten it. Yeah, that's it. Push your hip forward. More. More. More . . . You have to build up your arms and your leg. You have a very weak left leg. You need a good leg to walk."

Shamsi told Jackie to invest in ankle weights because Mrs. Jackson was going to need them for a long time. A few minutes later, he reconsidered and said Jackie could make them with socks and beans.

As Jackie watched, Shamsi tried to teach exercises to a reluctant Mrs. Jackson. He showed her how to build up her arms by lifting her cane to her chest like a barbell.

"Don't they have that kind of therapy at Schwab to give you the good arms?" Jackie complained, her irritation growing. Watching her listless grandmother go through the motions with Shamsi was disheartening to Jackie.

The last exercise Shamsi asked Mrs. Jackson to do was to tap her foot. She watched him tap several times and then slowly began to move her foot up and down.

"I want you to do this a thousand, thousand times," he said.

"Thousand times?" Jackie laughed skeptically. "She need some music."

As Shamsi was preparing to leave, he asked Mrs. Jackson to start tapping. "Like you're in church," Jackie urged. Mrs. Jackson tentatively lifted her foot from the floor; she was still tapping when Shamsi walked out the door.

Mrs. Jackson's three weeks in Schwab had been, by most accounts, a failure. First, the stump of her amputated leg did not truly begin to heal until her last week there. It bled so copiously that her second day at the rehabilitation center she was transferred across the street to Mount Sinai's emergency room for an evaluation. She was sent back that evening, but the problems continued.

She missed physical and occupational therapy sessions because of weakness and pain caused by her bleeding, swollen stump. When she managed to participate in the therapies later in her stay, persistent medical problems still interfered. At the beginning of her second week in the hospital, she had been attempting to stand between parallel bars during physical therapy when her blood pressure plunged. She had to be carted back to her room.

A physical medicine resident who followed Mrs. Jackson, Dr. Michael Shapiro, said she may have needed a longer stay at Mount Sinai, but her condition hovered in that gray area where hospital utilization reviewers are breathing down doctors' backs, questioning the necessity of keeping a patient in the hospital yet another day. "The bleeding could have stopped her first day [at Schwab], but it was a factor for three weeks," he said. "The problem is where do you put somebody." Deciding whether someone is sick enough for a hospital is not a hard-and-fast science, but if a discharge to Schwab is at all possible, it makes financial sense for patients to be there instead of Mount Sinai. That's because of the way Medicare reimbursement is designed. Acute care hospitals like Mount Sinai get paid under the DRG system; they receive a set fee for each patient according to diagnosis, regardless of the length of the hospitalization. Rehabilitation centers, however, are still paid under the old method and roughly recoup the costs of care. Since Schwab and Mount Sinai are affiliates—they share board members and some top staff—the rehab center does what it can to keep the hospital afloat.[1] For instance, Schwab's vice president of clinical operations, Jo-Ann Gruber, extolled her institution's stroke program at a 1988 meeting of Mount Sinai's Board of directors. "[The stroke] program will be of considerable benefit to Mount Sinai because most stroke patients are on Medicare, and often exceed the DRG allotted length-of-stay," Gruber said. "By expediting the transfer to Schwab, or another appropriate facility, Mount Sinai's length-of-stay can be reduced, thus increasing the profitability of the hospital stay."[2]

If Mrs. Jackson wasn't sick enough for Mount Sinai or well enough for Schwab, it would seem to have made sense to send her home for a while, and then bring her back for rehab. But in poor neighborhoods, doctors may be reluctant to do that, believing that patients don't have the resources or sophistication to get back to an institution once they leave. On top of that, Schwab's administrators do not encourage doctors to admit patients from home. "There's a sense in the rehab community that when you admit someone from home or a nursing home, the third-party reimbursers will scrutinize the chart more carefully," Gruber said. Careful scrutiny increases the chance that an insurer such as Medicare will refuse to pay for a patient, a chance the rehab center does not like to take.

Though Schwab is better off than its sister institution across the street, it operates on a tighter budget than many rehab centers because it serves very few commercially insured patients. Eighty-five percent of its patients are covered by either Medicaid or Medicare, compared to the Rehabilitation Institute of Chicago, located in a handsome building near the downtown Loop, where close to half of the patients are privately insured. The result is that a denial is far more costly to Schwab than to the Rehabilitation Institute. That institution's administrators have a sufficient financial cushion that they can risk admitting patients from home, or keeping them an extra week.

Mrs. Jackson also languished at Schwab because she was depressed over losing her leg—a fog that did not lift after she went home. Her psychologist at Schwab, Patrick Walsh, compared losing a leg to losing a close family member. In addition to that emotional trauma, he guessed that Mrs. Jackson was anguished over losing her independence.

Then, too, perhaps the longer Mrs. Jackson was confined to bed, with nothing to do but think, the more a lifetime's worth of hardships began to weigh heavy on her heart. According to Jackie, Mrs. Jackson had been ambitious as a child. "When she was supposed to go to the field and help, Mama would go to school," Jackie said proudly, repeating a family story. Yet Mrs. Jackson left school in the sixth grade, and, from then on, worked variously as a cleaning woman, cook, and nursing home aide. She and her first husband separated, and, as mentioned earlier, Mr. Jackson died from the burns he suffered in a factory fire. She outlived her beloved daughter, Nancy.

Walsh had to speculate about Mrs. Jackson's feelings because she did not speak freely with him. "Cora did not volunteer a lot," he said. "A lot of our interactions involved my trying to open her up." Walsh spoke with her four times during her three weeks at Schwab. She never attended a support group because they were held in the mornings and—when she was at all able—her physical therapist preferred to see her early because she was stronger then. Her motivation and manner were the same at the end of her stay at Schwab as they had been at the beginning: she had to be prodded to participate in therapy or to communicate.

An occupational therapist summed up Mrs. Jackson's condition a few days before she was discharged. During her entire stay at Schwab, the occupational therapist wrote, "patient has not been noted to smile."

The infrequency of Mrs. Jackson's sessions with Walsh is partially a reflection of the low priority rehab facilities in general put on psychological therapy.[3] For some patients, that emphasis may be appropriate, Gruber said, but she would prefer that Schwab better tailor its careplans to meet patients' needs. A greater commitment to psychology may well be impossible at Schwab, however, without an increase in staff. The Rehabilitation Institute has two times the number of beds as Schwab, but almost three times the number of psychologists.

Depression and medical problems having impeded her progress, Mrs. Jackson was released from Schwab. Medicare and other insurers cover only those patients who can show functional improvement, which in the case of an amputee usually means gains in physical therapy. Mrs. Jackson's discharge from Schwab may have been necessary: people who are mentally or physically unable to benefit from intensive rehabilitation should not be there. But once she got home, her despondency would never be effectively treated. She did not reach out for help, and meager insurance coverage and fragmentation of services kept help from pursuing her.

When she was discharged from Schwab, Walsh told her to call if she was interested in counseling. "The thing with Cora was that she wanted to go home and not come back," he said. To benefit from therapy, she had to want it, Walsh said. That is one of the operating principles of his field, but the problem was that her very illness, the trauma of losing a limb, and the depression and lack of motivation that accompanied it, seemed to prevent her from seeking help on her own. It would have been up to Jackie to get outpatient counseling for her grandmother, but Walsh said he did not have the chance to tell Jackie that Mrs. Jackson might benefit from seeing a psychologist.

Inpatient psychology may get relatively little attention at Schwab, but outpatient gets even less. Form follows funding, and even commercial insurers provide only minimal coverage for outpatient mental health services; public insurers are less generous. Medicaid, the health insurance program for the poor, does not cover *any* outpatient psychology in Illinois. Medicare pays for 80 percent of psychologists' visits for hospitalized patients, but it pays for only half of outpatient visits, not enough for Schwab to cover the costs of providing the service, according to the institution's chief psychologist. (Outpatient visits for *physical* illnesses are reimbursed the same 80 percent as inpatient visits.) Medicare expenditure data reflect the bias toward inpatient mental health care. Hospitalizations account for 63 percent of Medicare expenditures overall but 88 percent of mental health payments.[4] For the most part, the only people who receive outpatient counseling from Schwab are those who have the potential to return to work and who may be covered under special grants from the state Department of Rehabilitation Services.

Even if Mrs. Jackson had had the wherewithal to call Walsh, she still would have been stuck. He said he would have referred her to a city mental health center or to Mount Sinai's outpatient mental health department. Once again, she would not have had a reliable way to get to either place.

Mrs. Jackson's depression was severe enough that during the two-week hospitalization that followed her appointment with Dr. Gurevich, a psychiatrist diagnosed her as having a "major depressive disorder." Dr. Leonid Shvartsman was brought onto the case by Dr. Gurevich. Like his colleague, Dr. Shvartsman also emigrated to the United States from Russia, and his practice is based in the same northwest side office building as Dr. Gurevich's.

"Slowed down movements," Dr. Shvartsman wrote in his initial consultant's report on the case. "Decreased energy level, poor eye contact, does not want to talk." He visited Mrs. Jackson every day for several minutes, and the negative tenor of the notes continued. He put her on an antidepressant medication, Desyrel, and wrote that he provided her with "supportive psychotherapy." Three days before she was discharged, he wrote, "Still affect depressed, encouraged to vent her feelings."

Dr. Shvartsman's notes repeatedly say that Mrs. Jackson was "tolerating Desyrel well," and by the end of her stay he described her mood as "more stable." Nonetheless, he took her off Desyrel when she went home, after thirteen days on the medication. His decision is confusing considering that antidepressants are almost always given over the course of several months; drug trials of Desyrel, specifically, show that it often takes at least two weeks for it to have any effect.[5] If the Desyrel was working, or if Dr. Shvartsman wasn't yet sure of its effect, why did he take Mrs. Jackson off the drug? And if he decided to stop the drug because it was causing deleterious side effects, why didn't he note them in the chart?

Jackie would never have asked Dr. Shvartsman these questions; as far as she knows, no one else in her family has ever seen a psychologist or psychiatrist, and she is not well-versed on the treatment options for depression. Besides, Dr. Shvartsman never contacted Jackie to discuss her grandmother's treatment plan and never told her that she was taking the medication. The day before Mrs. Jackson was discharged he wrote in her chart, "with out-patient follow-up," but it is unclear what arrangements he tried to make for such follow-up because, again, Jackie said he never spoke with her about it.

Not surprisingly, when Mrs. Jackson was admitted to Mount Sinai with a urinary tract infection and other complications later that summer, Dr. Shvartsman again diagnosed a "major depressive disorder."

He did not put her back on an antidepressant but saw her for a short time every day. He received $39 for each visit, according to Medicare payment records. On his last visit with her during that hospital stay, he again wrote "will continue to follow." Jackie never heard from him.

Dr. Shvartsman did not want to discuss Mrs. Jackson's case, so the chief of psychiatry at Mount Sinai, Dr. Yogi Ahluwalia, who supervised Dr. Shvartsman when he was a resident, agreed to look over her record. He concluded that she had received "inadequate outpatient treatment."

"What is likely when the patient does not have follow-up is that she will relapse, and she did relapse," he said. "Depression is like rheu-matoid arthritis. You don't give up treatment. You need long-term outpatient treatment."

He speculated that Dr. Shvartsman decided not to follow Mrs. Jack-son because of the difficulties she would have had getting to his north-west side office. The decision to cease treating Mrs. Jackson's depres-sion might have been understandable were it not for the fact that Mount Sinai is one of the only hospitals in the state fortunate enough to have a home psychiatric program. Dr. Shvartsman might have ar-ranged psychological help for Mrs. Jackson simply by making a re-ferral.

A psychiatrist and social worker make up to twelve home visits to emotionally disturbed people, monitoring their medications and work-ing with their families. Designed primarily to serve people who live in the impoverished neighborhoods surrounding Mount Sinai, Home Psychare is funded through special grants from corporations and the Illinois Department of Mental Health. Without the grants, the program could not exist because few if any insurers cover psychiatric or psycho-logical care for homebound people.

Neither the social worker who administers Home Psychare, Sheila Curren, nor Dr. Ahluwalia could explain why Dr. Shvartsman did not refer Mrs. Jackson to the program. One reason some psychiatrists are reluctant to take part is that they perceive the program as "stealing" patients. A patient who builds a relationship with a home psychiatrist may stick with that person if she is subsequently hospitalized, meaning that the doctor who initially referred her loses out on relatively lucra-tive inpatient psychiatry visits.

One of the intentions of the ten-year-old Home Psychare program was to reduce overall medical costs by decreasing psychiatric hospital-izations, as well as those prompted by physical illness. Dozens of studies support such an "offset effect," where use of outpatient counsel-ing reduces the use of medical services.[6] The savings have been found to be especially strong for the elderly, whose depressions often mani-fest themselves in physical illnesses that require hospitalization. An-other reason the offset effect may be so pronounced for the elderly is that they respond well to treatment for depression.[7]

Dr. Ahluwalia guessed that some of Mrs. Jackson's repeat hospital-izations might well have been prevented had her depression been aggressively treated. "There is a direct correlation between her physical illness and her depression," he said.

Perhaps the best person to lift Mrs. Jackson's melancholy would have been not a psychiatrist or psychologist but Sister Mary Ellen Meckley, the social worker and nun who visited her through Mount Sinai's home health agency. But as usual, the question of who would pay for Sister Mary Ellen foreclosed the possibility.

Sister Mary Ellen's background does not suggest that she would have had any special rapport with Mrs. Jackson and the other black and Hispanic clients she visits. She is the only daughter of Italian-American parents, a beautician and a factory worker. She was raised far away from big city blight, in Phoenix, Arizona, in the 1940s, when Phoenix was more frontier than metropolis. Yet she has bridged the color gap in the most direct way possible: by living in the neighborhood surrounding Mount Sinai. For twenty-one years she has gone to church at an all-black parish a stone's throw from the hospital; she serves as an officer with the Douglas Park Advisory Council, which tries to breathe life into the beleaguered park. The first two floors of the red-brick three-flat she shares with another nun is devoted to Taproots, Sister Monica Cahill's thriving program for pregnant and parenting teenagers. Like most of the people who live on the West Side, Sisters Mary Ellen and Monica rarely leave it.

Sister Mary Ellen became one of the Sisters of Charity of the Blessed Virgin Mary at seventeen, after she graduated from high school. The Sisters of Charity was a teaching order, so from the 1950s to the mid-1960s, Sister Mary Ellen taught wherever her order dispatched her, in California, Kansas City, then Tucson, Arizona, and finally Chicago.

Once the Sisters of Charity loosened their rules and allowed nuns to do work other than teaching, Sister Mary Ellen began her social work career, first counseling prisoners, then black, college-bound teenagers who called her the "blue-eyed soul sister." "That was in the days of black power. [That nickname] was a real honor," she said earnestly and with pride. Nearly a decade ago she began work at the home health agency.

These days, she crisscrosses the West Side in a new gray compact

Chevrolet (her cars are always relatively new because she gets special deals from a family she helped as a prison social worker), not hesitating to slam on the brakes and swing into a U-turn when a quicker route occurs to her. "This is terrible," she apologized, turning the steering wheel with both hands, "but I have to get where I'm going."

Sister Mary Ellen was heading to the home of an elderly man who had fallen on a radiator and seriously burned his arm. He needed whirlpool treatments at Mount Sinai but did not have any way to get there. She sees about a dozen such people a week, all of whom are also visited by a home nurse or physical therapist. Her clients need all manner of help negotiating the system, much of it revolving around filling out forms, for special transportation, for Public Aid, for a state program that provides discount medications. They need equipment that will enable them to get into the bathtub, or alternatively they need Sister Mary Ellen to find out why a home helper from a state-funded program is refusing to help them wash.

Before getting out of her car, Sister Mary Ellen carefully arranged her canvas lunch bag on the seat. She left her turkey sandwich and homemade brownies poking out of the bag to deter any would-be thief who might be interested in it. Sister Mary Ellen has been mugged once, not on a home visit, but getting into her car to go home from Mount Sinai. She fought off the two young boys, but in the process fell hard on her knees, which still bother her sometimes.

Her old injury was not at all evident as she walked briskly to the front door of the stone building where the old man lived. She was dressed in a typical work outfit: a white blouse with blue pinstripes and a bow at the collar, a navy skirt, and low-heeled pumps. At five feet, one inch, Sister Mary Ellen is obviously no match for someone who really wants to do her harm, but she moves with a purposefulness that keeps most strangers at bay.

From the outside, the old man's building seemed in decent shape, though the two-flat next door was more menacing. Like many others on the street it was boarded up, and its front porch overflowed with garbage. The outer door of the man's building was unlocked, so Sister Mary Ellen pushed it open. Before she could press the bell in the vestibule, the door to the stairway opened. "Hello," Sister Mary Ellen called loudly, her voice tight and cautious.

"Hello," she called again.

Nobody was there. The rush of air from the outside had blown open the door. Sister Mary Ellen did not want to go up unannounced, so she rang the bell again. When there was no response, she hurried up the dark stairwell and knocked on the door at the first landing. "I thought he was on this floor," she said. Then she went up to the next floor—"Thank you, Jesus"—to the right apartment.

The old man's sister led Sister Mary Ellen into a living room, where he sat in a chair against the wall. In front of him three ashtrays rested on a rusty tray table. Unlike the Baneses' apartment, this one was practically bare. Other than his chair and table, the only furniture in the large front room was a sagging recliner and couch. A toaster sat on the floor, its cord snaking across the room. At Jackie's apartment, family photos, Mrs. Jackson's framed religious illustrations, and children's drawings decorate the walls; an oversized hemp fan covers a large hole. Here, no attempt had been made to camouflage. A felt hat hung from a nail in the way that a painting might, and two coats on hangers drooped from a wall sconce without a light bulb.

When he saw Sister Mary Ellen, the old man began to take off his tattered gold sweater to show her his wound. "What are you taking off your sweater for?" Sister Mary Ellen bellowed; the man was hard of hearing. "I'm not the nurse. . . . I'm going to get you some money."

The first order of business was to enroll him in the state "Circuit Breaker" program. Elderly or disabled people with incomes under $14,000 can either choose to receive an annual cash grant or a card that helps defray the cost of medications for certain chronic conditions. The "Circuit Breaker" was started by the Illinois Department of Revenue to assist people on fixed incomes that do not rise at the same rate as property taxes or rent.[8] (Mrs. Jackson had chosen the cash grant instead of the prescription card for 1989 because she was unaware that she would be put on the Medicaid spend-down program in March, leaving her without a regular green card with which to purchase medications.)

"Do you remember the address where you used to live?" Sister Mary Ellen asked, beginning to fill out one of the many forms that might give this man a lifeline to the world beyond his grim apartment.

He shook his head.

Sister Mary Ellen pivoted on the couch to ask his sister, who was eating her lunch from a plate on her lap. Sister Mary Ellen repeated the question loudly; the man's sixty-eight-year-old "younger" sister also was hard of hearing. It is common for the caretakers of Sister Mary

Ellen's clients to be old and somewhat disabled themselves. Nationwide, 35 percent of caregivers to the elderly are older than sixty-five; 10 percent are past seventy-five.[9]

The woman asked her middle-aged son, who had wandered into the room a minute before, to retrieve her address book. He went off and returned with a red-covered book. "Doesn't that look like the Bible to you?" she scolded, evidently giving up on finding her brother's old address.

After completing the Circuit Breaker form the best she could, Sister Mary Ellen moved on to the next program. "That security guard has been coming to take you to Mount Sinai, but we can't keep doing that," Sister Mary Ellen said. In a last-ditch attempt to provide some minimal transportation for its sickest patients, Mount Sinai had begun sending out its security guards to pick them up. This was not a long-term solution, and Sister Mary Ellen wanted to enroll the man in the Chicago Transit Authority's special services program, in which Robert participated.

Photo-identification cards are issued for CTA special services, so Sister Mary Ellen asked the man if he had a picture of himself; any snapshot would do.

"They're all down South," he mumbled. "I can't go on the bus anyway."

"No, they come right to your door," Sister Mary Ellen reassured him.

No one in the family had a camera, so Sister Mary Ellen offered to bring hers to Mount Sinai the day the man came for his whirlpool. She went on filling out the form, then tried to explain the transportation to the man and, more importantly, to his sister, who did not look up from her lunch.

"How much the doctor going to be?" she asked, jumping to a new subject.

"That's taken care of," Sister Mary Ellen said. "He's got that Medicare card, that red, white, and blue card."

"The day before you need the transportation," Sister Mary Ellen continued, trying to lock eyes with the sister, "you have to get up at five in the morning and call to reserve it."

"What *I* got to do with it?" the woman asked.

"Well, you, or some kind soul," Sister Mary Ellen cajoled, "need to make the call for your brother. You'll call, and it's going to be busy.

But you just have to keep calling. You keep getting a busy signal and finally you get through. They'll ask you your phone number and what time you need a pickup. Then you can go back to bed."

The woman smiled and nodded distractedly. In the abstract, booking a CTA car sounded so simple, if needlessly time consuming, Sister Mary Ellen thought, but sitting here with this sick old man and his sister, it became a Herculean task. (Robert did not have to book his car every day because he was a "prescription" rider; he was picked up at roughly the same time three times a week.)

"OK, OK," the woman sighed, as Sister Mary Ellen continued to ply her with the requirements of the CTA special services program.

"Sound good?" Sister Mary Ellen asked.

"Sounds good," the woman said without conviction.

Sister Mary Ellen steered the conversation on a different course. Now that her brother had moved in, was the landlord going to raise the rent? she asked the woman.

"If [the landlord] act like he ain't going to like it, we'll just have to get another place," the woman said, her affection for her brother becoming evident.

"Are you watching what you eat like the nurse told you to?" Sister Mary Ellen asked, turning back to the old man.

"Sometime," he responded.

"I see that little pork sausage sitting there."

His sister smiled with embarrassment, covering her mouth with her hand like a schoolgirl caught chewing gum. Processed pork, with its salt and cholesterol, is the forbidden but coveted food of the West Side's sick; health workers are forever cautioning patients to avoid it, without much success. No recent study has conclusively proved that poor blacks' diets are unhealthier than others, but those who care for them often point to pork and other salty foods as a possible explanation for blacks' greater rates of high blood pressure, stroke, and heart attack.

Sister Mary Ellen immediately switched tactics, admitting how hard it was to change a lifelong diet.

"Sure is because I came out of the country," the woman said, warming up to what seemed to be one of her favorite topics. "You ever been to Memphis?" Then she launched into her life story. Raised sixty miles outside of Memphis, she moved to Chicago to get a job when she was in her midforties. The year was 1963, the tailend of the Great Black

Migration to Chicago. Mrs. Jackson had come North at the same time, at the same age, and for the same reason.

Sister Mary Ellen had never been to Memphis but said she was soon going to Arizona to visit her parents.

"Sounds good," the woman drawled. This time with conviction.

Driving toward her next appointment, soothing classical music on the car radio, Sister Mary Ellen explained how she has had to get up at 5 A.M. to reserve CTA cars for people without phones. She understood why making the arrangements is beyond some of her patients. "It will be busy, busy, busy, and then when you're numbed to the busy signals, a clerk will answer and you have to be alert all of a sudden." Sometimes the clerk will say, "'Sorry. All booked up for tomorrow,' and hang up," Sister Mary Ellen explained. Then patients have to call another company that ferries disabled people for the CTA.

Her second client of the day was an old woman dying of cancer. Unlike the old man's barren, drafty rooms, she lived in a small garden apartment kept fastidiously clean by her sixty-year-old daughter who lived above. When Sister Mary Ellen arrived, the woman was sitting in a recliner in her robe and nightgown, a blanket with pink roses neatly covering her legs.

She clasped Sister Mary Ellen's small hand in her own, smiling and peering curiously at her from behind glasses thick as pop-bottles.

"Do you remember me? I'm Sister Mary Ellen."

"Hmmm," the woman said, who was not at all certain. "You're Catholic aren't you?"

"Yes, that's me," Sister Mary Ellen smiled.

She had come to fill out a "Talking Books" application for the old woman. In response to Sister Mary Ellen's question about her reading preferences, the old woman said she was only interested in Baptist religious material, but Sister Mary Ellen insisted on filling out a "Talking Books" questionnaire anyway. From personal experience, she thought it healthier to explore more than religious subjects. "Variety is the spice of life," she said.

"Do you like animal stories?" Sister Mary Ellen asked.

"No, no. I don't care about animals."

"Stories about people's lives?"

The old lady hesitated. "Well, some of them."

"Humor?" Sister Mary Ellen asked, telling the old woman about Norman Cousins, the mind-over-body guru. "He found that the more he laughed, the better he felt. He was very sick, and now he's up and around," Sister Mary Ellen said.

The old woman smiled sweetly but was not moved.

"It's probably just the religion then," Sister Mary Ellen conceded.

By this time, the woman's daughter had joined them, and the three women talked about applying for another benefit. Then they just talked.

"I gets up every morning, and I wash myself up. I clean myself," the old woman said proudly.

"She looks forward to doing it," her daughter added.

"I'm doing for myself now."

Before leaving, Sister Mary Ellen asked the woman to sign a form.

"I can put my 'X,'" she responded, smiling with pleasure at her ability to accomplish this small task.

These visits, which start with Sister Mary Ellen filling out forms and end with her providing a bit of good old-fashioned support, were common. But she rarely returned to give more directed counseling, even though she has been trained for it and Medicare will pay for counseling intended to help patients cope with physical illnesses. (Mrs. Jackson's depression, for one, seemed to fall into this reimburseable category.)

Sister Mary Ellen—and many home social workers—limit themselves to connecting patients with needed services because, although Medicare rules allow counseling, the federal insurer traditionally has emphasized nursing and other clearly "medical" care. In response, home health agencies tend not to promote counseling based on a lingering fear that Medicare will refuse to pay for it.

In addition, social workers themselves have been reluctant to start long-term therapeutic relationships. Medicare rules say that as soon as a patient no longer needs help from a home nurse or physical therapist, social work services will not be reimbursed. "Why try to even get a relationship started, when it has to be stopped?" Sister Mary Ellen asked. Sister Mary Ellen sometimes makes referrals to Home Psychare, but she usually does so only for patients who are suicidal or violent. Schwab's Patrick Walsh had heard of Home Psychare but did not know much about it; he had never referred a patient to it. Even professionals have a hard time keeping abreast of the patchwork of treatment options available to the poor.

Jackie knew her grandmother was acting differently, but she never sought psychological help for her. She was preoccupied with Mrs. Jackson's physical needs and baffled by her mood changes. She would have needed education and encouragement about mental health services from Sister Mary Ellen, or from the home health nurse, or from Dr. Shvartsman at Mount Sinai, or from Walsh.

Jackie noticed that for the first few days after her grandmother left the hospital, she seemed happier, more talkative. "The days when she first comes out of the hospital, yes, she talks. When I am washing and changing her up, she talks about what Jackie is doing for her, that she is healing the sores better than the hospital does," said Jackie, who sometimes switches into the third-person to pay herself a compliment. Mrs. Jackson would also talk about how she felt she was burdening Jackie. "Mama feels real bad about that," Jackie said.

Then a few days later she would sink into silence. "I get angry because she won't talk to me," Jackie said, a not uncommon reaction for relatives of depressed people.

Jackie also figured that if her grandmother refused to talk to her, the person to whom she was closest, she probably would not talk to anyone. "Seem like Mama is a hard piece of ice to break through. I thought I would be the perfect one for it. It seemed like when she shut me off, no one could even get close to her at all." That may have been true, but it was also true that Jackie was not familiar enough with psychological services to realize that sometimes they can help when family members cannot.

It was not that Jackie was opposed to counseling. Occasionally, she seemed to be casting around for something like it without naming it. "She just need somebody to really talk to her, get it out, see what is really bothering her," Jackie said one particularly bad day. "I guess I know what it is, the leg, but . . . well, she isn't talking to me."

6

The inner-city emergency room

G ive me my socks and shoes," wailed an old woman lying on a gurney in Mount Sinai's emergency room. "Give me my socks and shoes." As she struggled to sit up to better plead her case, her hospital gown drooped down from her shoulders, revealing her bare chest. She was confused, suffering from some form of dementia, and did not seem to notice her sad state of undress. Her long, snow-white hair was in disarray, her eyes far away, reflecting the unimaginable goings-on of her inner world rather than the events swirling around her. "Give me my socks and shoes."

None of the doctors or nurses had the time or inclination to pay much attention to an old woman's lamentations. At 6:30 P.M., it was still early according to inner-city emergency-room time, where the traffic of the sick and the injured and the otherwise undone peaks from 11 P.M. to 1 A.M.; but already the place was jammed. Diagnosed with pneumonia, the old woman had been there for hours, waiting for a bed to open up in the main part of the hospital. Mount Sinai's occupancy is on the high side,[1] especially in the critical-care unit, and patients requiring intensive care have spent as long as two days in the emergency room waiting for an open bed.

Any discussion of health care for the urban poor would be incomplete without an examination of the emergency room, where waits are long, doctors and patients are strangers, and continuity is nearly impossible. Yet poor patients continue to converge there for routine care, providing daily testament to the gaping holes in the broader health and social service system. The emergency room is where the inequities and distortions of a health-care nonsystem—one driven more by patients' ability to pay than by their medical need—are most obvious. The distortions are evident in the illness and injury that bring

West Side residents to the emergency room and in the relatively meager resources Mount Sinai has to treat them. The emergency room is also the place where the hospital collides hardest with the neighborhood around it, where the products of a broken-down inner city come to be put back together again.

The emergency room is divided into two sections, separated by a nursing station in the center. On one side, six beds are reserved for the most serious cases: patients who've been shot or stabbed, victims of car accidents, heart attacks, and drug overdoses. Nine beds on the other side are devoted to less serious problems, such as large-bone fractures, pneumonia, and high fevers. People who would be in a doctor's office rather than the emergency room if primary care were available are diverted to what is known as the "Fast Track" clinic. It adjoins the emergency room and is open from noon to 10 P.M., treating sprains, earaches, toothaches, and the like.

In the emergency room proper, beds sit a few feet apart, separated by thin beige curtains, so that patients have virtually no privacy, and doctors and nurses frequently trip over each other. (There are two small rooms for psychiatric patients, rape victims, and others for whom privacy cannot be sacrificed—unless, of course, these rooms are full.) On this night, every bed was occupied by 7 P.M., so an extra one had been pushed against the wall for the old lady. End-to-end with hers was another auxiliary bed, where a lanky fourteen-year-old boy lay still in a neck brace. He had been hit by a car while riding his bike and was whimpering with fear.

The emergency room's crowds have grown over the last couple of years, from about 32,000 patients treated in 1987 to 39,000 in 1990.[2] Mount Sinai is one of only six remaining hospitals in Chicago's trauma network, the system for routing people with life-threatening injuries to specially equipped emergency rooms. As has happened in large cities across the country, four Chicago institutions fled the network during the late 1980s, citing heavy losses incurred from treating severely injured patients who tend to be uninsured or covered by Medicaid. Though few hospitals expect to make money from trauma, they hope that the special designation enhances their reputations, pulling in top doctors and private-paying patients. Mount Sinai's ghetto location precludes it from taking advantage of those indirect benefits, but the hospital is trying to hang on, despite losses of approximately $4,700 per trauma case, a figure comparable to the other trauma centers in the city.[3] In 1989, the hospital lost $2.2 million on the 466 Level One (most seriously injured) trauma patients deposited at its doors.[4]

While the defections from the network certainly put an increased burden on Mount Sinai and the other hospitals that remained, the growth in emergency-room traffic cannot be attributed only to trauma. It is as much the result of people who trudge through the doors with less serious complaints and drop down in hard plastic chairs to wait. Studies in Chicago and nationwide have shown that Medicaid recipients, who comprise 40 percent of the West Side's residents,[5] are more likely to treat the emergency room as a doctor's office than the privately insured.[6] Researchers at the University of Illinois recently reviewed almost two thousand emergency-room visits by Medicaid clients at 20 large hospitals in the state and found that 58 percent were for what physician-reviewers classified as nonurgent conditions.[7] On the West Side alone, the Medicaid program could save $3 million if that nonurgent, primary care were given to its clients in doctors' offices rather than in emergency rooms, the Illinois Department of Public Aid has calculated.[8] That's because extensive, expensive medical workups are the norm in emergency rooms, where doctors are unfamiliar with patients and thus err on the side of caution.

Why do Medicaid recipients prefer Mount Sinai's raucous emergency room when they presumably could go to a doctor's office for the same care? Because they would rather wait hours than weeks for an appointment; so few physicians and public clinics are located on the West Side that it can take that long to get in. They prefer the emergency room because they do not trust the storefront doctors who have chosen to practice in their neighborhood. Or they prefer it because old habits die hard, and these people gave up going anywhere other than the emergency room years ago. The emergency room is always open, after all. It cannot turn you away. Its doctors can't be too bad if a hospital hired them.

A variation on these themes explained why Mrs. Jackson, whose main insurer was Medicare, used the emergency room frequently. First, she had a primary-care physician in name only. Jackie did not have any confidence that Dr. Gurevich would return her calls or answer her questions, so she took her grandmother to a place that she knew had to respond. And Chicago Fire Department ambulances, which Jackie learned to use as free transportation of last resort, do not take people to doctors' offices; they take them to emergency rooms. This is not to say that when Mrs. Jackson was transported to the emergency room she did not need to be there. Most of the time when she went she was admitted to the hospital, probably because by the time Jackie waited until her grandmother was sick enough to plausibly convince paramedics that the situation was urgent, indeed it was.

Following on the heels of the publicly insured are the uninsured, often in advanced stages of treatable disease, with undiagnosed diabetes attacking their kidneys, or even breast tumors large enough to break through their skin. Their conditions certainly are emergencies now but emergencies that, once again, did not necessarily have to be. They got so sick waiting, waiting, waiting, because they had no health insurance and did not think they could afford a doctor until they *really* needed one. And even when things got bad enough that they *really* needed one, they still feared they could not afford it—who knows how expensive a doctor's visit will be?—so they stumbled into the emergency room instead. There, the clerks ask if you have insurance but will not draw in their breath when you say you do not, will not ask you to wait while they confer with someone else, will not, cannot, turn you away.[9]

Finally, Mount Sinai's emergency room is swarming with patients because of supply-side problems. The nursing shortage and budgetary constraints keep city hospitals from staffing enough excess beds to quickly accommodate emergency patients who need to be admitted.[10] In addition, fewer institutions are open in poor neighborhoods these days: three hospitals have gone out of business on the West Side since 1986, as have two community health centers.[11] The emergency room, then, is at once a symptom of a diseased health care system and a makeshift, unreliable cure for what ails it.

Mount Sinai's director of emergency medicine, Dr. Karen O'Mara, tends to her emergency room in much the same way as many poor patients tend to their bodies. She does not try to persuade hospital officials to buy new equipment until she *really* needs it. No matter how desirable, expanding the cramped space is out of the question, as is setting up a satellite lab to decrease waiting times for test results. This penny-pinching mind set necessarily pervades the hospital; in an effort to offset its $1.9 million deficit in fiscal 1989, Mount Sinai saved $10,000 by washing windows less frequently and another $10,000 by changing to a cheaper brand of paper towels.[12]

Dr. O'Mara has her own tricks. One evening, another doctor

watched her wrestle to clean a young woman's lacerated ankle while at the same time protect herself from the splashing blood with a styrofoam cup. (Exposure to potentially AIDS-infected blood is a constant worry in the emergency room, where patients are strangers and invasive procedures are frequent.) Why not order some splash-guards from a medical supply catalogue? the doctor suggested. Dr. O'Mara rolled her eyes.

"We already have the cups," she said later. "There's no such thing as just ordering something. We have to research it for months." The emergency room's new electrocardiogram machine is an example. The old one had driven the staff to distraction because patients had to be tested repeatedly to get an accurate reading. Dr. O'Mara spent a year and a half to find a machine that would fit into the hospital's budget. Eventually, she bought a demonstration model that had been marked down several times. Bargain-shopping was new to Dr. O'Mara, who came to Mount Sinai from an affluent North Side hospital, where the $9,000 cost for a new electrocardiogram machine would hardly be noticed. "They wouldn't have even thought twice about that," she said. "It would be part of a routine hospital order."

"Give me my socks and shoes," the old woman continued to plead. She had been transferred by ambulance from a nursing home, and no one was sure whether she had been wearing shoes. One doctor offered her a pair of hospital booties as a substitute, but it did no good. Even if her own shoes had been located, it's hard to imagine that her plaintive cries would have ceased; what her tone seemed to beg for was comfort, someone to hold her hand, rather than something to cover her feet.

Another patient, a twenty-two-year-old man who had threatened to kill himself, was whistling like a bomb just before impact. He was hidden away in one of the private rooms, restrained with leather straps on his wrists and ankles, but he could be heard throughout the emergency room. The whistles alternated with regular calls for the nurse. "Heh, nurse," he barked. "Heh, nurse."

Sleeping through the whistles and cries and the *knock, knock, knock, beep, beep, beep* of the heart monitors was a young woman who had been given narcotics to ease the wrenching pain of sickle cell anemia. Dr. Bruce Tizes, an ophthalmologic surgeon and part-time emergency-room physician, said that he and the other staff had to watch out for people who use sickle-cell as an excuse to get high, but "we decided she was for real." A forty-seven-year-old man a few beds away was also for real, Dr. Tizes said. He had suffered a mild heart attack and was now being monitored for further problems. Neatly shaven with intelligent if tired eyes, the man looked better off than almost all the other patients in the emergency room, damaged heart and all.

Dr. Jerry Noble, a middle-aged veteran of Mount Sinai's emergency room who has managed to retain a compassionate, even tender, bedside manner, talked about what his colleagues mean when they used the word "real."

Heart attacks, for instance, are the mirage of urban emergency rooms, he contended. "In the inner city nobody comes in with a cold," he said. "Everybody comes in with chest pain and difficulty breathing." Dr. Noble put patients who inaccurately report heart attack symptoms into two rough categories: first are those who have not had much education or contact with the health care system. Unlike middle-class health care consumers who keep up on the latest diseases' signs and symptoms, they do not understand their bodies well enough to make good guesses as to what is really wrong. Their chests may hurt, but it's from the congestion of a cold, not a heart attack.

The second group understands the health care system perfectly well. "They know that if they come in with a cough and a cold, they are going to be put at the bottom of the list and have to wait for hours," Dr. Noble said. "If they have chest pain, people are going to take them a lot more seriously." As Mrs. Jackson's case suggested, they also may be following through with a story that started with the ambulance dispatchers. "If they call up 911 with a cough and a cold, they're not going to get an ambulance at all," Dr. Noble said.

In the bed next to the sleeping girl sat one of the clear-cut cases every red-blooded ER doctor appreciates: a twenty-two-year-old Hispanic man was gingerly cradling his right hand and wrist in his left hand. Its unnatural protrusions proved "real" injuries, bones snapped during a soccer match.

A couple beds away from him, however, lay an elderly black woman who fell into another of the amorphous nonemergency-emergency categories. She was a "social problem," Dr. Tizes said, a label used by doctors to explain their helplessness in the face of problems without an organic basis. "She wants to go to a nursing home because she doesn't like who she's living with, but there's nothing we can do for her now. She's got to go home."

In addition to Dr. Tizes, one other attending physician, Dr. Amarjit Singh, was working in the emergency room that night. Three residents also were on duty, one specializing in emergency medicine, two in surgery. Two medical students helped out with simple procedures, such as stitching wounds. And five nurses assisted the doctors, three of whom were on staff at Sinai and two from a nursing agency.

Mount Sinai has been hit hard by the nursing shortage plaguing the entire hospital industry. It cannot afford the large salaries wealthier institutions offer, and many nurses are turned off by the hospital's location. To fill the gaps, Mount Sinai turns to temporary nurses, who cost the hospital $20 an hour more than its own staff because of agency overhead and the higher salaries temporaries command. The nursing shortage feeds a vicious cycle: Mount Sinai's full-time nurses must cover many patients both because the total number of RNs staffing each shift is lower and because agency nurses are not familiar enough with the hospital's procedures to work at maximum efficiency. As a result, full-time nurses are more likely to become overwhelmed by their workloads and quit. Mount Sinai then must hire still more agency nurses, which wastes money that could be better spent on hiring new staff nurses or enhancing the salaries of the ones who have stayed. The hospital's chief financial officer estimated that Sinai could save $200,000 a month if agency nurses could be eliminated.[13]

The shortage has been severe enough that Mount Sinai has diverted ambulances to more distant trauma centers because its nursing staff was stretched too thin. The emergency room also has refused ambulances for another reason unique to poor hospitals: breakdowns of its CAT scanner, a diagnostic instrument that produces much clearer images than an X-ray. Mount Sinai's scanner is old, not designed for twenty-four-hour-a-day use, and malfunctions with some regularity. That affects the entire hospital. "Cannot do CAT scan due to machine being out of service," a resident wrote in the medical record of Mrs. Jackson's son, Tommy Markham, during his fourth week of hospitalization following his stroke. The scanner was slated to be replaced in 1992, but until then, Dr. O'Mara and the rest of the hospital were at its whim.

A little after 8 P.M., the "trauma phone" rang for the first time that evening. The head nurse that night, Gail Blazek, hurried to answer it. "We got a guy who walked into the fire house and drank a bottle of Wisk," she reported as she hung up the phone. (A dispatcher calls in paramedics' cases while they are en route to the hospital.) "So get your leathers ready, he's wild."

"Tsk, tsk, tsk," she added as an afterthought, parroting a television commercial for the laundry detergent. "Wisk, Wisk, Wisk." This kind of morbid joke is common in busy emergency rooms. Later in the evening one of the medical residents started a pool to guess the blood-alcohol level of a drunken bicyclist who had injured his head in a fall. Some commentators say such morbid humor demeans and dehumanizes patients. But others acknowledge that, while the language may be cruel, it relieves the pressure of making split-second decisions that can determine whether someone lives or dies. It also allows doctors and nurses to put some distance between themselves and the anguish they see each night.

Wisecracks aside, Blazek was the first one to the trauma phone when it rang. She has a round face, shoulder-length brown hair, and the solid presence of a nagging big sister. Her counterpart was Linda Ziarko. With ten years under her belt, Ziarko qualified as Mount Sinai's longest surviving ER nurse. "I like my trauma; I like the excitement," she said. Ziarko exuded straightforward tenacity. She often wore green scrubs to work—didn't want to fool around with anything fancy. She had lived on the same block all of her life and had no intention of leaving, though she was one of the few whites left in a Hispanic neighborhood fifteen minutes from the hospital. "This is my hospital," Ziarko said. "If I ever get injured or have a heart attack, they will bring me here."

While the Wisk-drinker was on his way, emergency medicine resident Dr. Joyce Rosenfeld treated a Mexican immigrant who had been hit by a bus. She treated him for internal injuries with a procedure called a peritoneal lavage. It involves pumping fluid into the abdomen through a catheter and then discharging it into a plastic bag; if red blood cells are floating in it, internal bleeding is likely. The procedure is painful. "You're going to kill me if you don't stop," the man told Dr. Rosenfeld in Spanish. He spoke no English, but fortunately for him Dr. Rosenfeld spoke fluent Spanish, acquired while she went to medical school in the patient's home state of Guadalajara.

As she watched the bag for telltale red blood cells, Dr. Rosenfeld talked about an omnipresent fear of needle-sticks and cutting herself. She said she made sure she purchased insurance that paid off if she committed suicide, which she plans to do if she gets AIDS.

The young man who'd drunk the detergent had arrived—with less fanfare than expected. Dr. Tizes walked across the room to show Dr. Rosenfeld the evidence of the patient's mental disturbance: an empty Wisk bottle paramedics had retrieved.

On his heels was surgery resident Dr. Elizabeth Faulk, who wanted to take a look at the Mexican patient. "I understand you got in the way of a bus," she said quietly, trying to lighten the gravity of the situation. He, of course, did not understand a word Dr. Faulk was saying. Dr. Rosenfeld reported that he did not seem to have any internal injuries, but he seemed to have a problem unrelated to his accident. "Take a look at his scrotum," she said. One of his testicles was enlarged.

The close inspection of his private parts shamed the man, who began to speak rapidly to Rosenfeld. "He fathered two sets of twins, one here and one in Mexico," she reported. "He wants you to know that."

On the other side of the nurses' station, the Wisk-drinker was now restrained at his ankles and wrists. Neither of the enclosed rooms was available, so he had no privacy. He was tall and attractive, wearing thin yellow drawstring pants and no shirt. "Heh, doctor, heh, doctor," he called louder and louder. No one paid any attention until the inevitable gastrointestinal consequences of drinking laundry detergent became impossible to ignore.

The nurse who had been assigned his case berated him for not letting her know he needed to use the bedpan. "I'm telling you, you will be lying in it," she threatened.

"I kept on hollering," he said.

"He did," interjected Dr. Singh, who settled the issue in favor of the patient with his matter-of-fact observation. Like Dr. Noble, Dr. Singh is an attending physician in the emergency room and has a quieter, more steady disposition than the younger residents and medical students. While they became jittery and excited when the trauma phone rang, Dr. Singh kept busy with more mundane matters. He had begun examining less serious patients in the waiting area because no space was left in the emergency room.

Emergency room gridlock is most severe and widespread in New

York City because of the extent of the AIDS epidemic there, the prevalence of drug abuse, homelessness, and mental illness, and the emergence of hard-to-treat tuberculosis. Hospital occupancy rates in New York are extremely high, well over 90 percent, which means patients can stall for days in the emergency room waiting for an open bed. A survey taken by the New York State Department of Health at midnight on 10 January 1989 found 599 patients in city emergency rooms waiting for a bed; 318 had been waiting more than eight hours; 108 had been waiting for more than a day.[14] Two years later the situation was worse: 1034 people waiting, many for more than 8 hours.[15]

In Chicago, ER backlogs are not yet as serious and are limited to fewer hospitals, Mount Sinai among them. But the outlook is not good. Close to 90 percent of Chicago and Cook County emergency rooms reported in 1990 that patients were waiting more than four hours to be moved into inpatient beds after being admitted to the hospital.[16]

The psychiatric patient who had been whistling like a bomb continued to cool out in the private room. This was not his first time in the emergency room, and head nurse Blazek admitted she had a certain fondness for him. (The deinstitutionalization of the mentally ill also has been blamed for the emergency room overload.) He had managed to squirm out of his wrist restraints, but Blazek did not feel compelled to do much about it. "He said he'd put them back on after he finishes his Coke," she said.

Her colleague Ziarko was trying to give discharge instructions to one of the few white patients to come through the emergency room that night. She was an old Russian woman who spoke no English. A younger relative served as her translator.

"What you basically got is an upset stomach," Ziarko said to the woman, who stared back sweetly but blankly from a wheelchair. "Tell her that," Ziarko said to the translator, who seemed confused herself but proceeded to say something in Russian.

"No greasy or spicy foods," Ziarko continued loudly. The translator looked on with concern but said nothing. "Tell her that. Don't fry anything." The translator responded with a few mumbled Russian words.

"She can have soft foods, juice, tea, 7-Up, soft pudding." Again, the woman listened intently but did not translate the nurse's instructions. "So tell her that," Ziarko said, her exasperation growing.

"Now does she have any questions?" Silence.

"Ask her," Ziarko commanded.

Evidently she did not have any questions, so Ziarko told the two women that they should follow up with their own physician on Monday. The translator nodded her head, and put her arm around the old woman, helping her toward the door. The chances that the old woman would get to a physician on Monday seemed remote.

A little after 9 P.M., a tall woman in tight jeans and high heels walked into the emergency room holding her young son's hand. The ten-year-old had been playing with his friends in the alley, she said, when a man started to pepper the children with a pellet gun from his second-floor back porch. "I've been shot," the little boy ran crying to his mother. His wound was a small dark mark on his cheek, not far from his eye. Dr. Tizes, the ophthalmologic surgeon, examined the boy.

He asked the child to follow his penlight with his eyes.

"You playing with me?" the boy growled. His eyes were hard. Whatever he was feeling, perhaps fear from being shot or bewilderment at the mayhem that now surrounded him, he expressed with belligerence.

Still relatively young himself, only thirty years old, Dr. Tizes did not seem to know what to make of the boy. Dr. Tizes breezed through medical school by age twenty, but no lecture could have taught him how to put a scared, sharp-tongued child at ease. Dr. Tizes told him to obey doctor's orders and insisted that he was trying to help. The boy scowled.

"What did you get hit with?" Dr. Tizes asked.

"A BB gun," he spat.

"He's a delightful little guy," Dr. Tizes cracked.

It did not appear that the pellet had entered the boy's cheek, but Dr. Tizes ordered an X-ray anyway.

At 10 P.M., the paramedics pushed another stretcher through the emergency room doors. The patient's blood pressure was quite low. Blazek, Ziarko, and Dr. Tizes pushed the man roughly from the stretcher onto a bed against the wall; time was of the essence. His eyes were swollen shut and blood was seeping from the back of his head. Ziarko began poking around his forearm with a needle; she needed to find a blood vessel, quickly, so as to force fluids into him through an IV. He jerked away in pain. "You have no blood pressure so you just cooperate with me, darling, and we'll be fine."

Meanwhile, Dr. Tizes examined his eyes with his penlight. Blazek readied another needle. "Another stick," Blazek said, "a little mosquito bite." She pushed the needle into his shoulder. "Awwww," he groaned.

"The biggest damn mosquito you ever saw," she laughed.

"You're poking holes in me," the man gurgled.

"What were you hit with?" Dr. Tizes asked, "Bottles, sticks?"

"I don't know; they probably hit me with the kitchen sink," he moaned. He began to shake uncontrollably.

"What do you do? Free-base, shoot-up?" Ziarko asked.

"Free-base."

"What's your birthdate?" She and another nurse wheeled him over to one of the curtained "rooms." (A man who had been given that space a few minutes before was asked to move to a chair. He had been stabbed superficially in the wrist and stomach by his girlfriend.)

Another nurse took over the questioning.

"What's your address?"

"I don't have one."

"You don't have a home?" she said flatly. "You live on the street?"

"Yes." He shook wildly, his eyes tearing.

"When did you last do coke? It's ten minutes to ten."

"Thirty minutes ago," he answered.

She pulled off his shoes. Then Ziarko was back. "Can you undo your pants for me?" she asked.

Still shuddering, crying, mumbling something about his sister, the man fumbled helplessly with his zipper.

"I'm here to take care of you," Ziarko said. "I don't know anything about your sister. Can you undo your pants for me?" she repeated. She walked away, and he lifted his pelvis from the bed, trying in vain to remove his filthy jeans.

The man eventually was admitted to the hospital for observation, then discharged the next evening. For him and other homeless people who stagger into the emergency room drunk or high, the hospital was a shelter with a one-night limit. A survey conducted in spring 1989 at one of the larger public hospitals in New York City, where homelessness is rampant, found that an incredible 42 percent of patients were homeless, 31 percent in the general hospital, and 60 percent among psychiatric patients.[17] In effect, homelessness and other "nonmedical" problems are forcing urban hospitals to rediscover their nineteenth-century roots as almshouses for the sick, lonely, and poor. "Like it or not," one commentator wrote, "[hospitals] are still the providers of last resort of shelter, food, and foster care as well as of medical care."[18]

"That guy in [room] One needs to leave," complained one of the nurses, eyeing the whistling patient's bed for another patient.

"It's going to be another hour for the ambulance on him," Blazek answered. He was being transferred to a psychiatric hospital, and private ambulance services can take hours for cases that are not deemed emergencies—another factor that contributed to the ER crush.

The trauma phone rang again. "We've got a gunshot wound—belly," Blazek blared. A minute later: "It's a thigh, not a belly, my fault."

Promptly, the paramedics rolled a stretcher through the door with a big-muscled, twenty-one-year-old sprawled out on it. "That's the thigh," Blazek said.

The paramedics pushed the young man over to the serious side of the aisle. He had been shot by a "male friend" of his girlfriend. "Hi, baby, I just saw you a little while ago," one of the paramedics greeted Blazek as he passed. She smiled a silent hello.

The trauma phone rang again. "Steering wheel in the chest, through the windshield," a voice called out.

A surgery resident began to get the gunshot victim's history as nurses peeled off his tight Lycra biking shorts. His thighs were red with blood. "How many times did you hear the gun go off?" the surgery resident asked.

"Three."

"How many times were you hit?"

A police officer walked up. "Hi, sweetheart," he called out to Blazek. He took advantage of a lull in the doctor's questioning to begin his own.

"Sir, what floor do you live on?" he asked the gunshot victim.

The officer backed off for a moment as the resident gave the young man a rectal exam. He moved back in.

"What's your girlfriend's name?"

Each trauma center in the city covers a certain region, and Mount Sinai's includes the tenth and eleventh police districts, the latter of which has one of the highest crime rates in the city. Among twenty-five police districts, the eleventh district's serious-assault rate is second highest, its murder rate fifth highest, its sexual assault rate third highest.[19] The district includes North Lawndale, where a violent crime occurs every three hours and a murder every twelve days.[20]

This epidemic of urban violence explains why Mount Sinai treats so many cases involving "penetrating" trauma—gunshot and stab wounds as opposed to the blunt injuries suffered in car accidents. Apart from the needless human suffering, victims of violent crime are less likely than other trauma victims to be insured, and their injuries cost at least as much, if not more, to treat. Not only is the number of shootings rising, but the injuries suffered are more severe, due to semi-automatic weapons. Cook County Hospital reported that in 1984, 5 percent of its gunshot victims had been shot more than once. In 1988, the bullet-riddled category had risen to 20 percent.[21]

The emergency room doors swung open again. The car accident victim's neck was in a brace. Drunk, he had collided with a tree, slamming his chest against the steering wheel and shattering the windshield. He was pushed over to the serious side of the ER, where Dr. Rosenfeld prepared him for an X-ray to determine if his neck or back was broken. She positioned herself at the end of the bed, took his hands and pulled, her face red with exertion. This allowed the harried X-ray technician to get a clear shot of his vertebrae. Because of the potential severity of his injuries, the X-ray was processed within minutes instead of hours.

"His neck *is* broken," Dr. Rosenfeld said with surprise. She complimented the paramedics on their good work. Patients with broken necks who are jostled around can end up permanently paralyzed. So far, this man seemed OK.

At 10:40, the trauma phone rang again. "We're getting a guy who jumped out of a second-floor window. Hearing-impaired," a nurse called out. "How's your sign language?"

Twenty minutes later, the "jumper," as he had come to be called, arrived. The paramedics had discovered the old man crawling around on his hands and knees, saying that he jumped out of the window when someone threatened him with a knife. "We didn't believe him," one of them said, "until we saw his ankles."

The old man's eyes were wide open with what seemed to be a combination of fear and pain. In addition to his swollen ankles, he was emaciated, sickly looking. Dr. Rosenfeld tried to ask him a few questions but his answers were incomprehensible. Then Dr. Faulk approached to give it a try. "What hurts?" she yelled. He moved his shrunken lips—he had no teeth—but his words were mush. Dr. Faulk looked at him sympathetically and ordered a full-body X-ray; she would have to use the pictures to find out what hurt.

Dr. Singh, meanwhile, had spent the last hour in the waiting room, referring two teenage girls, sixteen and seventeen, and a twenty-six-year-old woman to the labor and delivery clinic, where women more than five months pregnant are sent when they show up at the emergency room.

Ziarko phoned the intensive care unit for the third or fourth time that evening. "We need beds," she pleaded. "Could you please keep us in mind?"

A few minutes before midnight the paramedics showed up again. This time, they had picked up a drunken fifty-five-year-old who had fallen off his bike and hit his head. Dr. Rosenfeld began the examination. "Take a deep breath, Sir," she said. "And don't do it in my face, Sir. God!" She pulled back in disgust from the alcohol stench.

Blazek had come over to take the man's blood for laboratory tests. He reached up to push her away, his speech garbled by liquor. "You stop fighting now," she said, trying to maneuver the needle into his arm. "I'm fighting you, I am," the man snarled.

Battles more pitched than this one have become commonplace in urban emergency rooms as drugs, especially crack, increasingly infest poor neighborhoods. Another night, a heroin addict was rushed into Mount Sinai's ER after being shot in the leg. His blood pressure had dropped precipitously, and doctors tried to stabilize him but he would not stay still. He ripped a tube out of his nose and kept rearing up from the gurney. "You gonna fall your butt off the cart, goddamnit," a nurse yelled, shoving him back onto the bed and eventually restraining his legs with leathers. Commenting on incidents like this, a nurse in New York City told *Time* magazine that her days of playing "little Nancy nurse" were over: "You're tying people on top of stretchers, sitting on top of people and fighting with them constantly."[22]

The homeless cocaine addict had fallen asleep, but no one had gotten around to sewing up the laceration on the back of his head, which had clotted on its own. "Give it to Mike [one of the medical students]," Dr. Rosenfeld suggested. "He's hungry for a suture."

By 12:15 A.M., the sickle-cell woman's bed had been moved from one of the curtained rooms to the more public place against the wall.

"When is your ride coming?" Blazek asked. The woman raised her head, glanced around dully, and lay down again.

"Please keep us in mind," Ziarko said, once again on the phone begging the intensive care clerk to try to free up a bed. "We have a male and a female."

Though the emergency room was still full, the flow of patients seemed to be slowing. The paramedics showed up at 1 A.M. with submarine sandwiches for the staff. Ziarko sat at the nursing station and put her head down for a minute. The regular phone rang; she grabbed it: a mother wanted advice about her child's chicken pox.

Blood tests returned for the drunken bicyclist, which showed that his blood-alcohol level was four times the legal intoxication rate in Illinois. His blood sugar level was also high, indicating that perhaps he was a diabetic. Patients who come in with one problem and are found to have others are an everyday occurrence. Dr. Rosenfeld walked over to the man.

"Are you a diabetic?" she asked loudly.

"No," he screamed back. "I'm a Baptist."

At 1:25 A.M., the last serious trauma of the evening arrived. As all trauma patients do, he arrived feet first, pushed through the door by the paramedics. The bottoms of his white socks were muddy and covered with grass and twigs.

"We found him in the parkway [highway median strip], lying in the dirt," one of the paramedics said.

"We think it was his turn to buy [liquor], and he refused," chortled a police officer, who had showed up at the emergency room to ask doctors to examine the man to see if he had been sexually assaulted. When he was found, his pants were around his ankles.

He, too, would need X-rays; one of the medical students cut away his pants and boxer shorts. And once again, he spoke only Spanish. Obviously drunk, he told Dr. Rosenfeld how he ended up lying in the middle of the expressway. He met three men who asked him if he wanted to go for a drive and share their bottle of wine. The evening was progressing nicely, when, the man said, gesticulating with his bloody hand, they robbed him of $300, stabbed him, and pushed him out of the car.

He eventually was admitted to the hospital for observation and discharged the next day, as was the other Hispanic man, who had not been seriously injured in the bus accident (nor was he found to have the suspected testicular cancer). Both of these men were uninsured.

Every adult male mentioned was uninsured or self-paying (translation: nonpaying), except for the middle-aged heart attack victim, who had commercial insurance. If uninsured patients were hospitalized for a day or more, Mount Sinai tried to enroll them in the Illinois Department of Public Aid's General Assistance program,[23] which at the time provided some medical coverage for single adults who earned less than $165 a month. When that worked, the hospital recovered about half of its costs. But for Mount Sinai to attempt to enroll patients in Medicaid, they had to be sick enough to stay in the hospital for the interviews and evaluations that accompany Medicaid certification.[24] The two Hispanic men were considered "twenty-three-hour admissions," so Mount Sinai had no chance to recoup the costs of their care.

Here's what happened to the rest of the patients:

One of the pregnant teenage girls gave birth to a full-term baby that night; the other two women's contractions stopped, and they were sent home. Two of them were covered by Medicaid, one by an HMO.

Once the narcotics wore off, the woman with sickle-cell disease wandered aimlessly around the emergency room until 12:20 A.M., when a relative finally came to pick her up. She, too, was covered by Medicaid.

It turned out that the man who drove his car into a tree did not have a broken neck, only arthritic compression of the spine that made the bone look like it was cracked. He was hospitalized for five days with a bruised heart and chest.

The deaf man who jumped from the second-floor window had crushed bones in his feet, and he stayed in the hospital for nearly three weeks. A hospital social worker was not sure whether he should be discharged to his home, where the quarrel that resulted in his leap had occurred. He was sent home anyway.

The gunshot victim was observed overnight and released; the bullets had not severed any major blood vessels in his legs.

The little boy wounded by a pellet gun was discharged from the emergency room at 12:50 A.M. He'd had to wait so long because the X-ray technician was busy with emergencies until after midnight. Fortunately, the X-ray revealed that the BB had not lodged in his cheek.

The young man with the soccer injury had to be admitted for three days so doctors could repair his seriously injured hand; three of his knuckles had been wrenched out of their sockets.

The middle-aged man who had suffered a mild heart attack stayed in the emergency room until 1:45 the next afternoon; it took nearly twenty-four hours for a bed to open in the intensive care unit, the only other part of the hospital with machines that could continuously monitor his heart and vital signs. He underwent a cardiac catheterization and was discharged after four days.

The Wisk-drinker eventually fell asleep. He was kept overnight and discharged at 7 A.M. An ambulance came to take the other suicidal patient to a psychiatric hospital at 10:25 P.M.

The shoeless old woman stayed in the hospital for a month before returning to the nursing home. In addition to the pneumonia that prompted her admission, doctors treated cancer that was spreading through her body.

And the inebriated bicyclist picked up the tune that the old woman and the whistling suicidal boy had dropped.

"How are you all today?" he sang out again and again, having shifted from a surly to a gregarious drunk about 2 A.M. "How are you all today?"

7

One hospital's story: How treating

the poor is "bad" for business

Mount Sinai's emergency room may be a sorry substitute for a family doctor, but for many of the West Side's poor, especially the uninsured, it's the only option available. Its trauma center is indispensable in a neighborhood where so many residents are literally torn apart by violence. As Mount Sinai's chief executive Benn Greenspan told a Chicago newspaper, the hospital may lose a couple million dollars a year on trauma, "but we're the community hospital. It is not an acceptable alternative to stop serving the community."[1]

Maybe not, but unlike Mount Sinai, more and more city hospitals have chosen either to close money-losing operations like trauma centers, or to shut their doors altogether. Mount Sinai has survived not by working through the health care system, which is set up to reward hospitals that treat people with good insurance, but by working around it. Mount Sinai's means of survival is far from foolproof, however, or a model that could be replicated by other hard-up hospitals. For despite the determination and commitment of its leaders, every breath Mount Sinai took over the past two decades could have been its last.

The story of Mount Sinai, founded in 1911 to serve poor Jewish emigrants from Eastern Europe, is the story of Jews taking care of their own, as well as taking care of those who need them most. It is ultimately the story of this country's inability to care for the health of its poor. Two anecdotes tie the hospital's past to its future.

Bemoaning her grandmother's finicky diet, Jackie joked one day about getting takeout from Schwab, which shares food service with Mount Sinai. "Schwab feeds you like a soul food place," Jackie told the home nurse, Rose Murry. "They got greens, necks, everything."

Yeah, the food isn't bad, Rose agreed, but how would you like to go there on your *anniversary*? Rose said she talked to an elderly man at a bus stop near Mount Sinai who confided that he was taking his wife to the hospital's cafeteria to celebrate their twenty-fifth. Granted, the cafeteria had been redecorated in the mid-1980s in peach and mauve, with plants and abstract paintings for decoration, but a hospital cafeteria is a hospital cafeteria.

"I'd be so mad if my husband did that," Rose said, laughing along with Jackie.

Some time later, Greenspan, the hospital's chief executive, mentioned that he had visited his elderly mother in New York, where she works with two women who grew up in Lawndale in the 1920s. "Mount Sinai was the best place to eat on a Saturday night," they told Greenspan. What drew these women's families to Mount Sinai was that the hospital kept a kosher kitchen; few other places catered to the dietary needs of Eastern Orthodox Jews, who were new to the United States and struggling to establish themselves.

Today, North Lawndale remains a world apart, not because of religion or ethnic heritage, but because of generations of poverty. On the South Side middle-class black neighborhoods are common, but the West Side is an economic wasteland, and finding a place other than a McDonald's to have a cup of coffee can be a challenge. Mount Sinai's cafeteria may well be the most inviting restaurant around.

Not-for-profit, private hospitals such as Mount Sinai have taken center stage in American health care for a variety of reasons, not the least being the power of the medical profession. Hospitals rose in importance through the first half of this century as doctors demanded their own well-equipped, private "workshops" where they could practice as they saw fit. Organized medicine, later joined by the leaders of the many private hospitals that had sprung up around the country, strenuously resisted government interference, including attempts by a handful of reformers to make public hospitals anything more than institutions of last resort. Third-party payors such as Blue Cross and Blue Shield, commercial insurers, and, eventually, the government's own Medicare and Medicaid programs helped hospitals prosper by reimbursing them for whatever tests or treatments doctors deemed necessary. The funding gush only came to an end in the 1980s, as the payors who had once been so generous moved to staunch the hemorrhage of health care dollars, though the system they helped create remains.

Yet always excluded from this comfortable arrangement were public hospitals and some inner-city private ones like Mount Sinai, which never developed predictable sources of support from either benefactors or the government. As hospital historian Rosemary Stevens has written, "egalitarian expectations would require an egalitarian, universal insurance program."[2] And that the United States has never had.

The Eastern European Jews who founded Mount Sinai (originally called Maimonides Kosher Hospital) in 1911 were part of the second wave of Jews to settle in Chicago. Already in the city were German Jews who had emigrated in the mid-1800s and had acquired American ways and substantial wealth. The new immigrants did not feel welcome at the German-Jewish Michael Reese Hospital, located in an elegant neighborhood near Lake Michigan. Reading between the lines of an excerpt from a history of Michael Reese, the gulf between the Germans and their impoverished brethren is obvious: "Most [Eastern European Jews] were poor, having escaped with few possessions. And, though education was traditionally valued among Jews, these isolated groups were often ignorant of the world at large. For them, education was knowledge of the holy books and rabbinical law."[3]

A hospital for every group, and every faction of every group, was not unusual in the first decades of the twentieth century, as is evident by the names of the hospitals that still stand today. Chicago had fifty-nine hospitals in 1910, ranging from the behemoth public institution, Cook County, which then had 1,350 beds, to smaller places run by religious orders or ethnic groups, such as the sixty-bed German American Hospital, the forty-bed Swedish Covenant,[4] and the all-black Provident Hospital.

Despite the clamor for an Orthodox hospital, Maimonides went bankrupt a few years after it opened. It was revived and reopened as the sixty-bed Mount Sinai in 1919 by West Side businessman Morris Kurtzon, who had served on the original hospital's board and whose family still owns a lighting fixture company located just east of Mount Sinai on Ogden Avenue. "His parents were very, very Orthodox," his daughter Sylvia Koch remembered, "and he thought it was awful that his mother had to be treated by a Catholic nun." Mount Sinai also was a training ground for Eastern European Jewish doctors; most other hospital residency programs and medical schools set quotas for Jews well into the 1950s.

The new kosher hospital initially did not get much support from the city's dominant Jewish philanthropic group, the Associated Jewish Charities of Chicago, but gradually some of the barriers between German and Eastern European Jews began to crumble. The Charities commissioned a report on the hospital in the early 1920s as a preliminary step toward supporting Mount Sinai. (Michael Reese, the German-Jewish hospital, already was an affiliated agency.) The report foreshadowed the sometimes stormy relationship between Mount Sinai and some members of the Jewish community: "[T]here are persons active in the larger and long-established Jewish charities who appear to regard Mount Sinai as an unnecessary and sporadic venture."[5] Setting aside such reservations, the Charities began contributing to Mount Sinai in 1923.

Mount Sinai's first three decades were marked by steady expansion, though often in opposition to the Jewish Charities, several of whose biggest givers sat on the board of Michael Reese. In 1939, Kurtzon, still president of Mount Sinai's board, notified the Charities that the hospital wanted to add five new floors on top of its present building. The expansion was necessary, Kurtzon said, because Mount Sinai's occupancy was running 90 percent, very high, especially for that era.[6] (The Charities required that affiliate agencies get permission before soliciting money for such projects.)

The Charities' executive director, Samuel Goldsmith, fought the request, charging that Mount Sinai was treating too many paying patients as opposed to poor Jews, while Michael Reese was fulfilling its public service mission. "I believe that we should . . . decline to do anything with respect to the physical rehabilitation of the [Mount Sinai] building, and certainly in the physical addition of beds, until we are assured that . . . the institution [is] in effect a public service institution and not a medical hotel," Goldsmith wrote to his organization's Medical Care Committee.[7] He concluded that unless something changed, there was no sense in the Charities being "burdened" by two hospitals.[8]

Charities' statistics from that time show that both hospitals reported that about half of their days were "pay" and half "service," or free,[9] so it is not clear how Goldsmith decided Mount Sinai was more of a "medical hotel" than Michael Reese. Across the country, that label had been attached to the many hospitals unabashedly promoting a panoply of amenities to paying patients, while confining indigent patients to large wards. Historian Rosemary Stevens quoted a hospital administrator's summary of patient hierarchies: "If we could visualize the four divisions of the social strata as cream, milk, skimmed milk, and water, we could designate the private patient as 'cream,' the semi-private patient as the 'milk,' and the pauper or indigent patient as the 'water.'" As Stevens noted, to fund and justify their expansion, "all hospitals wanted a good dollop of cream."[10]

Today, the Charities' charge, that Mount Sinai ignored the poor, is strikingly ironic. In the 1980s, Mount Sinai became one of perhaps the most community-service-oriented institutions in Chicago, while Michael Reese could never quite reconcile itself to becoming something closer to what its location and the assimilation of Jews eventually dictated—a community hospital for poor blacks. Michael Reese came to the brink of bankruptcy before being sold to the for-profit Humana Inc. in 1991. The competition between the two Jewish institutions had been so keen that Ruth Rothstein, who led Mount Sinai from 1972 to 1990 and became one of the hospital's most influential leaders, could not hide her glee at Michael Reese's demise. "The fact that Sinai survived and Reese didn't, I love it! I love it!" she said, smiling shamelessly. She qualified that by noting that Chicago's poor will be the biggest losers if Humana reneges on its pledge to continue treating a significant number of Medicaid patients. But then she went on to gloat a bit more. "Michael Reese got up in the morning and said, 'Mirror, mirror, on the wall, who's the fairest one of all?' And the mirror answered, 'Michael Reese, Michael Reese, Michael Reese.'"

Back when Rothstein was still growing up in Brooklyn, the daughter of a Russian-Jewish emigré who worked in a shoe factory, the mirrors at *Mount Sinai* talked about Michael Reese, too, but Mount Sinai's board stubbornly refused to concede defeat to the wealthier institution. The hospital eventually received approval from the Charities for a three-story addition, which opened in 1942. And in the next decade, the hospital bulldozed past the Charities to build a new Nurses' Home and School, add two new floors, and build an outpatient and research facility.[11]

By the mid-1950s, Mount Sinai, and hospitals everywhere, bore little resemblance to their forebears. They had started the century as places for the penniless and lonely to die; medical science being unable to provide effective cures, people with means and family stayed home when they got sick. But led by the increasing expertise and power of the medical profession, hospitals began to promote real cures to the public, more and more of whom were covered by employer-sponsored health insurance. This shift was celebrated in 1949 in an essay written on the hospital's thirtieth anniversary: "[The hospital board] is imbued with the newer philosophy of hospital service which has for its premise that hospitals do not exist for the poor only, but that excellent equipment and facilities should be made available for the whole community, the well-to-do, the poor and those in moderate circumstances. . . . With this idea in mind, the Board takes every opportunity to add to the facilities and scientific armamentarium of the Hospital."[12]

The tension between Mount Sinai's commitment to serve the poor and its desire to court wealthier patients to fund the scientific armamentarium persisted in some form for the next three decades—as it did at hundreds of other nonprofit hospitals nationwide.[13] Running parallel to the debate about whether Mount Sinai's predominant mission was charity or medical progress was a second debate over serving Jews versus blacks, a controversial issue to this day.

Within two decades after it opened, the number of Jewish patients using Mount Sinai was dropping. A Mount Sinai board member had predicted the Jewish migration from Lawndale as early and perhaps presciently as 1922. "I have come to the conclusion that the present location for the institution is not adequate for its future needs," businessman Edward Katzinger wrote to an official at the Jewish Charities. "It is my opinion that a location further north would be much more adaptable for the present and the future, because of the Jewish population settling more in a northerly direction."[14] Obviously, Katzinger's recommendation was ignored.

Well into the 1970s, Mount Sinai annually reported its percentage of Jewish patients to the Charities, which was renamed the Jewish Federation of Metropolitan Chicago in 1958. In 1940, 86 percent of inpatients were Jewish. By 1946, that number had dropped to 71 percent; by 1950, it was down another 10 percentage points; and by 1963 only a quarter of Mount Sinai's patients were Jewish.[15] These decreases were largely the result of Jews moving from the West Side. They also reflect a trend that accelerated in the 1950s and 1960s—the lessening of discrimination at other hospitals against both Jewish patients and doctors.

Documents from that era show that the two Jewish hospitals and the Federation were as troubled by the increasing use of Mount Sinai and Michael Reese by blacks as they were by the attrition of Jews. "Negro" admissions were tracked as closely as Jewish ones.[16]

The first extended public discussion about discrimination against blacks in Chicago hospitals began in the mid-1940s. In 1947, admitting clerks at the University of Chicago's Billings Hospital submitted written testimony to civil rights groups about the methods they had been instructed to use to turn away blacks. "Shortly after being hired," Pauline Mathewson wrote, "I was told the Negro patients were not desired by the hospital Administration, and that they should only be given appointments in rare instances. Such cases would include a patient of teaching or research value."[17]

Mathewson described what happened when a clerk inadvertently made an appointment with a black patient over the phone. Clerks were to use the following methods to get rid of a black patient: "Quote the highest possible fee to discourage him. . . . State that no appointment is registered and that the patient might have contacted the wrong department. . . . THE DAILY SCHEDULE OF APPOINTMENTS IS HIDDEN UNTIL THE PATIENT LEAVES SO THAT HE WILL NOT BE ABLE TO SEE HIS NAME LISTED" (capital letters in original).

Another clerk testified: "On one occasion, when several appointments had been made for Negroes over a period of three days, I was asked to memorize the streets and boundaries of the Negro district on the South Side of Chicago."[18]

The Chicago Commission on Human Relations followed up with a report a year later that revealed that even the 50,000 Chicago blacks who had private health insurance could not get service at most hospitals and were forced to go to either Cook County Hospital, or the all-black Provident Hospital.[19] As racist as some of its policies were, Billings, along with Mount Sinai and Michael Reese, were commended in the Commission report for "greatly expanding services for Negroes." Other Chicago hospitals refused to admit blacks altogether.[20]

To address the problem, the Chicago Council of the American Jewish Congress worked closely with black groups in 1955 and 1956, first to pass a state law and then a city ordinance prohibiting racial discrimination by hospitals. But despite the Jewish community's advocacy on the part of blacks, discrimination did not disappear overnight at Mount Sinai, or anywhere else. In 1957, a Chicago Commission on Human Relations report praised Mount Sinai's "integrated employee force and the acceptance of one Negro physician on the medical staff," but then raised a concern about "retrogression."[21]

Commission members had interviewed Mount Sinai officials and found them less than forthcoming about the hospital's policies toward blacks. Their indirect answers were revealing, however. Hospital leaders explained that a perception might exist that black patients were being discriminated against because Jewish patients were indeed the institution's first priority. "No Jewish person will be turned away if at all possible," one Mount Sinai representative said. "Jewish patients will be catered to and wherever there is a problem we will favor the Jewish patient."

Hospital administrators denied a charge that black patients were segregated to two floors—well, sort of. "If we have a little wing set aside for ritzy patients you shouldn't worry about that," one official reportedly said, describing a practice that was common in many hospitals that needed to coddle benefactors and VIPs. "We just do it to cater to big contributors. We're 99 . . . percent pure and we don't worry about a small temporization." Another comment that the commission considered noteworthy was: "Basically, we can't push integration too fast."[22]

As late as the 1970s, racial segregation had not been eliminated at Chicago hospitals. A group of medical students at the prestigious Rush-Presbyterian-St. Luke's Medical Center protested in 1973 that black obstetric patients, those with good insurance as well as welfare recipients, were relegated to an old, deteriorating building, while white women gave birth in a modern wing of the hospital.[23] Hospital officials contended that only black *Medicaid* recipients were excluded from the new rooms because Medicaid would reimburse only for the cheapest accommodations. The students countered that the price differential existed solely to promote segregation since the charges for the new and old rooms were only a few dollars apart.

Though overt racial segregation largely was eradicated by law and public condemnation, Mount Sinai and the Charities continued to face a conundrum: How could a hospital favor Jews without discriminating against other groups? The question became irrelevant by 1960, as Jews no longer lived in Lawndale; by 1980, virtually the only Jews who traveled to the hospital were staff members and newly arrived Russian-Jewish immigrants. This population shift raised another question, however, asked repeatedly by various board members, administrators, and doctors at Mount Sinai, as well as by the Jewish community at large: Why should a Jewish hospital, supported by Jewish money, stay in a community that is mostly black?

This question was posed as early as the mid-1950s, as Lawndale rapidly "turned," block by block. In 1950, 13 percent of the neighborhood's residents were black; by 1960, an astounding 91 percent were black.[24] Journalist Nicholas Lemann describes Lawndale's transformation in his book about black migration to Chicago, *The Promised Land*. "Sleazy realtors known locally as 'panic peddlers' would move a black family into a neighborhood, often subjecting it to the familiar terrifying round of fire-bombings and snarling crowds. They would go around to the white families and warn them that they'd better move out before it was too late, thereby obtaining their houses at rock-bottom prices. Then they would rush in new black residents, gouging them in the process. Apartment buildings were cut up into overpriced and undermaintained kitchenettes. . . . The West Side quickly became overcrowded (while Lawndale was changing from white to black, its population was growing by 25 percent), and it began to become physically dilapidated."[25]

The upheaval shook Mount Sinai. A consultant hired to study the hospital in 1961 concluded that Mount Sinai had drifted without developing a long-range solution to its problems because "it has been caught between the impact of dwindling usage from its original service group on the one hand and its hope, on the other, that changes in transportation, ease of accessibility and urban renewal of the local area would occur in sufficient time to redirect the original supporters to its doors."[26]

Meanwhile, the hospital's relationship with the Jewish Federation certainly did not encourage Mount Sinai's doctors and administrators to put much faith in its future. Goldsmith, who led the Federation from 1930 to 1966, wanted to merge Mount Sinai and Michael Reese. Several times, it almost happened, but in the end, one or another of the institutions always got cold feet. Mount Sinai was worried about being treated as the poor cousin, said Dr. LeRoy Levitt, a retired psychiatrist and one of the hospital's most respected former physicians and leaders. "Mount Sinai thought Michael Reese would be the east campus and get all the rich Jews, and they would be the west campus and get all the blacks," he said. That may have been uncomfortably close to the truth since Michael Reese officials made no secret that, as the merger evolved, they expected their better-equipped institution to take over most of the research and surgery, leaving Mount Sinai as a West Side community hospital.[27]

In addition, the age-old animus between German and Eastern European Jews bollixed the deal, according to Dr. Levitt and others. "The boards of Michael Reese and Mount Sinai, they hated each other," he said. "The German Jews against the Russian Jews."

The last straw for the merger plan was Mount Sinai's insistence that it be allowed to construct a new facility, a demand opposed by Michael Reese and the Federation. "We knew that Lawndale was going down the drain, and to put so many millions of dollars in another pavilion that would not be used by the Jewish community was wrong," recalled Abram Davis, the president of the Federation's board from 1965 to 1967. To Mount Sinai, that cold assessment meant that the merger was a prelude to the hospital's extinction.

The intense pressure to merge subsided only when Michael Reese turned toward the University of Chicago Medical School, in another doomed affiliation attempt. At the same time, James Rice, who had replaced Goldsmith as the Federation's executive director, gave up on what had been a time-consuming effort to push the hospitals together. Each hospital was more or less left to its own devices.

Ground was broken for Mount Sinai's long-sought-after addition, the 208-bed Olin-Sang building, in 1967. It was completed three years later, adding its own distinctive mark to the hodgepodge of architectural styles that are inevitable at an institution that grows slowly. Olin-Sang resembles a large honeycomb, six stories of wide windows running eleven across in white concrete casings.

Despite the investment that had been made in the new building, Mount Sinai officials continued to discuss the possibility of moving the hospital to the northern suburbs, where most Chicago-area Jews now live. It's easy to scorn Mount Sinai doctors and administrators who "wanted a clean suburban hospital where patients were more like them," as a board member committed to staying in Lawndale put it. But during the late 1960s, much of white America was, at the very least, uncomfortable with blacks' new militance. Rothstein speaks proudly of not missing a day of work during the West Side riots that followed Martin Luther King Jr.'s assassination in 1968. She remembered a phone call from her now-deceased husband, a labor lawyer. "He called and said, 'You better get out of there. Everybody says the West Side is burning,'" Rothstein chuckled. "I said, 'Wait a minute, let me look out the window.'" Rothstein pulled back her blinds, as she had done twenty years before. "It's not burning here," she told her worried husband. (Today, the view from Rothstein's office is of Cook

County Hospital's main entrance on Harrison Street; Rothstein left Mount Sinai in late 1990 to try to revive this larger, infinitely more troubled institution.)

The riots were a turning point for North Lawndale. Most of the remaining businesses bolted, taking 25 percent of the area's jobs with them, according to one report.[28] The few whites who still lived in the neighborhood fled, as did many middle-class blacks. Mount Sinai, however, did not budge. According to a statement repeated again and again in hospital literature, Mount Sinai made a "bold, irrevocable decision: It chose to stay, to continue to provide private health care to the medically underserved and to improve the community environment."[29]

Mount Sinai's reasons for staying in Lawndale were more complicated than the community commitment the hospital stresses in its annual reports; that idea only gained deep, widespread support in the 1980s. At first, Chicago Medical School kept Mount Sinai where it was, according to Rothstein and others. Mount Sinai wanted to stay close to the West Side school to maintain its teaching and residency programs, though in truth, Chicago Medical School's reputation had never been strong enough to attract a full cadre of residents to the hospital. Nonetheless, a so-so medical school affiliation was better than none at all.

Rothstein, who ascended to the chief executive's job in 1972, is often credited with Mount Sinai's rediscovery of its mission to serve the disadvantaged. A former labor organizer, Rothstein, according to the lore that has grown up around her, would never have allowed the hospital to abandon the West Side. But for at least the first five years of her tenure, the hospital's board continued its search for a site for a northern hospital, one that might or might not replace the West Side hospital altogether. Some former board members insist that Mount Sinai only wanted to open a satellite on the North Side and never intended to leave North Lawndale. Others, among them Burton Olin, a lifetime trustee of the hospital (whose grandparents are the namesake for the Olin-Sang building), presented a different version of events. "We tried desperately to move," he said. "What we were trying to do was build a branch out there and gradually phase out of the West Side. We kept trying to follow the money."

Conflicting views about the board's ultimate intentions for the Lawndale hospital aside, Mount Sinai's tight budget foreclosed the possibility of purchasing land on the North Side. And by the end of the 1970s, the hospital probably could not have moved even if it had received a windfall. With public concern about medical costs and an oversupply of hospital beds at a new height, Illinois and most other states had started certificate-of-need programs that regulated the construction of new hospitals. They were only permitted in areas with a shortage of beds, and that certainly was not a problem in the northern suburbs.

Ironically, Chicago Medical School announced in 1974 that it was moving to Downey, Illinois, in the far northern exurbs near the Wisconsin state line. Mount Sinai administrators and doctors perceived the move as a massive betrayal, as the school had led the hospital to believe that it planned to stay on the West Side for good. The chairmen of Mount Sinai's clinical departments, who also had faculty appointments, resigned from the school. They did not want to abandon the hospital where they had built their practices, and moreover, the doctors predicted that the school would never find a sufficient number of hospitals in which to train its students. They were right. Certificate-of-need laws ultimately prevented Chicago Medical School from building its own hospital in Downey, and in 1987, its leaders asked to renew the affiliation with Mount Sinai. Mount Sinai readily accepted. Though Rush Medical College had agreed to place some residents there, the hospital was still struggling to fill the positions on its house staff. The chance to once more become the *primary* teaching hospital for a medical school was too good to pass up.

Depending on whom you talk to, Mount Sinai settled on the West Side as its permanent home in 1967 when ground was broken for the Olin-Sang building, in 1974 when a potential land deal on the North Side fell through, or in the late 1970s when certificate-of-need laws began to be enforced. Whatever the precise date, Mount Sinai has remained on the West Side in presence, but not always in spirit.

As anyone with even a glancing knowledge of medical care knows, hospitals today look more like businesses and less like charities than ever before, with "product lines," "marketing strategies," and "profit centers" as crucial as public service. That trend accelerated in the 1970s when not-for-profit hospitals looked around and saw that for-profits were making no pretense toward charity and were stealing their patients. The not-for-profits' reaction was to act more like their competitors, and Mount Sinai was no exception.

But Mount Sinai's business—tending and mending the poor—is unprofitable business. Lawndale's poor were its natural patients, and they are not well insured if insured at all. Faced with that inescapable fact in the early 1970s, Mount Sinai took a deep breath, and did what most hospitals were doing: it tried to draw paying patients. Throughout that decade and well into the next, Mount Sinai worked to shift its "patient mix," or replace patients who were uninsured or covered by Medicaid with those who had commercial insurance. Another way to look at it is that the hospital tried to keep people from the surrounding community from using the institution, and, at the same time, attract outsiders. A more charitable way to judge the strategy is that the hospital attempted to offer services to the middle-class Jewish community that had supported it for so long. "We thought if we built a shiny new building [Olin-Sang], patients and doctors would flock back to the hospital," said Harold Sherman, another lifetime trustee and board chairman during the 1970s.

For the hospital *not* to have tried to reduce its reliance on Medicaid would have been "absolutely crazy," given the hospital environment that existed at the time, added Mount Sinai's director of grants and government affairs, Roberta Rakove. "What hospitals were being told was that if you don't diversify your patient base, you're going to be dead meat."

Yet Mount Sinai, shoestring budget notwithstanding, also began some of the more creative, substantial ventures to rebuild the local community that the hospital industry has seen. In partnership with one of the few large companies left in the area, steel distributor Joseph T. Ryerson & Son, the hospital provided seed money for housing rehabilitation and construction. Hospital leaders also badgered their counterparts in city government to demolish several dangerous abandoned buildings on Ogden Avenue and to repair parts of that decaying street.

But the two actions held an inherent contradiction. While Mount Sinai might help local residents rehab their homes, it also might try to discourage them from occupying its beds unless they were adequately insured. The contradiction would begin to fade in the mid-1980s, when the hospital all but gave up trying to lure privately insured patients. Instead, Mount Sinai concentrated on becoming an almost *public* private hospital, so enmeshed in government programs that state and city bureaucrats and politicians would go to some length to prevent its demise. Government officials could not make it easy for Mount Sinai to survive—only a changed national policy could do that—but they were willing to pull it back from the brink.

One reason Mount Sinai got into such bad shape can be found in the Congressional legislation that created Medicare and Medicaid in 1965. It required that hospitals be paid at cost for providing care to the elderly and poor, with no cushion for bad debt or other overhead expenses. Such a reimbursement scheme was feasible for hospitals in middle-class and well-to-do areas. These institutions could raise the prices of commercially insured patients to subsidize the care of the small number of uninsured or publicly insured patients they treated. Hospitals such as Mount Sinai had fewer private shoulders to carry the load of charity care and more of that burden to bear. In 1973, for example, fewer than 20 percent of the hospital's patients were commercially insured; more than 40 percent were covered by Medicaid.[30]

Not only did Mount Sinai have few patients with adequate insurance, it had few patients of any kind. Its patient population had declined by the early 1970s, partly as a result of doctor flight to the suburbs, which accelerated after the 1968 riots. One study showed that while more than one hundred physicians had been practicing in Lawndale in the 1940s, only twelve had offices there by 1972.[31] Without doctors to admit patients, Mount Sinai could not fill its beds.

One group of doctors whose allegiance to Mount Sinai had survived population shifts was the Chicago Medical School faculty, but their attachment to the hospital was weakening in the early 1970s. For years, the academic doctors had been salaried by the hospital and medical school, giving free care to clinic patients in exchange for using them as research subjects. Such arrangements were considered obsolete with the advent of Medicaid and Medicare—the government now paid for patients who traditionally would have needed free care—and Mount Sinai's doctors wanted to earn incomes that more closely approximated those of their peers.

To boost physicians' incomes and curtail the hospital's losses, Mount Sinai closed its outpatient clinics in 1972 and reorganized the Chicago Medical School faculty into private group practices.[32] Under the new setup, Mount Sinai (or the school) continued to pay faculty physicians a stipend to conduct research and to supervise medical students and residents, but the doctors also began to earn income from Medicaid and Medicare for patients who were formerly treated for free.

The private practices had the added attraction of eliminating parts of the two-tiered system of care. Patients would no longer have to wait all day to see a doctor whom they typically did not know, as had been common at the clinics. Still, one group of poor patients lost out under the "Doctors-for-People" plan. Uninsured patients had particularly benefited from the long-standing bargain that teaching hospitals had struck with the poor, but Mount Sinai's new "private" doctors would not treat anyone without third-party coverage—except for emergency cases and Jews, who can never be turned away under hospital policy.

"We will continue to take care of the crisis patient," Rothstein told the *Chicago Daily News* in 1972, "but we are going to have to send some patients to County."[33] (When asked about that decision today, in her present post as chief of Cook County Hospital, and so on the opposite side of the issue, Rothstein deadpanned: "Did I say that?") Dr. Levitt, dean of Chicago Medical School at the time, explained it this way: "We cannot be that noble as to provide care to all the people who cannot pay anything. We would not be able to stay open if we did."[34]

In fact, for years Mount Sinai and all Chicago hospitals had quietly been transferring uninsured patients to County; indeed, public hospitals are considered by many experts as the government's way of greasing the wheels for private enterprise. According to this view, Cook County's existence has been predicated on its willingness to absorb patients that private hospitals do not want: those who are poor, minorities, or victims of chronic or incurable diseases. Periodically, County doctors complain that, in their eagerness to be rid of uninsured and, in recent years, Medicaid patients, hospitals transfer people who are too sick to be moved. One influential study found that a quarter of patients dumped at County in late 1983 and early 1984 were medically unstable.[35] Hospitals' definition of "stable" had been reduced to "basically alive," one County physician charged at the time.[36]

In order to put Mount Sinai's decision to close its clinics into perspective, Rush-Presbyterian-St. Luke's took a similar route five years later, in 1977. The same year, Rush's president announced that the hospital's assets had more than doubled over the previous decade to $163 million. This was the result of a massive construction and renovation project, the likes of which Mount Sinai could only dream of. Two floors were added to a patient care building, giving it fifteen stories; six floors were added to the outpatient professional building; a $4.5 million, fifteen-hundred-car parking garage was constructed and then expanded; and a $24.5 million academic facility was erected. And this was only the beginning. "The Decade of Achievement" that ended in 1977 was to be followed by a "Bridge to the Twenty-first Century," a five-year master plan to raise a whopping $154 million for still more building and refurbishing.[37]

If a massively endowed medical center like Rush did not think it could afford to take as many charity patients, how could Mount Sinai have been expected to? Those who believe Rush has forsaken its responsibility to care for the poor might scoff at that comparison[38]— Mount Sinai should never use Rush as a yardstick! One Chicago hospital observer pointed to Rush's soaring atrium lobby, which must be heated through Chicago's long, bitter winters, as an example of that institution's damnable priorities: "That's wasted space. They're running a not-for-profit institution in a city that is desperate for health care, and they're throwing away money."

As unfair as Rush-Presbyterian's unrelenting growth may seem, it illustrates a simple business axiom: in the health care industry, as in all others, it takes money to make money. Only by constantly updating its facilities, acquiring new technology, and hiring the biggest names in medicine can a hospital such as Rush, which is also on the West Side—about three miles from the Baneses' apartment—hope to attract a significant number of commercially insured patients.

Closing the clinics reduced the financial drag on Mount Sinai somewhat but not enough. Hospital board minutes from the 1970s through the early 1980s are studded with references to the hospital's need to woo more physicians with larger practices of commercially insured patients. Rothstein's quote from a September 1973 board meeting is typical: "At present . . . we hope to obtain a new patient population, with other kinds of insurance."[39]

To this end, the hospital opened offices for its faculty group practice in a posh high-rise on Chicago's Magnificent Mile and in two blue-collar, well-insured communities on the South and Southwest sides of Chicago. The hospital also opened an office in a middle-class Jewish neighborhood on the North Side of the city, which demonstrated

Mount Sinai's commitment to the Jewish community more than it attracted well-heeled patients.

Though working to broaden its reach, Mount Sinai could not afford to ignore state Medicaid policies. Along with other Illinois hospitals, Mount Sinai periodically pressured the Illinois Department of Public Aid to raise its rates. One time, the hospital announced that it would refuse any new Medicaid patients.[40] In the 1970s, Public Aid supposedly still paid hospitals at cost, but at times it would delay payments or freeze rates, two tactics that became common practice in the next decade. In 1976, Mount Sinai joined the Illinois Hospital Association in a suit against Public Aid for its "illegal, unconstitutional freeze on our rates."[41] And for the first time, the association issued a list of hospitals in danger of closing, which it defined as those with Medicaid patient loads of 36 percent or more, a category that included Mount Sinai and 12 other urban hospitals.[42]

Both strategies—bringing in private-paying patients and nagging Public Aid—worked for a time. For the fiscal year ending in June 1977, Mount Sinai reported a $600,000 surplus (with Public Aid paying close to cost),[43] and in fiscal 1980 the hospital had $1 million left over after the bills were paid.[44] Then, in the early 1980s, Mount Sinai was hit by a nearly lethal combination of economic recession and drastic reductions in government reimbursement for the poor and, to a lesser extent, the elderly. The hospital once more tried to grasp those elusive saviors: privately insured patients.

Administrators developed detailed analyses of admissions from each clinical department, separating them by insurance source, then broke out the data by individual physician. They sat down with key doctors in each department to "engender [their] commitment to balance the patient mix."[45] Members of the faculty group practice were asked to reduce by 15 percent the time they spent treating patients at the hospital's campus and instead work at satellite offices outside of the neighborhood.[46]

The Chicago Medical School faculty had never pulled in as many privately insured patients as the hospital thought it should, said Dr. Henri Havdala, a faculty member and the longtime chairman of anesthesiology at Mount Sinai. "If somebody wants to be making a lot of money in private practice, they wouldn't stay here in the first place. But those same people when you push them to do private practice, they don't want to do it. Kling [the out-patient building on the hospital's grounds] is convenient. You just walk over there and supervise the residents. When you go out to the satellites, it takes all day, and you have to see the patients yourself."

Persuading nonfaculty physicians to admit private patients to Mount Sinai was nearly impossible for another reason. "A lot of patients, Jewish and not Jewish, thought going to the West Side was like entering Lebanon," Dr. Levitt said, explaining that the hospital built its parking garage largely so patients would feel more safe. "Ruth and I would hear about so-and-so doctor who had a big practice. If a patient didn't have enough to pay, they'd take him to Mount Sinai. If they had enough to pay, they'd take him to Skokie Valley." Trying to beat this system was futile, Dr. Levitt said. "Ruth had a short fuse about that and so did I, but doctors are never going to say to their patients, 'You don't want to go to Sinai? Well, then find yourself another doctor.'"

Between 1981 and 1985, Mount Sinai laid off hundreds of employees and put beds out of service; Medicaid reimbursements were dropping too drastically to be offset. While Medicaid was not overly generous in the 1970s, federal rules at least required states to pay hospitals for the cost of care. But in the 1980s, with medical inflation far outpacing the overall inflation rate, Congress gave states far more leeway to cut hospital reimbursement—and they did.

In addition, Medicare had become less lucrative. Because minority populations are younger than the white population, Mount Sinai treated relatively few elderly patients, but the hospital had fared well with the Medicare patients it did treat. When the federal government began using the DRG system, paying hospitals a predetermined fee for each Medicare patient based on illness rather than the amount of resources used, the elderly stopped being as profitable.

Despite its creative budget-slashing and marketing efforts, Mount Sinai lost money or just barely broke even every year from 1981 to 1985. Hospital admissions were in a free fall, and the patient census, or percentage of beds filled, hit the low 60s by the end of 1984.[47] The hospital's administrators and board had to find a way for Mount Sinai to survive.

One problem they had to confront was that fewer patients were being admitted from the blue-collar communities where Mount Sinai had pinned many of its hopes. Greenspan, in charge of ambulatory care at the time, attributed the drop to two factors. First, many manufacturing workers had lost their jobs—and their health insurance—during the recession. Second, hospitals in the working-class neighborhoods that Mount Sinai had targeted began to pull back local patients.

As for the West Side blacks and Hispanics for whom the hospital was supposedly hanging on, they were not beating down the doors, either, Greenspan said. "When we put resources outside the community, people in the community realized we were taking away resources that they needed. They stopped coming. We had chosen a path that seemed like an easy route to survival, that was less of a radical confrontation with the views of our peers. The temptation was that if we can just shift the patient mix by 10 percent. . . . That's how the industry as a whole works."

In the mid-1980s, however, the hospital changed course. It made, in the words of its 1986 annual report, a "formal reaffirmation of our commitment to serve West Side residents. . . . To do so, we have directed more resources to this area and focused our marketing efforts on three groups who live here: the disadvantaged, including those on public aid and the uninsured; the elderly, the majority of whom are also disadvantaged; and the blue-collar workers, who include blacks, Hispanics and ethnic Europeans."[48]

Marketing to the poor and *uninsured?* To gauge the unconventionality of such an approach, consider the 1982 recommendations of an ambulatory care expert from the American Hospital Association. Hospitals should explore "selective demarketing" techniques, the AHA official advised, including intentionally creating long lines in emergency rooms, eliminating primary-care clinics for the poor, and shunting nonpaying patients to waiting areas with "few seats, poor lighting, few signs, and no food or drinks."[49]

Rejecting that kind of strategy, Mount Sinai embarked on dozens of new ventures guaranteed to attract poor patients. The groundwork had been laid a few years earlier when the institution began its neighborhood revitalization projects and sought government grants to fund family planning and home psychiatric services for West Side residents. The major difference between the beginning and the middle of the decade was that the hospital stopped trying to sell its core service, namely hospital days, to people other than the local poor and working classes. "It wasn't until that time that we said we are who we are; our patients are our patients, and we better concentrate on being here," said Dr. Maurice Schwartz, the chairman of medicine at Mount Sinai since 1979. "I think the change brought an institutional sigh of relief."

In accordance with its new priorities, Mount Sinai stitched together a system of a dozen clinics in poor neighborhoods, most within two to five miles of the hospital. Three of the clinics, called Sinai Family Health Centers, were housed in high schools. Because they treat people who receive insufficient medical attention, the clinics were designated as federally qualified health centers in late 1991. The federal designation shored up the clinics' finances, allowing them to be paid at "reasonable cost" for treating Medicaid patients—$70 for a standard office visit instead of the $22 the Illinois Medicaid program usually paid.[50]

In keeping with its renewed West Side focus, the hospital jettisoned a few programs designed to appeal to affluent patients, including an in-vitro fertilization program, the first to open in the Midwest. The hospital decided it was not worth the $250,000 it cost to run the program. (In addition, by the time the program's first baby was born in 1985, high-technology fertility services were available in hospitals more to the liking of the financially secure couples who tend to seek them.) "You've got to ask yourself, 'Why would you do that kind of exotic fertility in this community?'" Greenspan said. "We're concentrating on high-risk maternity services instead."

The hospital continued to try to reach beyond the West Side, but it seemed motivated by a desire to subsidize its operations there, not abandon them. For example, Mount Sinai acquired a 20 percent interest in the North Side's Bethesda Hospital in early 1988, hoping to capitalize on its ties to the Jewish community. The hospital was renamed Mount Sinai Hospital North, but it was closed within a year because the company that owned the largest share of the institution pulled out of the deal, blaming a continued decline in Medicare payments.

To make its embrace of Lawndale's destitute possible, Mount Sinai jumped into the arms of state government. The hospital pursued nearly every special state government grant or project that came along. Currently, Mount Sinai runs a Department of Public Aid demonstration project to link Medicaid recipients with primary-care doctors as a means of controlling costs and promoting early, regular treatment. Notable among the other government projects at Mount Sinai is one of Chicago's largest Women, Infants, and Children (WIC) nutrition programs and Pediatric Ecology, an inpatient unit where IDPA and the state child welfare agency send abused children for assessment.

Mount Sinai also distanced itself from other private not-for-profit hospitals. Instead of joining the Illinois Hospital Association in 1991 on its annual trek to the state capital to lobby for higher Medicaid rates, Mount Sinai scheduled its own day in Springfield. "We didn't want to be with the *industry*," Greenspan said, dismissing wealthier hospitals that continue to fret over their bottom-lines.

The former director of the Illinois Department of Public Health, Dr. Bernard J. Turnock, said Mount Sinai's strategy has not only provided needed service to the local community but has helped ensure the hospital's survival by raising its stock in the eyes of politicians and bureaucrats. "They are a symbol," said Dr. Turnock, a measured man who does not make such pronouncements lightly. "This is a hospital that stuck with the community and slugged it out."[51]

The symbol Mount Sinai's leaders have chosen to represent it is an anchor. With its primary-care network, community development, and provision of jobs to local residents, the analogy works well—Mount Sinai keeps the West Side from drifting into more dangerous waters. That has garnered support from foundations and corporations, money that is essential if the hospital's facilities and equipment are not to become hopelessly outdated. With $3 million in grants, Mount Sinai built a new cancer treatment center that houses a linear accelerator for radiation therapy. "If we were a suburban hospital, we would have bought the new machine six to eight years ago," said Mitchell Balk, the hospital's development chief. Health planners interested in a more rational system may ask whether it makes sense for every hospital to possess such technology, but in the current environment, the question may be moot. "It's one thing to say equal care for rich and poor," says Mount Sinai's director of public affairs, Diane Dubey, "but unless we have a linear accelerator for cancer patients, we can't give care equal to Rush."

Mount Sinai depends on corporate and foundation grants partly because it still does not get many large donations from Jewish philanthropists. The source of the problem does not lie with the Jewish Federation: Rothstein patched things up with that organization some years ago. Rather, individual donors shun the hospital. Consultants who interviewed nearly 100 prominent Jews for a study commissioned by Mount Sinai observed that despite the hospital's help for Russian-

Jewish emigrés, "many people insisted—some rather strongly—that the Hospital is essentially a 'black' hospital because of its location. . . . One refrain which carried through from interview to interview was that Mount Sinai seems to stand in the shadow of Michael Reese Medical Center, both socially and medically."[52] Yet not much Jewish money was diverted to Mount Sinai when Humana purchased the other Jewish hospital. Several of Michael Reese's biggest donors passed over Mount Sinai in favor of tonier institutions like Rush-Presbyterian and Northwestern Memorial.

Another impediment to Mount Sinai's fund-raising is the much-discussed tension between Jews and blacks. The acrimony cannot help but fetter the hospital's fund-raising with both groups. (The consultants' report concluded that wealthy blacks were unlikely to contribute much to Mount Sinai because they tend to reserve their dollars for black-run institutions.)[53] And although the Jews who run the institution have for the most part accepted the situation, the distrust of blacks and disdain of Jews remain frustrating.

A Chicago newspaper once compared Mount Sinai to a "medieval monastery . . . for half a century, a center of healing and teaching for the community."[54] That tenacity is admired by many, including another venerable institution, the reigning activist of Chicago health care, Dr. Quentin Young. The sixty-nine-year-old internist/radio commentator/health reformer has seen hospitals come and go, and he respects Mount Sinai's achievement. But his enthusiasm is muted. "Ruthie [Rothstein] understood one crucial thing, that to survive you had to have all kinds of anchors in the community," Dr. Young said. "But I can't tell you Sinai won't go down in a year. Springfield [the state capital] could do it, a lot of things could do it."

Only Dr. Young would dare call Rothstein, who is nearing seventy herself, "Ruthie." At Mount Sinai and now at Cook County Hospital, Rothstein is known for being sharp-tongued and demanding. As one colleague said, "She's done a lot for Mount Sinai, but it's not because she's sunshine and roses." Her successor, Greenspan, whom Rothstein brought up through the ranks, has a different style. His sense of social justice is as passionate as Rothstein's, but he is more contemplative and, at least in private, seems more saddened by the inequities he sees.

It may be more that he is not easily satisfied, that he is a pessimist.

Settling down to talk in his office one day, he repeated a story he'd likely told before. It was about the day he and his wife lost a baby at Evanston Hospital, a well-funded institution located in the affluent northern Chicago suburb where Greenspan lives.

"I was extremely impressed and grateful for the support we were getting, but all I kept thinking was that [Mount Sinai] could never do this," Greenspan said, sounding tired. "We had three nurses who spent that day with us. There is no way Mount Sinai can ever deliver that kind of care, that kind of personal support for people who need it a lot more than I do. The system will never allow us to do for people what we want to do."

8

Who's responsible for

Tommy Markham's health?

Mrs. Jackson's middle-aged son, Tommy Markham, could easily be stereotyped as the kind of patient who frustrates Mount Sinai's best efforts: a poor, uneducated black man who can't—or won't—follow health advice to save his soul. Before a stroke left him partially paralyzed at age forty-eight, Tommy smoked, drank heavily, and stopped taking high blood pressure medication because it made him impotent. Since his stroke, he's sworn off his worst habit, alcohol, but he still smokes, devours fried meats and other fatty food, and rarely exercises.

Lawndale Christian Health Center, and particularly its founder, Dr. Arthur Jones, might be Tommy's best hope. With his dress shirt, tie, and suspenders, Dr. Jones looks the part of the small-town physician. More importantly, he acts it. He makes house calls; he comforts patients who are hurting and dying, holding their hands, tenderly stroking their foreheads. One early morning, making rounds at Bethany Hospital, a couple of miles north of Mount Sinai, he stopped to visit a woman suffering from pneumonia and asthma. He found her window wide open, a cold breeze gusting through the room.

"How about closing your window?" he suggested. "The cold might be making it harder to breathe."

"I have to have air," she said, seated on the edge of her bed. Her eyes were fearful; her chest trembled as she struggled to breathe.

"Well, honey, there's plenty of air in here," Dr. Jones reassured her.

"But it gets so closed in."

"I'll leave the door open for you," he said, moving toward the window to close it. The woman still seemed agitated, so Dr. Jones sat down next to her and put his hand on her knee.

"Don't get discouraged. We'll get you better. You were doing OK and you just had a little set-back." She started to cry.

"What's the matter?"

The woman confessed that what was bothering her most was her schizophrenic adult son; she worried about what would happen to him were she to die. Dr. Jones sat on the bed comforting her for about five minutes—a very long time, by doctors' standards.

Dr. Jones was not always so gentle. He adjusted his manner to fit the situation, and when Tommy visited him at Lawndale Christian, he was kind but no-nonsense. Still, Dr. Jones often failed to reach Tommy. The interaction between these two men shows the limits of health education and, ultimately, the unfairness and futility of any health system predicated on holding people morally responsible for getting sick.

More than most facilities, Lawndale Christian and other community health centers are designed to reach across the divide between health professionals and poor patients, to give care in such a way that the poor will take advantage of it. They are run by local boards, which often have deep roots in the neighborhood. One of the conditions for employment at Lawndale Christian, located almost directly behind the Baneses' apartment, is that its doctors live near the clinic. ("How can I say to someone who is black, 'Now you've made it, come back to [North Lawndale],' unless I'm here?" Dr. Jones said. "The only way we're going to change the community is to hold onto the leadership.") Most community health centers have night and weekend hours to accommodate the working poor, and the uninsured pay for care according to a sliding fee scale. Community health centers often go out and get their patients. Lawndale Christian hired a lifelong neighborhood resident to track down children who miss checkups and immunizations.

But despite a proven record of providing high-quality, cost-effective care, community health centers are few and far between, and underfunded.[1] The first centers opened in 1965 as part of the War on Poverty, but the federal government subsequently sank most of its health care money into Medicaid, choosing to give (some) poor patients insurance rather than establish special clinics for them. Insurance better served the medical world's most powerful players—doctors and hospitals—argued sociologist Paul Starr in his influential book, *The*

Social Transformation of American Medicine. "[Medicaid] covered what would otherwise have been bad debt for hospitals and raised no challenge to private interests in the medical sector," Starr wrote.[2] Today, there are about 600 community health centers—thousands were originally planned—and one study estimated that they reach only a quarter of the 43 million Americans who need their help because they can't get care either in the private sector or from other public programs.[3]

With federal funding stagnant throughout the 1980s, Lawndale Christian was not designated as a federal health center until 1991 (a designation similar to the one given to Mount Sinai's Family Health Centers). Before then, Lawndale made ends meet with private foundation grants and its doctors' willingness to work for next to nothing—Dr. Jones made $8,000 his first year running the clinic. And although the federal designation qualifies Lawndale Christian for higher payments for Medicaid patients, no government money was available to help the health center defray the cost of treating its many uninsured patients.

Tight budget notwithstanding, Lawndale Christian does not look like a facility for poor people. Dr. Jones purposely chose to call it a "center" rather than a "clinic," a term that has become associated with poor service for poor people. The building's white cement exterior is trimmed with mint-green and mauve paint, in contrast to the ugly brown brick of most health care and social service offices in the neighborhood. In addition to doctors' offices, the facility houses Lawndale Community Church. And adjoining the health center's waiting room, visible through large glass windows, is a full basketball court, with a gleaming wood floor.

A young man was shooting baskets the first time Tommy visited the health center. Dissatisfied with the progress he'd made since his stroke, Tommy had scheduled an appointment with Dr. Jones on a recommendation from his uncle, Mrs. Jackson's only brother. "Hey, man," Tommy called out as he limped slowly through the health center's front door, "let me shoot some." The basketball player chuckled and faked a pass toward Tommy. Tommy smiled, pleased that his joke was appreciated.

Whenever Tommy gets out of the house—to cash his disability check, to buy lottery tickets, to visit a doctor—he incessantly teases whoever crosses his path. To the nurses who take his blood pressure, it's "Heh, baby, check that arm out; that's a nice arm." Or, "You know, it's womens who get my pressure up." To the elderly woman waiting in line behind him at the currency exchange, he gushes, "How you doing this morning? You lookin' mighty fresh." But when the wordplay gets beyond a superficial level, especially when Tommy is asked about himself, he shuts down. Having spent seven years in the state penitentiary, and most of the rest of his life prowling the West Side's streets, he trusts virtually no one.

In the waiting room that day, a man who appeared to be in his late thirties took a seat next to Tommy. "Don't I know you from somewhere?" the man asked in a pleasant voice. Tommy did not turn his head toward the man; he stared straight ahead.

"I used to live over this way," Tommy responded icily.

"Whereabouts?" the man asked, still friendly.

"In Lawndale," Tommy said, falling back into stony silence.

The man looked puzzled and leaned back in his chair. Evidently he got the message: Tommy was not talking.

After a half-hour wait, a nurse's assistant called Tommy back for his appointment. "I don't want nobody recognizing me," he muttered under his breath as he followed the nurse. "I don't know where they're recognizing me *from.*"

Dr. Jones greeted Tommy at the examining room door. He took his jacket, then showed him to a chair a few feet away from his own. "How can I help you?" he asked, meeting Tommy's eyes with his own.

"Every way," Tommy said. Tommy's beefy arms were folded across his lap, the partially paralyzed left arm resting on the right one. He wore tight, faded jeans and a silvery polyester shirt, a pack of cigarettes stuffed in his pocket. Because his bad arm got in the way of dressing, his shirt was buttoned wrong; the simplest tasks required major effort since his stroke—shaving, clipping his fingernails, even zipping his pants.

"Can you be more specific?" asked Dr. Jones.

"I feel like I should have improved more than I have since I had the stroke," Tommy continued. After his stroke, he had spent two months at Schwab Rehabilitation Center and attended outpatient physical therapy for two more months. Then he was on his own. Since he was disabled, Tommy qualified for monthly Supplemental Security Income payments and Medicaid, but neither the health insurance program for the poor nor for the elderly cover periodic therapy to ensure that people like Tommy maintain their strength.

It's not that Tommy was telling Dr. Jones that Schwab was mistreating him. He complained about soreness in his arm and leg and seemed vaguely dissatisfied with the rehab center, but whenever Dr. Jones pressed him about what he needed, he evaded the question. "Do you feel like people are not talking to you, that you're getting the runaround at Schwab?" Dr. Jones asked.

"I feel like I've been blessed. I've come a long way," Tommy said, refusing to engage on the subject.

Dr. Jones abandoned that line of questioning for the moment. "Do you follow a low-salt diet?" he asked Tommy.

"I do," Tommy said smiling slyly, "and I don't."

"Come on," Dr. Jones answered, leaning closer to him, "you have to work with me."

"I really don't follow a low-salt diet," Tommy conceded. Tommy lived with his girlfriend of sixteen years, and Dr. Jones asked him if he had ever requested that she cook with less salt. Tommy said he had not.

"How many eggs are you eating?" Dr. Jones continued, probing for more specifics on his diet.

"Three or four a week," Tommy answered.

"How about getting that down to two. Is that realistic?"

"I can get it down to one or none," Tommy responded.

And the cigarettes, had Tommy ever considered quitting? Dr. Jones asked.

"I could if I wanted to."

"How come you don't want to?"

"It's just something I do."

"Do you know why specifically they're not good for you?"

Tommy mumbled incoherently, so Dr. Jones told him that cigarettes increased his chances of heart attack, lung cancer, and emphysema.

"Very true, yes," Tommy said, rubbing his unshaven chin.

Dr. Jones leaned toward Tommy again. "It's a waste of your money," he said. "I can get anyone to stop once they've had their first heart attack, but it's too late then. Even though smoking may not feel bad now, when it does, it may be too late."

"You know what, Doc. Anything I need to stop doing, I can do it. I used to love whiskey, and I stopped that," Tommy told Dr. Jones.

However, Tommy continued to use salt, eat eggs, and smoke.

Tommy's responses were no different at Schwab. He said he would do, could do, whatever doctors asked, but then he didn't. At Dr. Jones' prodding, he eventually returned to Schwab for a checkup and was fitted for a new leg brace because the old one did not provide enough support. The new brace would fit higher on his leg and be more uncomfortable than the old one, a doctor told him, but he should resist the urge to go without it. "My main objective is to walk better. I don't care if the brace comes up to my neck," Tommy said.

A month later, Tommy went to pick up the brace. The bracemaker strapped it on for a test run in Schwab's lobby, and Tommy took a few awkward, evidently painful steps.

"Pretty soon I'm not going to need no brace at all," Tommy said, leaning on the receptionist's desk for a rest after he had walked no more than five feet.

"The odds are pretty high that you're going to need at least a knee brace for the rest of your life," the bracemaker said.

"Knee brace, hip brace, I don't care," Tommy retorted, "as long as I'm part of the living."

For months, Tommy declined to wear the new brace.

It would be easy to accuse Tommy of refusing to take responsibility for his health. Similarly, Mrs. Jackson could be blamed for getting so sick. When she was recovering from her stroke in 1987, she attended classes on proper diets for people with diabetes and high blood pressure, but Jackie said she pretty much ignored the instructions. "Mama would be the worst person to go on a diet. She would always get the smoked meats and the salt pork and just load up on it." While the accusations may be true, it is also true that complying with health advice is harder for the poor than for the middle class, which has more choices.

Perhaps because of the greater obstacles they face, but more likely in spite of them, poor minorities like Tommy and Mrs. Jackson have been the targets of recent campaigns by federal health agencies to urge people to take responsibility for their health. The individual-responsibility movement gathered momentum during the Republican presidential administrations of the 1980s, reaching its peak under the leadership of Dr. Louis W. Sullivan. Appointed by George Bush as secretary of the Department of Health and Human Services in 1988, Dr. Sullivan crisscrossed the country, in his words, "summoning our nation to a new culture of character, one that empowers the individual to influence his or her own health."[4]

Dr. Sullivan rarely discussed the disparities in health status between blacks and whites without beating the drum for individual responsibility. Typical of his campaign were the remarks he gave at a meeting of the National Medical Association, a group of black physicians: "Each American must feel a sense of urgency—the need to stop poor health practices, and to maintain good health practices in the days, months and years ahead. . . . We must remember that good health is a responsibility we really have to each other."[5]

Dr. Sullivan's comments imply that health choices are completely voluntary—an assumption that's difficult to accept. First, while his federal health agency anointed health education as one of the primary solutions to the 42 percent excess death rate among blacks,[6] statistics show many do not get close enough to doctors and nurses to get educated: 21 percent of blacks and 33 percent of Hispanics under sixty-five do not have health insurance.[7] In addition, urban poverty may refuse to accommodate the simplest healthy habits.

For example, during Tommy's second checkup at Lawndale Christian, Dr. Jones told him that he needed to walk regularly so he wouldn't lose the ability.

"I do not want to be no prey," Tommy answered, shaking his head slowly. He did not like the idea of hobbling through his neighborhood of West Garfield Park on a cane. The community adjoins North Lawndale and is equally poverty-stricken and violent.

Since Dr. Jones lives with his wife and two young daughters two blocks away from the Baneses, he could immediately empathize with Tommy's concern. As an internist, Dr. Jones's main job was to monitor Tommy's medical problems—high blood pressure and a mild heart condition—but he figured if he didn't pay attention to Tommy's rehabilitation, nobody else would.

"I don't want to see you get jumped," Dr. Jones continued. "Do you have someone you can walk with?"

"I know what I need," Tommy responded, pausing.

Dr. Jones looked at him hopefully.

"I need me a nine-millimeter."

"No, no," Dr. Jones said, unable to resist smiling at Tommy's street-smart, smart-alecky answer. Dr. Jones could understand why a gun might seem the only solution, but he was not about to start prescribing firearms.

Maybe Tommy's neighborhood was too dangerous to walk, maybe his girlfriend couldn't afford to fix healthier meals—fresh vegetables are hard to find and expensive in poor neighborhoods—but Tommy could have tried to quit smoking. There, it seems, he ignored his individual responsibility. The next question is: So what? Should he be denied medical care, or have to pay more for it? And should the same restraints be put on the privately insured?

Though outright denials of care or medical surcharges for unhealthy behavior may sound extreme, public pleas for people to take responsibility for their health cannot avoid those connotations. As University of Wisconsin medical ethicist Daniel Wikler wrote, "Health promotion is frequently said to proceed from the premise that *individuals are responsible for their health.* Fine—but what does it mean? Perhaps nothing more than that people will usually be healthier if they try to take better care of themselves. However, if that is all it means, it is too simple an idea to serve as the philosophical foundation for a comprehensive approach to health and health care. To fulfill the latter role, it must be understood as having moral and policy implications, and must involve ethical and even juridical concepts . . . fault, blame, and excuses, guilt, punishment, and compensation. Even when one who uses the slogan intends no such message, those who hear it may do so."[8]

Accordingly, Dr. Sullivan's individual responsibility campaign could not help but look like an elaborate disguise designed to mask the Bush Administration's indifference toward health care reform. Dr. Sullivan did not discourage that interpretation. Individual adoption of healthy behaviors, he said repeatedly, "would have a far greater impact on preventing disease, increasing lifespans, and reducing the cost of health care than would reform of the national health care system."[9] In the end, the emphasis on "individual responsibility" may be more dangerous than a diversion. It has the potential to undermine any attempt at all to reform the health care system to benefit the poor. Because, after all, if these poor folks make themselves sick, why should we waste our efforts helping them out?

The middle class and affluent are not immune to the individual-responsibility movement, however. Some companies are requiring employees to pay higher premiums if they smoke. Others have gone further. One Minnesota business reduced its employees' insurance premiums by $700 if they scored well on a health risk appraisal that measured cholesterol levels, body fat, blood pressure, heart rate, flexibility, and tobacco use.[10] (Cholesterol and blood pressure, at least, are thought to have strong genetic as well as lifestyle components.) That practice may strike some as fair, but pegging rates to health risk appraisals may be no more than a back-door means of "risk rating," where commercial insurers charge higher rates to the sick compared to the well, eventually pricing chronically ill people out of insurance altogether. While that might raise an uproar when the sick person is an "innocent" child, it's easier to justify for people who could be blamed for getting sick.

Even if "it is fair, . . . it is just, [that] persons in need of health services resulting from true, voluntary risks are treated differently from those in need of the same services for other reasons," as Robert Veatch, a Georgetown University medical ethicist wrote, determining "true, voluntary risk" may be nearly impossible.[11] It might change one's view of Tommy's situation, for instance, to read what a psychologist noted on his discharge from Schwab. Tommy would struggle to "set and maintain realistic goals," the psychologist wrote, because "he has difficulty with an emotional comprehension of his deficits and alternates between expecting/desiring total recovery and stating that he is not looking for miracles." If one of Tommy's problems is denial that he has one, it seems unfair to punish him for not doing everything he could to solve it.

Or in another case, is it a voluntary choice when people who hold religious or folk beliefs that conflict with modern medicine do not follow doctors' advice? Folk beliefs can harmlessly coexist with medical concepts: Jackie said her grandmother took laxatives before every appointment with Dr. Marino, believing they lowered her blood pressure, but at the same time faithfully took medication to control the disease. (She only skipped pills when she lost her predictable Medicaid coverage, and Jackie began to ration the medication to make it last.)

Folk beliefs are not always so benign. In a small study in New Orleans, two-thirds of elderly and middle-aged black women who blamed their high blood pressure on folk illnesses did not take their medication regularly, compared to only a quarter of the women who believed in the medical concept of hypertension.[12] One of the folk diseases was "high blood," characterized by "hot," "rich," or "thick" blood. It could be prevented by avoiding spicy, greasy foods and by drinking liquids such as lemon juice. The other was "high-pertension," where the blood was thought to "shoot up" to the head in times of stress. Women who professed that belief tried to stay away from emotionally charged situations.

Tommy, who was a bartender at the time of his stroke, knew about the latter disease. Here's how he described what caused high blood pressure: "Stress, you strangle everything up. The blood rises to the brain; you shoot that blood up. I was under a lot of stress in the lounge dealing with all sorts of people. You don't want to hurt anybody, and you don't want to get hurt."

But Tommy said he stopped taking blood pressure medication not because he thought he had a better cure for "high-pertension" but because he disliked the side effects of the medication, namely, impotence. He also said he skipped the pills because he took his health "for granted." Perhaps Tommy's belief in the emotional cause of high blood pressure interfered with his ability to take the drug treatment seriously.

After the stroke, Tommy put stock in another kind of folk belief: magic. Part of his resistance to doctors' advice about preserving his remaining health and strength seemed rooted in the notion that all would be well were a spell lifted from him. He never told Dr. Jones about it, which apparently is not unusual. In the New Orleans study, only two of fifteen physicians knew their patients' beliefs about "high blood" and "high-pertension."[13] In another study, a middle-aged black man told Detroit researchers that he used sassafras and tea leaves to treat his slightly elevated blood pressure but was not about to tell his doctor. "If I tell him I'm using herbs, he'd think I was silly."[14]

Tommy may have been similarly embarrassed. Although asked repeatedly about the causes of his stroke, he did not mention black magic until Jackie suggested specifically asking him about being "fixed, voodoo-wise." At that, he said he suspected that a relative of his girlfriend had cursed him. Usually, he said, people are protected from spells by "shields." But if they commit many "evil deeds," which Tommy believed he had, the shield can be penetrated. "I may have let down my guard," he explained.

Tommy had considered paying a spiritual advisor to lift the spell,

Jackie said. She told him he was getting conned—one healer asked $1400 for the service—and she marveled at how her father could reconcile voodoo with his professed Christianity. He kept his radio tuned to a Christian radio station day and night and proclaimed his belief in "the Master" to anyone who would listen. Jackie, for one, considered her father's stroke as a kind of Christian retribution. "You hear my father say that if you've been a bad person all your life you cannot think you can leave this world with curly white hair," Jackie said. "You're going to have to reap what you sow. So I feel like now he's reaping."

Loudell Snow, an anthropologist who has studied health beliefs of poor blacks, concluded in an article in the *Western Journal of Medicine* that doctors need to understand folk diseases and remedies to effectively treat those who believe in them. Understanding, according to Snow, does not mean denying that "high blood" and the like exist.[15] It would have been foolish for the New Orleans' doctors to try to debunk the beliefs of the women who stayed away from fatty or spicy foods to keep their blood from thickening; after all, low-fat, low-salt diets are part of modern medicine's recommended treatment for hypertension. The trick would have been to bring traditional medicine into the mix, to help patients realize that medication can make a difference, too.

Culturally sensitive doctors were only part of the answer to Snow. Racial oppression feeds superstitions and supernatural beliefs, he wrote. "The ultimate cause of the curse lies in economic, racial and political inequality, not in the hands of the sorcerer. It lies in unemployment, poverty and negative self-image, not in a bag of roots and graveyard dirt. It rests in a social environment so hostile that the individual would be a fool not to believe in the evil intentions of others. The real cure lies not in medications or mojos, then, but in a restructuring of American society which would truly result in equality for all."[16]

But short of restructuring society, aggressive public health programs can help poor, less educated patients live healthier lives. One of the largest high blood pressure studies ever conducted is proof enough.[17] Research teams at fourteen university medical centers across the country studied 11,000 hypertensive patients to discover whether the high rates of sickness and death associated with low socioeconomic status could be ameliorated with aggressive care. Half of the group was referred to local doctors for traditional high blood pressure treatment, and the other half was called back to the universities for an intensive program called "stepped care." The university patients received free medication; they were reminded of appointments by telephone. Health educators counseled them at the end of each medical checkup, even counting their pills in an effort to find those who were not taking medication as prescribed.[18]

After five years, the results were in. In the group referred to local doctors, people with less than a high school education died at twice the rate of the better educated. No such difference was found for those who received care from the university program.

"These findings on ability among hypertensive patients to reduce the adverse effect of low socioeconomic status have importance for both clinical practice and public health," the researchers concluded.[19] Indeed they do. Because after all, if the goal of health care is to preserve and restore health—and what else can it be?—affixing blame is beside the point. Medical interventions must be developed within the confines of real human behavior, whether it is judged responsible or not.

9

Jackie Banes's "patient"

Jackie emerged from her grandmother's bedroom carrying Mrs. Jackson's used absorbent bed pads. She walked back to the kitchen holding them out in front of her, as far away from her body as possible. Her face was expressionless, but her body language betrayed her understandable distaste for this task, which she performed four to five times a day.

Jackie's daughters were squeezed together on the vinyl recliner sharing a bowl of corn flakes. Their four-year-old brother, considered the big eater of the household, was also busy with his breakfast. DeMarest sat across from his sisters on the couch, scooping soggy cereal from his own bowl. Applause erupted every few minutes from the game show on the television outside of Mrs. Jackson's bedroom door, but as was often the case, no one was watching it.

Jackie passed by her children once more and disappeared into her grandmother's room. She carried a glass of cranberry juice with a straw in it. Because Mrs. Jackson slips down from the large pillow that Jackie uses to prop her up, it is easier for her to drink through a straw.

When Jackie came out again, she bent over near the apartment's front windows to inspect her plants. It had rained hard that morning, and the sun was trying to break through the clouds and make its way through the grimy windows. Jackie picked up the plants' tangled vines, pulling them apart. "Latrice, get me some tacks," she said.

Eleven-year-old Latrice was her mother's shadow. Like most children, she pouted when she got mad, but she often obeyed her mother without a murmur of complaint. A gangly girl whose legs seemed to be growing faster than the rest of her body, she tagged along after Jackie even when she was doing something as simple as tacking vines to the window sill.

Latrice's attention to her mother was not unappreciated. Jackie valued her eldest daughter's company, so much that when she felt overwhelmed caring for her grandmother, she sometimes kept Latrice home from school. Jackie could discuss more adult topics with her oldest daughter, and the two had forged a special bond in the five years they lived alone with Mrs. Jackson before Robert and Jackie married.

Brianna waddled up to the front of the room to join her mother and big sister. She whined for attention. "What's a matter, pooch?" Jackie asked, turning away from the window to placate her youngest child.

Before she could say anything else, the phone rang.

"If that's my father, tell him I left the planet," Jackie grumbled. Tommy called her at least once a day to chat. "That's my heart," he says of the daughter he rarely saw when she was growing up. "She is number one. Anytime I call her, if I need anything, she's right there." Though Jackie did not want to be bothered by her father right then, she often expressed sympathy for him. Since Tommy's stroke, he and his girlfriend had not been getting along too well, and Jackie worried about where her father would go if they broke up. Jackie took the phone from Latrice. She was right; it was her father. The conversation was brief.

Jackie returned to the kitchen to start her grandmother's breakfast. With the sausage sizzling on the stove, she rejoined her children, bringing them a small glass jar that held a grasshopperlike insect. The family had been collecting bugs that summer.

Jackie sat down between Brianna and Latrice on the couch, and they peered through the jar at the bug, which Jackie thought might be a locust. "Isn't there a page in the dictionary with all the insects?" she asked.

Latrice jumped up and pulled a thick dictionary from a stack of books and papers that sat next to the couch. They found the right page but were not sure from the drawings which creature they had caught.

"Monday a holiday, ain't it?" Latrice asked, bored by the locust.

"Ain't it?" Jackie scolded.

"Isn't it, I mean," Latrice corrected herself.

Monday is Labor Day, Jackie told her. Jackie sometimes reminded her children to speak standard English, though she frequently injected slang into her own speech. Even if Jackie were ever-vigilant about

CHAPTER NINE

correcting Latrice and DeMarest, changing their speech patterns would
be a challenge since almost everyone they knew usually "talks black,"
as Jackie puts it.

Back in the kitchen, Jackie fixed a plate of sausage and grits, the
breakfast Mrs. Jackson had requested. Jackie had stopped paying careful attention to her grandmother's dietary restrictions. "When I bring
Mama food the way Rose [the nurse] say to fix it, she don't want it,"
Jackie said.

That morning, Mrs. Jackson also decided she did not want the very
breakfast she had asked for a half-hour before. A few minutes after
Jackie gave her grandmother her plate, Mrs. Jackson called for Latrice
to take it away. Jackie overheard.

"Are you through eating?" she called into her.

"Yes," Mrs. Jackson said.

"Why didn't you try to eat more?"

"I didn't feel like it."

"Don't tell me you want something else later on," Jackie warned,
now standing by Mrs. Jackson's door.

"Jackie, I stop eating something when it makes me sick," Mrs. Jackson snapped.

"That's all you had to say, Mom," Jackie said quietly.

"I want something else," Mrs. Jackson continued. Jackie walked away
muttering. A few minutes later, she sent Latrice and DeMarest to the
store to buy a tomato.

At thirty, Jackie was mothering the woman who once mothered her.
But it was harder to care for an old, sick woman than a little girl, Jackie
thought. She could not tell her grandmother to eat what was in front
of her or go hungry. Her grandmother needed food for strength, and
Jackie knew the old woman might feel fine one minute and queasy the
next. She could not console herself with the knowledge that one day
her grandmother would stop needing so much help; her dependence
seemed permanent.

Since physical therapist Talha Ahmed Shamsi's visit nearly three
months before, Mrs. Jackson had not had any at-home physical therapy. She had returned to the hospital in late July and stayed through
the first week in August. In the four weeks since she had been home,
only Rose had visited her.

The physical therapy supervisor at Mount Sinai's home health
agency, Bob Prischman, reviewed Mrs. Jackson's case some months

later. He was troubled that Mrs. Jackson had received so little physical therapy, considering that she had not even mastered moving from her bed to her wheelchair. He attributed the void primarily to restrictive Medicare policies. Even though Mrs. Jackson might have benefited from more therapy, he said, the home health agency had to consider the possibility that Medicare might not pay for it because Mrs. Jackson's chances for substantial improvement were slim. "We are being looked at all the time for over-utilization of services," Prischman said. "If Medicare turned around and said the service was unnecessary we're out thousands."

Mrs. Jackson was unfortunate to require home care at the tail end of a conservative era in the home-health industry. Agencies that were once quick to provide services had become wary of taking on Medicare clients. The chill came about because of a marked increase in Medicare's denial of home-health claims, a trend spurred by 1984 Congressional legislation intended to curb fraud and abuse in the home-health industry. Medicare refused to pay home-health bills on many grounds: services were not medically necessary, too frequent, or exceeded medical treatment plans.

A General Accounting Office study showed that nationwide, denials of home-health bills increased from 3.1 percent of all bills in 1985 to 9 percent in 1987.[1] The number of denials varied across the country because in each region bills are processed by different "fiscal intermediaries," insurance companies the Health Care Financing Administration hires to handle Medicare billing. The Chicago region experienced one of the highest denial rates: nearly a fifth of Medicare claims processed in the second quarter of 1987 were rejected.[2]

The denials were viewed by many as no more than a sneaky method of cost control, and in late 1988, a federal judge ruled that a large group of them were "arbitrary" and "contrary to law."[3] Subsequently, an organization that took part in the suit, the National Association for Home Care, was allowed to help write new rules for Medicare's home program. The changes made the rules more specific and broadened coverage. For example, physical therapists now can provide more services to help patients maintain their functioning. For the first time, they are allowed to visit invalids like Mrs. Jackson once a month to assess such things as their compliance with exercise plans.

The new rules were issued in July 1989, but home-health agencies were so gun-shy that it was some time before they began to take full advantage of them. "We were afraid of getting burned," Prischman said. An internal hospital report reflected that initial hesitancy; it showed that Mount Sinai's home health agency made 36 percent (or 437) more Medicare-funded visits in March 1990 than it had in July 1989, Mrs. Jackson's second month home from Schwab.[4]

Medicare restrictions aside, overworked home nurses sometimes simply forgot to request physical therapy for their patients, Prischman said. "The nurses are so busy teaching patients how to take their medications, how to do their dressing changes, that they don't always cue into the need for physical therapy." The nurses' workload had increased in the winter of 1989, when Mount Sinai administrators directed home nurses to visit more patients each day.[5] Many hospitals rely on programs like home health to subsidize their operations. Notwithstanding the spate of denials in 1987, home health is reimbursed relatively well by Medicare.

Whatever the reasons Mrs. Jackson's physical therapy was cut short, Prischman regretted that it had happened. "The more somebody's in bed, the worse everything gets. Everything slows down. You need to increase blood flow to the extremity as much as possible to prevent further amputation. You also want to get people up to feel like they're making progress." Better mobility for Mrs. Jackson would have made Jackie's job easier, he said. "Once the family sees nothing is happening they don't want to help as much because they're not seeing any change. They give up hope."

Sometimes, Jackie did feel hopeless. When her grandmother first got sick and part of her foot was amputated, Jackie delighted in watching her gradual improvement. She progressed from a walker to a cane, and occasionally even set that aside. "We would whisper to each other, 'Look, look at her. She's going without the cane,'" Jackie remembered.

But when Mrs. Jackson's leg was amputated, the light at the end of the tunnel—some degree of recovery—became dimmer and dimmer. "Mom never moves her own self forward in her wheelchair," Jackie lamented. "She won't even make a couple of rolls forward to answer the phone."

So Jackie did the rolling. And just about everything else.

Once a day, Jackie washed the wound where her grandmother's leg was amputated and changed the dressing on her foot ulcer. Before meals, she tested Mrs. Jackson's blood sugar with a home kit. She tried to remember to give her a high blood pressure pill in the evenings. She gave her sponge baths, changed the pads in her bed, and emptied her catheter when Mrs. Jackson was given one in the fall. She washed her grandmother's soiled sheets and nightgowns and fixed her a plate of food when she called. She dragged her out of bed once a day so she could sit in the living room. She collected bills from hospitals, medical suppliers, and ambulance companies so that her grandmother might meet her spend-down and become eligible for Medicaid.

And of course, Jackie also mothered her own three children and her ailing husband.

That Jackie was still caring for small children when she took on responsibility for her grandmother is not unusual for black and Hispanic women.[6] Poor minorities are debilitated by chronic diseases earlier in life than whites, which means their caregivers will be younger, too. Other factors make black and Hispanic women of any age more likely than whites to become responsible for elderly family members: more minorities suffer from chronic diseases; many cannot afford outside help; and a smaller proportion live in nursing homes.[7]

Blacks fill fewer nursing home beds than whites mainly because they are more likely to be poor Medicaid recipients, and that group is no more lucrative for nursing homes than it is for hospitals and doctors. But Medicaid's relationship to nursing homes is more complicated than it is to other health care providers. First, neither commercial insurers nor Medicare pay for much nursing-home care. Medicare pays only for high-skilled care for a limited time, covering less than 5 percent of the country's total nursing-home bill. Commercial insurers pay even less. Medicaid, however, covers anyone who needs custodial care, high skilled or not, as long as they're poor enough. It has become the nation's de facto long-term care insurer, covering a whopping 45 percent of national nursing home costs.[8] With nursing home rates running at least $30,000 a year, many people who enter them as members of the middle class eventually exhaust their savings and become eligible for Medicaid. Blacks' chances of being admitted to nursing homes are worse than whites because they are more likely to be poor from the start. And some nursing homes, especially the best ones, require potential residents to prove that they personally can afford to pay for at least one year of care—before reverting to the lower, slower paying Medicaid. Ann Hilton Fisher, an attorney who represents nursing-home residents for Chicago's Legal Assistance Foundation, said one local *non-profit* nursing home requires residents to show available assets of $140,000 before admission.

Latrice pushed open the front door and threw her book bag onto the recliner. She was dressed in school clothes, red stretch pants and a black and red striped shirt. Jackie came from the kitchen to greet her, Brianna resting on her hip. The little girl had just been rousted from her nap. Her eyes were still puffy from sleep, which made her resemble her father before his dialysis treatments, when his face is sometimes swollen from fluid retention.

Latrice, who had just started sixth grade, handed her mother a notice about an upcoming meeting to discuss the new local school councils. The councils are part of a Chicago school-reform program started in 1989 to give parents more control over their children's educations. Jackie used to serve as secretary for the Parent Teachers Association. Would she attend the meeting? "She can't," Latrice answered for her mother, "not with grandma here."

When Latrice took standardized tests later that school year, she was just at grade level in math and six months behind in reading. That was the first time she had tested below grade level in reading, and the gain she registered in math between fifth and sixth grades was her lowest ever. Latrice may have faltered in the sixth grade because of the turmoil at home, but the turmoil at her grammar school, Paderewski, probably had an equally profound effect. She was in a split sixth- and seventh-grade class, and her teacher left midway through the year, putting the children in the hands of a succession of substitutes. The school, which goes through eighth grade, had no regular sex and health education course, despite being located in a neighborhood where sexually transmitted diseases are rampant and infant mortality all too common. The Chicago Public Schools have a program that allows students with decent test scores to attend better high schools outside of their area, but two-thirds of Paderewski's graduating eighth-graders go to the local high school, Farragut Career Academy, where 90 percent of graduates test below average in reading, and 88 percent are behind in math.

"Jackie," Mrs. Jackson called out.

"Yes, ma'am," Jackie answered as she walked toward her grandmother's room, leaving Latrice to watch Brianna.

Mrs. Jackson was lying in the middle of her bed with a pink blanket wrapped around her and crossed in front, making her look like an old Navajo woman. Without opening her eyes, she asked Jackie to turn off the small fan on her dresser. She had been sick to her stomach that day but had declined Jackie's offer to call an ambulance to take her to the hospital.

Jackie returned to her children who were playing in the rear of the living room, where the family spent much of their time. Sometimes Jackie and the children stayed in back so as not to disturb Mrs. Jackson in the front bedroom; other times, they stayed there so as not to be disturbed *by* her.

With her grandmother asleep and Robert away for the afternoon, Jackie was enjoying some time alone with her children. She showed Latrice how to do a card trick, then helped her with math homework. She pulled out the dictionary and tried to identify another insect the children had caught.

Jackie did not even flinch when DeMarest leaped onto the couch brandishing Brianna's tiny shoe, intent on smacking a roach that was crawling up the wall. She and her daughters joined in the attack in what seemed almost like a family ritual.

"Here, use Latrice's shoe," Jackie said.

Latrice quickly pulled off her shoe, long enough to give DeMarest room for error, and handed it to her brother. DeMarest watched the bug's progress up the wall, then whacked it. Jackie handed him a piece of paper to wipe away the remains.

"That's one I don't have to worry about," Jackie thanked him. DeMarest smiled proudly and walked to the kitchen with his kill, a hunter carrying his vanquished prey.

Later, as Jackie walked into her grandmother's bedroom to straighten it up, she paused before Mrs. Jackson's dresser and picked up a snapshot-sized photo album. She began to flip slowly through it, stopping at a picture of her and Latrice, taken on the little girl's third birthday. "That's the way it should have been," Jackie sighed, "just me and Latrice."

It almost was just Jackie, Latrice—and Mrs. Jackson. Jackie first met Robert when she was eighteen, at a birthday party for his mother.

What she remembered most about their first encounter was not Robert, whom she considered "kind and nice," but the yellow-brick bungalow where he lived. It was decorated with gold-trimmed mirrors, a marble-topped table that hung from the ceiling on gold chains, and an illuminated picture of a French village. And it was a *home;* Robert's mother owned it. "These are people with lots of cash," Jackie thought to herself as she surveyed the gilded living room. "Everybody had a nice job." Robert's mother worked in an office; Robert had a job at a nearby hospital.

Right away, Robert and Jackie began spending much of their time together. "The very first week he was buying me gifts and what not, clothes and rings and stuff." Within a few months, Jackie was pregnant, and as quickly as it began, her new relationship ended.

Jackie refused to see Robert because his mother let it be known that she thought the baby wasn't her son's. Robert continued to call on Jackie, imploring her to ignore his mother, but Jackie would not let him any further than the front steps. She was stoic about the matter. When Jackie feels she is in the right, she will not try to win others over with pleas or persuasion. It's as if such acts are beneath her. "I just let it go," she says.

But soon after Latrice was born, Mrs. Jackson saw Robert on the bus and told him he was a father. Then one morning Robert's mother came by and asked if she could see the baby. Jackie was in the midst of going through Latrice's baby clothes. "Everyday I took [the clothes] all out and smelled them, touched them, planned what I was going to put on her on Monday, Tuesday . . ."

Jackie invited Robert's mother in, pleased that she would see all of the baby's finery, proof that Jackie did not need Robert or her. Robert's mother took one look at Latrice and burst into tears. "She was pointing to different parts of her face, 'I can see Robert here and here and here.'"

Amends were made, and Jackie and Robert resumed seeing each other daily, though Jackie continued to live with her grandmother. The couple married five years later, in 1983.

Now, Jackie was wishing she had stayed single. Robert, Jackie strongly suspected, was back taking drugs. In mid-September, he had been fired from his security guard job because scrap metal had been stolen during his watch, and he had been accused of the crime. Jackie had no idea whether he had had something to do with the theft because when Robert used drugs, there was no telling what would happen. One thing always happened, though, and this time was no exception. Robert stopped giving Jackie money to pay the bills. She was broke.

At the same time, Jackie had become increasingly frazzled being at her grandmother's beck and call twenty-four hours a day. When the old woman awoke, she had asked her granddaughter for a plate of greens and became annoyed when she had to wait while Jackie warmed them.

"Jackie did them greens heat up?" Mrs. Jackson called out from her bedroom.

"Come and get them," Jackie said in a rare display of spite.

"I can't," Mrs. Jackson said.

Mrs. Jackson remained in a foul mood. When DeMarest climbed up onto her bed, she gruffly ordered him out of her room. Sometimes DeMarest and Brianna wandered into their great-grandmother's room on their own; other times Jackie sent them in to keep her alert. DeMarest's great-grandmother was alert all right; he scurried out of the room.

A few minutes later, though, he and Brianna followed Jackie back in when she brought her grandmother the greens. They lingered, played with the pill bottles on her dresser. "Put them pills back on the dresser," Mrs. Jackson said. But almost immediately she relented and told the children they could play with a couple of the empty bottles. Once more, DeMarest crawled onto her bed, but this time Mrs. Jackson did not seem to mind his presence, until she began to slide off her pillow. "Pull me over, DeMarest," she barked. "Grab me by the arm and pull me that way."

DeMarest stopped his play, a perplexed look on his face. "I can't," he said, realizing that he was too small for the task.

"Get off the bed, then. If I slap you, you're going to feel it."

DeMarest disappeared.

In the late afternoon, Rose arrived to check on Mrs. Jackson, whose combativeness could be transformed into pleasant talkativeness with strangers, something Jackie had a hard time understanding. "In good spirits," Rose wrote in Mrs. Jackson's progress note for that day.

Before she left, Rose asked Jackie if she had tested her grandmother's blood sugar.

"No, you want to do it?" Jackie asked. She handed Rose the test kit so that the nurse had no other choice.

That was typical of Jackie's attitude as the fall wore on. She only gave her grandmother sponge baths on the three days a week that Rose visited. She cleaned Mrs. Jackson's foot ulcer once a day, though she thought she was supposed to do it more often. And when she got a muscle spasm in her back, Jackie stopped taking her grandmother out of bed.

"DeWayne tell you what I wanted," Mrs. Jackson called from her bedroom immediately after Rose left.

"You mean DeMarest," Jackie said. DeWayne is Jackie's cousin; Mrs. Jackson every once in a while confused him with DeMarest.

"Get me a piece of watermelon."

"Cool down, Mama," Jackie sighed.

Both the Illinois Department on Aging, and to some extent, Medicare, pay for homemakers who might have relieved Jackie. But her tight budget and confusion over how the system works have prevented her from taking advantage of them.

In February, when part of Mrs. Jackson's foot was amputated, a hospital social worker told Jackie about the Department on Aging's homemaker service. Through what is called the Community Care Program, the department provides homemakers to the elderly in an attempt to prevent inappropriate placement in nursing homes.[9]

Mrs. Jackson qualified for four hours of help each weekday, according to a needs assessment administered by the social worker in early March. A homemaker could bathe and dress her, help her get in and out of bed, do her shopping, fix her meals, and launder her clothes. A state-contracted agency called Staff Builders sent a homemaker to the Baneses for two weeks before Jackie cancelled the service. She decided she could not afford the homemaker's help, which cost $110 a month, a fifth of her grandmother's $619 Social Security check. Then, too, in March, Jackie had not realized how demanding the care of her grandmother would become. She assumed she would not need any extra help—she always had cooked and cleaned for her grandmother—and preferred not to have another stranger in her home if she could help it. Still, the decisive factor was the $110 monthly fee.

The Department on Aging did not always charge for homemakers. Before 1982, they were free to anyone sixty and older. But a long waiting list developed because the state agency could serve only a small number of clients with the fixed budget set by the Illinois General

Assembly. By the time many elderly people got to the top of the list, they were already in nursing homes, or dead. In response to a lawsuit, a federal court ruled in 1982 that all eligible clients must be served. To comply without increasing costs, the state required a copayment from anyone whose income was more than $426 a month, $74 below the federal poverty level for one person in 1989.[10]

The theory behind the cost-sharing was that by requiring less-poor elderly to make copayments, the Community Care Program presumably could serve more people. The problem, however, is with an income cutoff of $426, many of the elderly required to make a copayment are still quite poor. They may desperately need help around the house but cannot spare $100, or even $50 of their small fixed incomes. A third of elderly black women in Illinois have incomes at or below the poverty level, and another 20 percent are in Mrs. Jackson's situation, with incomes between 100 percent and 150 percent of the poverty level.[11]

The state's short-term savings may translate into long-term waste. More than half of the clients who withdrew from the Community Care Program did so because of the fee, one study found. The fee was expected to weed out elderly who could get by without a homemaker, but the study showed that people who needed help—judging by their high scores on a disability needs' assessment—still withdrew because they could not afford the copayment. Many of them ended up in nursing homes.[12] The state and federal government spend $16,000 a year on each of the nearly 50,000 nursing-home residents eligible for Medicaid in Illinois. In contrast, though elderly people living at home may use other government money, the Community Care Program spends about $4,000 a year on each of its clients.[13]

After Mrs. Jackson dropped out of the homemaker program, a Staff Builders' case manager offered Jackie another option. If she completed a twelve-hour class, Jackie could earn about four dollars an hour for the twenty hours of care that had been authorized for her grandmother.

At first Jackie was intrigued, but she worried that if she lost her welfare grant, AFDC, her children would no longer get Medicaid. Few employers provide health insurance for part-time workers, and in low-paying industries such as home care, even full-time employees often do not receive health benefits. No one knows how many women stay on welfare primarily to retain Medicaid coverage, but policy experts say that stories like Jackie's suggest that the group may be quite large. "It's the number one thing women say they fear they'd lose out on if they left AFDC," said Kathryn Edin, a sociologist conducting research on the subject. "National health care and subsidized child care . . . are essential in any package of benefits these women would need to make it in a low-wage job."[14]

The reasons Jackie chose not to become a homemaker for her grandmother—low pay, no health benefits—account for the rapid turnover in the industry as a whole.[15] The Department on Aging's Community Care Program contracts with agencies like Staff Builders, paying them about $7 for each hour of service their homemakers provide. That means, after subtracting administrative costs, homemakers themselves earn at most $5 an hour. The owner of a home care agency south of Chicago explained the dilemma which the state's low rate created for him and his workers, who were almost all women. "It's not enough money for them to survive; we pay a trash hauler better than we pay people to take care of our mothers," Larry Lee said. "They have to go back on Public Aid because they have to have the green card if their kids get sick." The situation had gotten so bad, he said, that he was offering his homemakers an option to work for wages *or* health insurance.[16]

Although Jackie feared losing her medical benefits if she worked part-time, that might not have happened. Her income would have been about $320 a month; Illinois and some other states have a medically needy program that allows some families whose incomes are a shade higher than welfare grants to continue receiving Medicaid. The AFDC payment for a family of four in Illinois is $386 a month, but same-size families who earn up to $517 can still get green cards. (In July 1988, new federal laws began to be implemented that required states to give Medicaid to pregnant women and infants in families with somewhat higher incomes. So even if Jackie made more than $517, Brianna might have been eligible for Medicaid under these changes, although Latrice and DeMarest would have been too old.)

But Jackie's cash-grant definitely would have been reduced or eliminated since the program in Illinois and elsewhere takes away nearly a dollar for each dollar increase in earnings, a policy that welfare expert David Ellwood, a professor at Harvard University's John F. Kennedy School of Government, compared to an almost 100 percent tax on welfare recipients' work.[17] For Jackie, the situation was even worse because caring for her grandmother was not steady work. "With Mama in the hospital so much, a lot of times I wouldn't have had a patient, so I wouldn't have had any income."

Ellwood says part-time work is irrational for women on welfare. "A woman is crazy to try and work part of the time and stay home with her children [and grandmother in Jackie's case] part of the time. She gets into even more hassles with the welfare system because she must constantly report her earnings; she must arrange for day care; and she must cope with work, children, and sometimes several forms of welfare. Her reward for all this is a tiny amount of extra income and often less medical protection."[18]

There was still one other program that could have helped Jackie, but she did not understand that it would have been free, paid for by Medicare. Again, Medicare does not pay for long-term custodial or nursing-home care, but in a limited number of situations, the federal program will pay for home health aides, who perform many of the same tasks as Department on Aging homemakers, such as bathing, dressing, changing bandages, and preparing light meals. Medicare only covers home health aides when patients are sick enough to require visits from a home nurse, a category that included Mrs. Jackson.

Mount Sinai's home health agency offered one of these aides to Jackie after her grandmother's leg was amputated, but Jackie assumed that someone who performed the same tasks as the Staff Builders' homemaker would cost the same $110 a month. No one told her differently. "I don't know if we ever say [home health aides] are 'free,'" said Joyce Kaires, the director of the home health agency. "Maybe [Jackie] just didn't understand." In fact, Jackie has never been quite sure how government programs intersect, although she has been using them for much of her life. "For a long time, I was thinking Medicaid and Medicare were the same thing," she said.

Her confusion is not unusual. An expert on women and poverty who works in Philadelphia summed it up this way: "Show me the poor woman who finds a way to get everything she's entitled to in the system, and I'll show you a woman who could run General Motors."[19]

Mount Sinai's home health agency may not have been exactly forthcoming about the homemaker benefit, however. The agency was just emerging from the period when it had sharply curtailed home visits in response to Medicare denials, a time when one hospital administrator concluded that staff had "probably become too conservative and [were] not rendering as many visits as may be allowed by third party payers."[20]

It was the first week of October, and Jackie had not taken her grandmother to the doctor since she had been released from the hospital nearly two months before. Part of the reason was transportation; Mrs. Jackson's Medicaid spend-down coverage had expired at the end of July. Jackie also was angry at her grandmother's doctors; she did not think they were trying hard enough to cure Mrs. Jackson, or that they understood the family's plight.

The two weeks Mrs. Jackson had spent in the hospital after Jackie persuaded Dr. Gurevich to admit her had been a washout as far as Jackie was concerned. She thought her grandmother had been admitted so that the darkening sore on her left heel could be treated. But doctors subsequently discovered a bigger problem. The bypass graft that had been inserted in Mrs. Jackson's right thigh in a vain attempt to save her leg had become infected. The graft was surgically removed, and Mrs. Jackson's condition improved.

The Friday her grandmother had been discharged, Jackie was told that if she remained concerned about the heel, she could take her grandmother to Dr. Steinberg's podiatry clinic on Monday. The podiatrist had not debrided the wound (surgically removed infected tissue) because he was not sure the procedure would help, but he was willing to consider it again. That seemed absurd to Jackie. "Why didn't they clean it out while she was there?" she complained. "They make me feel so helpless." For their part, doctors did not feel they could justify keeping Mrs. Jackson in the hospital over the weekend simply because of her heel; wounds can be debrided as an outpatient procedure.

While Jackie indicted the doctors for what she thought was foolishness, she also felt judged by them. She thought doctors talked about her behind her back. "I look like the bad granddaughter to them. Every time she goes to the hospital they tell me not to worry about her heel, then when we get home, it's a problem," Jackie complained, her voice rising. "Now I might go in there and they'll say the whole root of the problem is that I haven't brought her back. I don't even want to talk to those doctors, they make me so mad."

Jackie's resentment toward Mount Sinai and its doctors had magnified in August, when once again she complained that her grandmother had been sent home before she was well. Mrs. Jackson had stayed in the hospital for two weeks while doctors tried to treat a urinary tract infection and determine the cause of her persistent vomiting. Several tests were inconclusive, and efforts to take a CAT scan of her abdomen were thwarted because barium which Mrs. Jackson had retained from an earlier test interfered. So Dr. Gurevich decided to discharge her. "We will bring her back as outpatient in 1 wk. to assess [her kidneys, ureter and bladder] at that time," a medical resident wrote in her chart.

Of course, the doctor would not bring her back. That was Jackie's job. And since Mrs. Jackson had not met her Medicaid spend-down for August, Jackie would have to spend $70 she did not have for the round-trip ride to the hospital. "That's stupid," she said. "I'm not bringing her back. Forget it. I'll bring her back when she's sick." And that's what happened.

Mrs. Jackson was readmitted to the hospital two months later on October 8 with sharp abdominal pain and diagnosed with acute diverticulitis, an inflammation of the small pockets in the wall of the large intestine. It's impossible to know if the missed CAT scan would have detected the disease before it reached a serious stage, but it seems likely. Complicating the diverticulitis were two other conditions: Mrs. Jackson's umpteenth urinary tract infection, as well as a stomach ulcer.

Mrs. Jackson sat in a chair next to her bed with a dinner tray in front of her. She had taken only a few bites of the beef, mashed potatoes, and spinach; she was swallowing a lot, as if she felt sick to her stomach. "Feeling a little rough," she said.

Her skin sagged from her cheeks as if weighted, almost seeming to drag her prominent lips downward into a frown. It was obvious that it had been a while since Jackie had done her hair; a few braids poked out from the gray frizz that framed her face. Her hospital gown was awry and did not cover the stump of her right leg; amputated well above the knee, it looked like a sack of potatoes sewn up at the end by a zigzagged scar. Her other leg was as skinny as a bird's. A quarter-sized black sore had developed on her shin, similar to the one on her heel.

Having had more than enough of her dinner, Mrs. Jackson called for the nurse's aide, who appeared a few minutes later. "I'm done," Mrs. Jackson said.

"I'll move you as soon as I get me some help," the large, good-natured aide responded.

Jackie had witnessed the same scene many times, nurses' aides declining to move her grandmother by themselves, but on one occasion, an aide had started to lift Mrs. Jackson on her own.

"No, baby, you can't do it," Mrs. Jackson had said. "It takes more than one of you to move me."

Jackie was surprised.

"What about Jackie? There's only one Jackie," she said to her grandmother, miffed that Mrs. Jackson had never acknowledged to her how hard she was to move. Mrs. Jackson did not respond. "She just stare at me," Jackie said.

Jackie did not know what to make of the flashes of anger she felt toward her grandmother. How could she get mad at a woman who was so sickly, who was a pale shadow of her former self? In a book about caregiving, one woman recounted the frustrations of coping with her husband's Alzheimer's disease: "He seemed to be more incontinent when I was around than when he was around other people. One morning, he said he had to go to the bathroom. I interpreted that to mean that he had to have a bowel movement. So I got him ready . . . and he stood there with a urinal two feet away from him and just urinated all over the floor. I really got mad and I yelled at him."[21]

The aftermath of anger for caregivers can be guilt. Jackie frequently talked about feeling guilty for all manner of supposed sins: for wanting time away from the old woman, for not taking her to the doctor, for considering putting her grandmother in a nursing home, for *not* putting her in a nursing home, for using part of Mrs. Jackson's Social Security check for household expenses, for not visiting her enough at the hospital. "I got a guilt streak running down the middle of my back," she said.

Eventually, the aide found some help, and after much pushing and pulling, Mrs. Jackson sat upright in bed.

"What day is it?" she asked dejectedly. It was the tenth day of Mrs. Jackson's October hospitalization, the ninetieth day she had spent in Mount Sinai that year. The answer did not seem to mean much to her.

"I want to go home," she pleaded somewhat uncharacteristically. Mrs. Jackson rarely said much to anyone other than Jackie and her children, and it was extraordinary for her to express such heartfelt sentiment. Over and over again in her medical chart, nurses had written that she refused to use the call button when she needed something. Once, when asked why she so often watched the hospital television without sound, she replied, "I'd listen if somebody turn it on." But she never asked anyone. One of the hospital social workers suggested that such pronounced passivity explained why she sometimes got so surly. By the time she asked for something, she had waited so long—and become so resentful that nobody had provided it—that she lashed out.

This October evening, Mrs. Jackson was more morose than mad. The other patients on the floor certainly did not help to lift her spirits. For the first time, she had been put on Mount Sinai's geriatric floor, which was reserved for the sickest elderly patients, many transferred from nursing homes.

The floor was extremely quiet; no resident physicians stood outside patients' rooms animatedly discussing cases. New doctors were not assigned to the geriatric unit because the hospital had decided that patients with such chronic, long-standing illnesses did not need the constant medical attention residents provide. (Patients with acute illnesses make better "teaching material" for residents, anyway.) For the same reason, only a registered nurse, two licensed practical nurses, and two nursing aides were assigned to care for twenty patients. Which leads to another reason the floor was so subdued: the few aides were uneasy about their ability to control some of the demented patients, so they tied them down, whether a doctor had ordered it or not. To do this is a violation of state law, but the law is hard to enforce.[22]

As Mrs. Jackson looked through her open door, an old man on a gurney rolled slowly by, pushed by an orderly. His shrunken head was thrown back, his mouth open. He looked closer to dead than alive. Mrs. Jackson turned away.

The old woman seemed lonely. Jackie had visited her three days before, on a Sunday. She used to take the bus to Mount Sinai every day, but it was the ninetieth day of Mrs. Jackson's hospitalizations for her, too. In addition, the hospital was enforcing a rule that forbade children younger than sixteen from visiting patients, which meant Latrice could not come with her mother anymore. Jackie sometimes had considered the bus ride to the hospital with her daughter as a break from her usual routine, but going alone was not as appealing.

Jackie had expected her grandmother to come home the day after she visited her, on a Monday, but Mrs. Jackson was not discharged that day because her ulcer flared up. Four days later, however, on a Friday, doctors again thought she was well enough to return home. This time, the Baneses were not ready to take her back.

When the ward clerk called home, Robert told her that Jackie had gone out of town. "There's no way we can take her," he said. Robert lied because Jackie wanted to go to a suburban mall with his sister on Saturday. Robert's sister had a car, and the two of them were planning to do some early Christmas shopping. Jackie was excited about the day away.

Mrs. Jackson's social worker during that hospitalization, Marion Garmaise, later said she had suspected Robert wasn't telling the truth but chose not to confront him. "There's no point in getting people all riled up if you're not going to change the situation," she said. "It might have gotten [Jackie] mad, and then her grandmother would have ended up staying even longer."

Jackie did not like lying and had tried the straightforward approach in August, when her twenty-eight-year-old brother died of pancreatic cancer in Mississippi. It had not worked.

Jackie had hoped to drive south for his funeral with some cousins, but her grandmother was to be discharged from the hospital the day after he died. She asked the hospital to keep Mrs. Jackson a few extra days, but Mount Sinai refused because Medicare would not pay for such custodial care. "It's a problem because no one can do what I do," Jackie said. "I don't guess the hospital would go bankrupt keeping her an extra day, but I guess they couldn't keep her all the days I wanted them to."

Jackie did not get much help from her family. Mrs. Jackson's younger sister, Eldora, lived nearby, but she was blind. Tommy, of course, could not provide much help; Jackie ran errands for him.

Had she not been so poor, Jackie might have been able to put Mrs. Jackson in a nursing home for a few days, or perhaps contacted Kin Care, a private agency in Chicago that arranges respite in homes. As Mount Sinai's social worker, Garmaise, pointed out, money makes caregiving easier in many ways. "You can hire help. You can hire taxis. You can get a car with a wheelchair lift. You can go traveling."

No one told Jackie about a $69,596 federal grant that had been given to Chicago's Department on Aging to provide free respite care. The money was to be doled out through agencies like the one that had arranged a homemaker for Mrs. Jackson. But the grant was so small that the city did not openly promote respite, fearing the demand would be too great, said Mary Lou Budnick, the Department on Aging's grants management director. Ironically, half the money was not spent and was therefore transferred to the fiscal 1990 budget.

Solely responsible for her grandmother, Jackie experienced what is known as "caregiver burnout." Dozens of studies have reported on the factors that take the greatest physical and emotional toll on caregivers. Among them are other family stresses, of which the Baneses had no shortage: a high level of dependency on the part of the disabled person; little potential for improvement; the inability of the sick relative to communicate with her caregiver by, for example, expressing gratitude; and lack of help from other family members or from formal respite services.

Much of the literature about caregiving is obviously written with middle- and upper-class women in mind. One publication offered a "checklist/guide" to help potential caregivers assess whether they have the "physical and emotional resources" to keep a relative at home, or whether they should consider a nursing home. Here are some of the questions caregivers are supposed to ask themselves:

—Is the home large enough: Are there stairs outside and inside the house? Can you hire help, is outside help available?

—Finances: Can you afford to pay for attendants, nurses, physical therapists, and are they available?

—Transportation: Can you drive or do you have transportation for daily needs?

—Family and personal services: Do you have family members who can share the burden or can afford to hire trained reliable help/[22]

If Jackie had used these questions as her guide, Mrs. Jackson would have been put in a nursing home immediately after her leg was amputated. Caregiving is a strain no matter how affluent one is, and Jackie certainly never had the financial flexibility or family support that the checklist suggests are necessary. Did Jackie make the wrong decision in keeping her grandmother at home? Mrs. Jackson certainly did not think so.

But the old woman was becoming ever more pessimistic. "It look like my body just getting black things all over it," she told Jackie one day after she came home from the hospital in October. Her grandmother's continued deterioration distressed Jackie, too. She considered a nursing home. "That might be best for her. They would do better than me. I guess she gets depressed just laying in here." She considered her grandmother dying. "Sometimes, it seems like Mama might be better off dead," she said. "You want it, but you don't."

Jackie's passing thoughts about her grandmother's death were mixed with a desperate desire for her to live. The feeling peaked early in the morning, before another long day of caretaking had begun. Sometimes, as soon as Jackie awoke, she shook DeMarest, who slept in a trundle bed beside her.

"Go in there and see how your Nana's doing," she told him. DeMarest, who eagerly helped his mother by performing such tasks as reporting on the level of urine in his grandmother's catheter bag, hurried off to perform his "grown-up" chore. He returned.

"She didn't say anything," he said.

"What?" Jackie demanded, her voice rising with fear. "Go back there and ask her how she's doing."

DeMarest turned and ran to the front of the house. He was back. "She said she's doing all right."

Jackie threw off her bed covers. "Thank you, DeMarest," she said.

10

Empty promises: Preventive care
for the Banes children

By the time the summer had faded into fall, Jackie had collected more troubles than all of her soap opera characters combined. Her grandmother continued to deteriorate; her father, Tommy, always seemed to need her to run one errand or another; and, worst of all, Jackie was haunted by the possibility that the police might come after her husband. Since Robert's employer had accused him of theft, Jackie's ghastliest nightmare was that an officer would march up the stairs, handcuff her husband, and cart him away in front of her children. Robert's binges had turned her life upside down before. Right after Brianna was born, he had spent $400 on drugs—money the couple had saved to buy a crib and baby clothes. And he had never shown up at the hospital to take Jackie and his new daughter home. On other occasions, Robert had come home broke on payday, claiming he had been robbed. "My husband done been robbed more than any man in this city," Jackie says

Jackie kept her growing apprehension about Robert to herself and retreated into the house. She refused to give her husband a key to the apartment for fear it would get into the wrong hands when he was high. "I feel like I want to draw back in a shell and hide," Jackie said. "I want to lock all the doors, put steel on the windows. A lot of times the doorbell rings and I don't let anybody in."

While Jackie was trying to hide from the world, the worst measles outbreak in Chicago in more than two decades raged outside her door. Two thousand Chicagoans contracted the disease—most of them poor minority children who had not been immunized[1]—and nine people died, including two children from North Lawndale. Jackie, however, failed to get measles shots for Brianna.

The little girl had been scheduled for a combined measles, mumps, and rubella immunization at Mount Sinai's pediatric clinic in October, but Jackie skipped that fifteen-month appointment—the first time she had ever missed one of Brianna's checkups. The shots would have been paid for by Medicaid, but Jackie simply was not thinking about the potentially dire consequences of not getting Brianna immunized; measles can cause brain damage, deafness, and, of course, death.

But to say that Jackie and other poor mothers "fail" to immunize their children is not the end, only the beginning, of the story. If government child-health programs are to work, they must reach out to poor parents, or at the very least ensure that getting care is relatively straightforward. They do neither, and the blame stretches from the city, to the state, to Washington, D.C. In Chicago, the most visible culprit is the city clinic system. The fourteen clinics provide free care, but they are too overburdened to meet poor children's needs, and their policies block efforts to prevent deadly childhood diseases.

In 1989, the city's own report, "Clinics in Crisis," said the clinic system was "unable to maintain the quality of care provided to those it is able to see." The last few words in that sentence—"those it is able to see"—are crucial. When the report was issued in 1989, pediatric patients waited an average of forty-seven days for an appointment. By the end of 1991, they were waiting a day longer.[2]

The long waiting times, which discourage people from getting any care, never mind preventive care, are symptomatic of a system buckling under increasing demands and decreasing resources. The number of people with AIDS and without adequate insurance has soared. Meanwhile, a large clinic and eight Chicago hospitals located in poor neighborhoods have closed since 1986. Federal grants for city health services have declined in real dollars every year since 1980, and the city's contributions to all of its departments, health included, have been squeezed because of reductions in other kinds of federal aid.[3]

As a result, the health department lost 900 employees during the 1980s—about a third of its staff.[4] In fiscal 1992, the department liquidated another 230 of its unfilled positions. About 80 percent were secretarial and laboratory jobs at the clinic level, and, while no doctors' or nurses' spots were eliminated, five of the department's fifteen dentists were laid off.[5] Cutting clinic clerical workers forces the skeleton medical staff to answer telephones, make appointments, and pull medical records, further diminishing the number of patients who can be seen.

A year after the 1989 epidemic had peaked, the director of the health department's immunization program, Edward Mihalek, reviewed immunization procedures at the seven largest health department clinics. To prevent an epidemic of the kind that happened in 1989, it is generally thought that at least 70 percent of children must be fully immunized by the time they are two. Mihalek found that the clinics just barely met this standard—69.7 percent of their patients were "age-appropriately" immunized, according to more than 1,000 charts checked.[6]

While that sounds almost adequate, it is not. This percentage applied only to "registered" children, those who had been enrolled as clinic patients prior to getting immunizations. A significant number of shots are given to walk-in clients, whose records are poorly maintained and were not reviewed by Mihalek. It was not worth the time. The department had done little to change its practices for walk-in patients since an April 1990 review by the Centers for Disease Control (CDC), a federal health agency headquartered in Atlanta, found that *none* of forty-nine walk-in children were fully immunized.[7]

That CDC review uncovered other problems as well, which health department officials took steps to correct but with only mixed success. The department's new policy is to immunize children whenever possible. That means minor illnesses should not stand in the way of shots, and clinics should inoculate children against several diseases at once so they do not have to make repeat visits. Both practices are considered safe and are recommended by national medical groups.

Mihalek's review found, however, that two of the seven major clinics still list illnesses as a reason to defer shots, and at a third, "doctors *refuse* [emphasis original]" to simultaneously give vaccines against meningitis and measles, mumps, and rubella. "This is a recurring problem," the report added.[8] Doctors at these clinics may not have been aware of the city's policy, but more likely they chose to ignore it, clinging to the outdated notion that it's dangerous to immunize mildly ill children, or to give them several shots at one time.

Considering the virulence of the 1989 measles epidemic—and city officials' prediction that another will occur in the next several years— the clinics' uneven adherence to their own policy is astounding. According to department rules, if a mother brings in her child without an appointment, he or she should be "shot-on-the-spot," with the shortest waiting time possible. But an informal survey conducted in 1991 found that only three of fourteen clinics could give immunizations on the day they were called. Four others required complete checkups, with three- to seven-week waits for appointments. Each of the seven major clinics is supposed to have an immunization-express service on Fridays, but only two tell patients about it, one warning that the "express service" required a daylong wait.[9]

When asked why such barriers persist, Mihalek threw up his hands. "We can only point out to clinic administrators what we find," he said. "I have no control over the clinics." Though Mihalek runs the immunization program, he is a federal government assignee, employed by the CDC, and clinic workers do not take orders from him. They are overseen by a separate bureau of the health department, led by a city official, for whom immunizations are only one of many priorities.

The clinics' reluctance to inoculate children without complete checkups has its roots in their tradition of giving comprehensive care to all patients, which may be ideal but impossible considering their limited resources. "The best is the enemy of the good," said one immunization expert, quoting Voltaire.[10]

In addition to recommending changes in clinic practices, CDC officials had suggested that the department start immunization-only sessions at low-income housing projects and at WIC sites, where poor mothers pick up food and milk coupons (a study of the children stricken with measles in 1989 found that 61 percent had visited WIC offices in the previous six months).[11] The CDC also recommended that nurses be assigned to regular clinics to expand express-lane hours, as walk-in patients—if accepted at all—must wait hours to be seen.

The city started a demonstration project at selected WIC sites, with a $404,000 CDC grant, but it ignored the rest of the federal health agency's recommendations. The city clinics were hesitant about abandoning their comprehensive-care philosophy in favor of immunization-only clinics; more importantly, with such severe staff shortages, nurses could not be spared to run the special clinics. The city might have been able to surmount the last obstacle had the CDC put its money where its mouth was. CDC rules said federal money could not be used to hire nurses to give shots; it was reserved for disease surveillance, coordination, evaluation, and education.

But even these activities, which are certainly important considering the renewed outbreaks of measles nationwide, have not been fully funded over the past two decades. The federal immunization budget has grown dramatically, from $5 million in 1976 to $185 million in

1991, but the vast majority of that increase has been devoured by huge jumps in vaccine prices.[12] Fiscal 1992 marked the first significant increase in funding for program operations, about $40 million, since childhood immunizations were introduced in 1963. (And, for the first time, the money can be used for vaccine administration, so that communities can pay nurses to immunize babies in clinics or housing projects, for example.)

One last piece missing from the Chicago health department's immunization program shows why it is callous, not to mention counterproductive, to blame poor families for the city's low immunization rates. Chicago's clinics do not have a system to track children's immunization records and remind parents when shots are due. This is true even for children enrolled in comprehensive care, who supposedly get better service. So while it is safe to say that poor families may well need more encouragement to get their children to the doctor than their middle-class counterparts, they in fact get less.

Jackie hasn't used the city clinic system for years. The maternal/child health outpost where she took Latrice, located in Tommy's neighborhood, West Garfield Park, has closed. Now, the clinic closest to her apartment is in Hispanic South Lawndale, where Jackie does not feel welcome. "It doesn't seem like black people should be going over there," she said. Jackie once had been referred to a dentist in South Lawndale, but after she checked out his office, she decided not to visit him. The receptionist spoke Spanish, the brochures were in Spanish, and not a single black sat in the waiting room.

Jackie used another alternative to city clinics for the poor: Medicaid, the state and federal health insurance that allows poor families to visit private doctors who agree to participate. Jackie's children were eligible for a Medicaid program called Early and Periodic Screening, Diagnosis, and Treatment (EPSDT), which is supposed to ensure that children get immunizations and other preventive care. But in many ways, it, too, has failed.

EPSDT is not a "program" in the sense that the welfare offices that run Medicaid give medical checkups to children. State Medicaid programs have some flexibility to choose which medical services they cover, but to get federal matching money, the government requires them to pay for a package of EPSDT services that includes children's immunizations, hearing and vision tests, dental checkups, and regular physicals. They also must pay for any treatment needed to correct problems detected during such health screens. Finally, rules promulgated by the Health Care Financing Administration say that, if necessary, state Medicaid programs must help families get their children to doctors.

Some common criticisms of EPSDT are fundamentally criticisms of Medicaid as a whole. First, Medicaid's rates are so low that few doctors practice in poor neighborhoods, and consequently mothers may not be able to find doctors for their children. A 1991 study by the Physician Payment Review Commission found, not surprisingly, that the government program for the poor paid doctors significantly less than Medicare, the program for the elderly. In Illinois, Medicaid payments were 48 percent of Medicare's; only New York, West Virginia, and New Jersey were more tightfisted.[13]

With a dearth of doctors to choose from, Medicaid patients tend to be concentrated in a small number of large practices where the quality of care is questionable. Jackie took DeMarest and Latrice to see Dr. Marino for several years; yet one of the major criticisms cited in the Illinois Department of Public Aid's quality review of Dr. Marino was his apparent failure to immunize children under his care. Of the fifteen cases the peer review committee evaluated, four were children, and none had received a full complement of shots.[14] Patients are not informed when their doctors essentially fail Medicaid's peer reviews, and Jackie never suspected that Dr. Marino might have been lax in the care of her children. She switched to Mount Sinai's pediatric clinic because she wanted a tubal ligation after Brianna was born. Saint Anthony Hospital, the Catholic hospital where Dr. Marino delivered DeMarest, will not perform sterilizations.

Medicaid's second general shortcoming is that it covers so few of the poor. Working poor families are often excluded, and, the argument goes, if EPSDT purports to ensure that poor children receive preventive care, it should not leave so many of them out. That should change—eventually. Congressional legislation enacted in 1989 requires that states phase in Medicaid coverage for all children in families under the federal poverty level by the year 2002.

But the next task is to make sure Medicaid fulfills the underlying promise of EPSDT, to keep children healthy and treat them promptly when they're ill. This goal has so far proved elusive. Two-thirds of the children covered by Medicaid nationwide did not have a single EPSDT visit in 1989.[15] As the National Vaccine Advisory Committee noted in its report on the 1989 measles epidemic that struck cities from Chicago to Houston to Los Angeles, "The failure to adequately vaccinate many children currently enrolled in public assistance programs suggests that many of the potential benefits gained by [granting] Medicaid eligibility to a much larger group of poor and near-poor children may not be realized."[16]

At the same time Congress made more children eligible for Medicaid, the federal legislators enacted several fairly significant reforms in EPSDT. States had been stingy with the number of periodic health screens they covered, so Congress required them to pay for enough to meet reasonable medical standards. States also had refused to pay for needed follow-up care if it was not part of their regular Medicaid plans; the new law eliminated that loophole.

But reforms are irrelevant if the mothers who are supposed to use EPSDT do not know about it, and despite federal rules that require state welfare departments to inform clients about the program, getting information about EPSDT in Chicago can be next to impossible. A poster behind the check-in desk at Jackie's Public Aid office epitomized the problem. It advertised "Healthy Kids," Illinois' name for its EPSDT program, and showed an illustration of a doctor examining a child over the words "Call for More Information." There was a white box for the phone number underneath those words; it was blank.

When asked about Healthy Kids over the phone, one worker at Jackie's office confused it with child support, another with a program for pregnant women. They asked a supervisor to field the call, but she, too, had not heard of Healthy Kids. After conferring with several of her colleagues, she returned to the phone. "Thank you so much for waiting," the supervisor said. "We don't have that program here. You'll have to call Family Focus."

A call wasn't necessary; Family Focus, a social service agency several blocks away from the Public Aid office on Ogden Avenue, has nothing to do with Healthy Kids.

Chicago's Public Aid offices are supposed to tell new Medicaid recipients that Healthy Kids covers preventive care for their children and, if necessary, help them arrange doctors' appointments and transportation. But just as prevention may be low on the priority list of poor mothers, Healthy Kids gets short shrift among Chicago's Public

Aid caseworkers, whose primary task is to determine who is poor enough to qualify for cash grants and food stamps. "Chances are, maybe 5 percent of Chicago caseworkers know about Healthy Kids," admitted Ben Behrent, one of two administrators who oversaw the program for the entire state. "The caseworkers have sixty to a hundred people sitting in the waiting room all day. They don't have the time or the inclination to discuss it."

The problem went beyond a caseworker shortage. From the top down, Healthy Kids was riddled with holes. For at least five years, the central office of the Department of Public Aid in Springfield sent cards to all new Medicaid recipients asking them to check a box if they needed help finding preventive care for their children, but it was official department policy not to respond to the cards from Chicago mothers, said Diane Hayes, the other Healthy Kids' administrator. The Chicago offices were too busy for the extra work, she said.

Still, Public Aid's main office went through the motions. The state received about two hundred cards each day, and a secretary dutifully compiled lists of people who had asked for help—only the Chicago lists never left her desk.[17] It's not quite true that *no* Chicago mothers received the help they requested. Perhaps the supreme irony is that while the program is designed to provide preventive care for well children, the only Chicago cards that got any response were those in which mothers penned in an extra plea for help in getting care for a very sick child. Those cases Hayes felt compelled to handle herself.

Why conduct such a farce? One possibility is that Illinois officials needed the cards to show federal reviewers that they were following EPSDT's outreach provisions. One federal official, who reviews state Medicaid programs out of HCFA's regional office in Chicago, suggested that Illinois' poor promotion of Healthy Kids had an even more cynical design: a deliberate strategy to control Medicaid costs. "Illinois' general approach to handling programs has been if you don't tell clients about them, they won't use them, and the state won't have to spend money," the reviewer said.[18]

But HCFA has come under fire, too, for going easy on states. Illinois' EPSDT program was cited by HCFA in the summer of 1986 for "suppressing" the lists of Chicago clients who requested help, but HCFA obviously did nothing to stop it.[19] Child-health advocates in Pennsylvania got so frustrated with HCFA's oversight that they went over the agency's head and sued that state in federal court in 1991. The suit alleged that Pennsylvania's Medicaid program had ignored federal EPSDT requirements and set doctors' fees so low that poor children had less access to health care than others, which is in theory forbidden under federal law.

In Illinois, there is one special EPSDT program to give children the care they are entitled to receive, but it falls far short of need. In Jackie's neighborhood, Bethel New Life, a well-known, community-based social service organization, was contracted by Public Aid's central office to help children enrolled in Medicaid get regular care. Ten other agencies across the state, in places where children are considered at particular risk of not getting care, received similar "case-management" contracts.

What is hard to believe is that no one at the local level, at the Ogden IDPA office, mentioned Bethel New Life when asked about the Healthy Kids program. Even harder to believe, a Bethel Healthy Kids worker is stationed *next door* to the Public Aid office, at the Lawndale Christian Health Center.

Bethel's target population is the 54,000 children enrolled in Medicaid in the three zip codes it serves, including much of North Lawndale. With a budget of $120,000, Bethel could afford to hire only four caseworkers, who follow about 800 children—less than 2 percent of its "target" group. So IDPA set that goal with a wink and a nod, realizing it could not be met.

Yet Bethel was overloaded even with 800 children, or about 200 children for each caseworker. Getting women to the doctor's office who do not have cars or child care, who are drug-addicted, or poorly educated, can be a time-consuming task involving lots of counseling, cajoling, and carrying. It frequently takes more than a phone call, especially since many of Bethel's clients do not have phones. The program was so full that one Bethel worker said she and her colleagues probably would prefer to remain anonymous at the Ogden Public Aid office. "We can't handle more people," she said. "Getting more people from Public Aid offices would just make things worse."

Even so, Bethel and the other contract agencies were expected to increase their caseloads by 15 to 20 percent in fiscal 1992, although their budgets would not increase.[20] It might have helped ease the strain if the agencies had been able to track clients with computers that

IDPA gave them in December 1990. But as of July 1991, the $6,000 computers sat idle because IDPA had not assigned anyone to program them properly.[21]

Though the state has not put much money into case management—only a handful of Illinois' Medicaid-eligible children are even theoretically followed by an agency such as Bethel[22]—it is generally considered one of the more effective methods of getting children into preventive care. South Carolina's EPSDT program, one of the models for the country, depends heavily on home visits and case management. The state doubled its number of EPSDT visits over several years, and as of 1989, had 83 visits per 100 children, the best record in the United States.[23]

One reason case-management agencies may work is that they have a measure of independence from state welfare departments. Many Public Aid recipients, including Jackie, loathe and fear the welfare office. She avoids putting herself in situations where she will have to push Public Aid workers for information about health care or anything else. In public health jargon, welfare workers tend not to be "culturally sensitive." It is not that they are a different color than Jackie, or speak a different language, it is that, from her point of view, the culture of welfare offices is at best brusque or nitpicky, at worst capriciously cruel and punitive. Secrecy also pervades the culture; welfare recipients, Jackie among them, sometimes withhold information to protect their interests. In sum, welfare offices seem about the worst places imaginable to station a health care program. Jackie's main goal when she walks through the door at the squat, brown-brick office is to give away nothing that might reduce her welfare payment, to make as few waves as possible.

An image problem among the poor is only one of the many crosses Medicaid bears because of its connection to welfare. One of the leading medical sociologists in the country, Paul Starr, calls Congress's decision to link Medicaid to welfare and Medicare to Social Security the "original sin of American health policy." "Medicare enjoys the political protection created by a span of eligibility that includes the middle class; Medicaid suffers from the political vulnerability created by identification with welfare and the poor," Starr wrote. "The hospital benefits of Medicare are additionally protected by financing that comes from an earmarked payroll tax, whereas Medicaid must compete for general revenues—at not only the federal but the state level."[24]

Indeed, state budget shortfalls are the latest threat to children's Medicaid coverage. States generally went along with the federally mandated expansions of Medicaid that started in 1984—after hundreds of thousands of people were cut from the program during the early 1980s. They saw helping pregnant women and children as a worthy social goal, as well as a cost-effective one. A dollar spent on immunizations, for example, will eventually save more than ten dollars.[25] The reforms also enabled states to get Medicaid matching funds for maternal and child health programs that state and local governments previously had paid for themselves. But with health care costs continuing to grow at a rapid rate, governors increasingly resisted Congressional mandates for children. Making Medicaid coverage available to all poor children will cost much more than previous reforms, they complained.

The real frustration is that poor women and children are relatively cheap groups to cover. Nationwide, children make up half of Medicaid recipients but account for only a fifth of expenditures.[26] In contrast, the elderly and disabled comprise 27 percent of Medicaid recipients but are responsible for 73 percent of expenditures.[27] A large part of that money goes for nursing-home care. As mentioned, while Medicaid was intended to provide health care to poor women and children, the middle-class elderly take advantage of its nursing-home coverage as much as anyone. Nursing-home costs truly impoverish some middle-class people, but others have become adept at Medicaid "estate-planning," using various legal maneuvers to qualify for the public program without actually becoming poor.[28]

Jackie often made comments to signal that she was a conscientious mother. One time, she boasted that she had not been to a bar or party in months. "I got three reason not to go out: Latrice, Brianna, and DeMarest. I'm always called the old maid, but I don't care. The squarer I am, the more I get done." Under trying circumstances, Jackie managed to be a good mother.

Her strong sense of responsibility for her children shows just how far-reaching are the failures of the health system for poor children. There are many Jackies in poor neighborhoods. If their children aren't being immunized, whose will be?

In all likelihood, Jackie would have responded to fairly simple public-health measures. A personal letter from a doctor or clinic that explained the dangers of not having Brianna immunized against measles might have worked. Such a letter might have pointed out that adverse side effects from immunizations are extremely rare, since Jackie had heard rumors about children being brain damaged by the shots. If not a letter, a phone call might have reached her, explaining that children in her neighborhood were getting sick and dying from a preventable disease. (Middle-class pet owners get more prompts from their veterinarians.)[29]

A responsible neighborhood doctor or well-staffed clinic could have provided this type of one-to-one outreach; Lawndale Christian personally contacts mothers whose children miss appointments, but the center can only handle so many patients and Brianna was not enrolled there. (Jackie and her children were members of a Medicaid-HMO and so were restricted to using Mount Sinai's pediatric clinic.) The family needed what one public health professional called a "health care home." Roger Bernier, an assistant director for science at the CDC, described how health care delivery works in Sweden. "When you're born, you fall onto a conveyor belt; your number gets sent to the local community health center. If you don't show up with your baby, they send a home visitor. You're part of a social net. Here [in U.S. cities], it reminds me of being in Africa where the women just hunched down and had their babies on the ground."

But even some Third World countries have aggressive, coordinated national vaccine campaigns, as well as more universal access to health care, and as a result, their children fare much better than blacks and Hispanics who live in U.S. cities. According to the World Health Organization, almost 90 percent of children in Algeria are vaccinated by their first birthday, 76 percent in El Salvador, 77 percent in Uganda, and 98 percent in Cuba, Chile, and Antigua.[30] In Chicago, less than half of poor minority children are fully immunized by their *second* birthday.[31]

Fortunately, Brianna did not get measles, but no thanks to the health system. Some will say that the kind of health care program that could have given the little girl her measles shots, the kind that Bernier suggests, is too labor intensive, too expensive. They, then, must concede that the United States is not able to give to all its children what Third World countries give to theirs.

11

Robert Banes plays the transplant game

R obert Banes and a half-dozen other kidney dialysis patients were watching—or trying hard not to watch—the spectacle of Isaiah. Wearing dark sun glasses and jeans with the back pocket ripped away, Isaiah strutted through the waiting room at Neomedica Dialysis Center, ranting about the way he smoked cocaine in the hospital, about how he could score drugs for anyone who was interested.

"My heart is ticking just fine. I'm better off than all of you," he spouted to his fellow dialysis patients. The next minute he asked a visitor to the dialysis unit if she could get him a kidney to replace his failed organ. The answer, of course, was no; kidney distribution is regulated by a government-chartered agency. "I'm going to kill all of you in here," he bellowed over and over again.

No one on Neomedica's staff emerged to quiet Isaiah. The patients waiting for rides home from the North Loop center to their mostly poor neighborhoods shrank into their seats to avoid him or rolled their eyes at his antics. The only exception was a rakish middle-aged man, known as Candyman. He was waiting to be called back for the afternoon dialysis shift. "I'll take this stick across your ass," he playfully warned Isaiah, slapping his cane across his open palm. Isaiah ignored him, but a couple of other patients laughed at his bravado. "Hey, Candyman," a feeble woman called from her wheelchair, "you aren't gonna hurt nobody after you get done with that machine." Candyman may not have been physically imposing, but his teasing disarmed Isaiah. He sputtered out, and a low murmur filled the room as the patients took up their usual conversations of special diets, medications, and family matters.

Robert ambled over to the pay phone to call Jackie. He usually checked in with her after dialysis to see if she wanted him to pick up something for lunch.

"You know you got to make that phone call," Candyman razzed Robert, his new target. "You know you got to report in every morning or the key not gonna fit the lock." Robert grinned ruefully as he dialed the phone. The truth was he did not have a key because Jackie did not trust him with it.

Jackie blamed drugs for Robert's rejection of his transplanted kidney. When he was high, she said, he sometimes skipped taking the immuno-suppressive medication that prevents the body from attacking a "foreign" kidney in the same way it does a virus. For that reason, active addicts are excluded from transplant waiting lists, but drug use did not enter into the University of Illinois program's deliberations about whether to list Robert for a second time. He did not talk about drugs with anyone outside of his immediate family, and although he liked the transplant coordinator, Patricia Barber, he was not about to bare his soul to her. On the way home from Neomedica the day of Isaiah's outburst, Robert mentioned he had heard that Isaiah had been waiting for a kidney for five years. "Doctors don't like talk like that," Robert said knowingly. "That's why Isaiah don't get a kidney."

Barber and another nurse work with surgeon Raymond Pollak to assess patients' suitability for transplant and provide follow-up care for anyone who receives a new kidney. "Trish," as Robert called Barber, had more direct contact with patients than the doctor. Slender and pretty with long prematurely gray hair, she had the calm demeanor of someone who has raised a big family and seen it all. She knew the fixes transplant patients could get into, and little shocked her. She scolded Robert and others for missing appointments or indulging in foods that upset their blood chemistries, but her disapproval was fleeting. She gave her charges the benefit of the doubt.

Whether or not drug use had anything to do with Robert losing his first kidney is uncertain, but Barber said she had no reason to suspect that it was a problem for him. To listen to her stories of patients consumed by drug use is to understand why Robert did not stand out. Take Isaiah. He hadn't, in fact, been waiting five years for a kidney; he wasn't even on the transplant list. Barber had refused to list him because he "used every drug he could get his hands on." She had nothing to do with Isaiah's dialysis treatments, but she still heard from him occasionally. She once received a call from a doctor who had written Isaiah a prescription for narcotics after he claimed Barber was his physician.

Barber had no shortage of tales about patients unable to curb their appetites for drugs. There was the guy Barber caught stealing syringes from the clinic; the one who called for advice because he could not remember whether he had taken his antirejection medication while he was wasted; the one who told Barber he smoked a bag of marijuana a day but still insisted he should get a transplant. Some of her war stories are decidedly tragic—one young man suffered a massive stroke and died after ingesting prodigious amounts of cocaine—while others are tragically comic. After a patient persistently begged for codeine-laced Tylenol, a transplant surgeon gave in and prescribed a bottle of the mild narcotic for him, only to receive a call from the police a few days later. Why was the doctor doling out pills to a guy who was peddling them on the street? the officer asked.

Then there was the other inquiry from police, who had nabbed one of Barber's transplant patients robbing a drug store. Was it true, an officer asked her, that he could not be jailed because of his medical condition? "You could hear this little voice in the background, 'I didn't do it. I didn't do it,'" Barber remembered, laughing. "We told them by all means to lock him up because then we would know where he was and could make sure he took his meds."

To Barber, Robert seemed an "exceptional" patient, an exceptionally good patient, that is. "He's brighter than most. He's been married I don't know how long. He holds a job." His first kidney lasted for a relatively long six years. She put him in a category of patients who, after a while, neglect their medications because they feel so healthy they forget that immunosuppressants keep them that way. Then, too, Barber figured some drug use was almost unavoidable for many of the urban poor enrolled in her transplant program. "Drugs are common," she said. "You walk down the block and people try to sell stuff to you."

Robert was well aware of the power Barber wielded. He wanted another chance at a transplant and courted her approval to get it. That extended from judicious reporting of drug use—Robert said he smoked a little marijuana—to providing Barber with examples of how well he followed doctor's orders.

When Barber met with Robert to determine whether he was a good candidate for a second transplant, he told her that when he had a boil a while back he had it checked out right away. Barber nodded her head in approval. "If you would have sat home on the boil for a few days it could have ruptured, the bacteria would have disseminated, and you could have died."

As Barber skimmed Robert's medical history, she mentioned offhand that focal glomerulosclerosis had caused his kidney failure. His eyes widened in surprise. For the past ten years he had assumed he lost his kidneys to high blood pressure, when, in fact, hypertension had been a symptom, not the cause, of his renal failure.

"No one ever told me that. They didn't *tell* me that," Robert said edgily. From the distance of a decade, it's hard to know how well doctors initially explained Robert's kidney disease, but somehow he hadn't understood, which angered him. But he did not dwell on that in front of Barber. Any expression of discontent—the kind of thing taken to an extreme by Isaiah—might diminish his chances of getting a kidney, Robert thought, or at least extend the waiting period.

Indeed, as Robert sat facing Barber, he seemed to be fishing through his mind for some way to mute his mild complaint. He tugged nervously on his baseball cap. "The [hospital] food was good, though," he said, replacing his scowl with a smile.

Robert had reason to be anxious about his chances. He could expect to live for another two years with the chills, the anemia, the fatigue, the three-times-a-week dialysis treatments that are a corollary of kidney failure. That is the average waiting time for patients with Robert's blood type, Barber told him.

"I had a feeling it was going to take a long time," Robert replied with characteristic acceptance. "Everybody has been telling me how long they've been waiting."

When Robert received his first kidney in 1982, only 255 people were on the transplant waiting list in Illinois. He was listed in the spring and transplanted in the summer. Close to 700 people were waiting seven years later. In the 1980s, the number of people waiting for kidneys nationwide doubled and then trebled to 18,000 by the end of the decade; meanwhile, the number of organ donors stalled at about 4,000.[1] The demand for transplants burgeoned with the introduction of more sophisticated drugs to prevent or reverse rejection, as well as better techniques to gauge compatibility between donors and potential recipients. Because transplants interfere less with living a normal life than dialysis does, many patients prefer them. "You ain't got to worry about going three times a week," Robert said. "You can eat anything you want to."

"It's a blessing not to be confined to a machine," Jackie added, "knowing that if you miss, it's a life and death situation."

While the long wait discouraged Robert, in some ways he was fortunate simply to be standing in the organ queue. Several large national studies have shown that the poor are less likely to receive kidney transplants than others,[2] and the process that squeezes them out starts early—preventing them access to transplant waiting lists in the first place. The situation is exacerbated for poor minorities. In Illinois, whites are nearly three times as likely to be on transplant waiting lists as others. As of December 1988, 40 percent of nonblack dialysis patients were on waiting lists compared to 15 percent of blacks. (Income data were not available.)[3]

Transplantation cannot escape the income-based inequities that permeate the larger medical care system. "Since the poor do not have the same access to high quality primary care as other members of our society, the chances are good they will not be referred for consideration [for transplant] at the same rate or at the same stage of disease," explained Arthur Caplan, a University of Minnesota medical ethicist who has written extensively on transplantation. Too poor to pay for care, they may become too sick to be good transplant risks.

Though Medicare provides substantial medical coverage for most Americans once they suffer renal failure, gaps in the program may keep the poor on dialysis. Medicare pays for dialysis for as long as patients need it, but the expensive immunosuppressive medications that are necessary after transplant are covered for only one year. With that in mind, nephrologists, who supervise dialysis, may not refer patients for transplant who seem too poor to afford antirejection drugs. Patients themselves may balk at the $6,000 annual expense. One study found that 90 percent of transplant patients had private insurance to supplement Medicare, but less than half of dialysis patients reported additional coverage.[4] While placement on one transplant waiting list may elude the poor, the more affluent can afford to jet around the country and claim spots on several. A study of more than 23,000 people on transplant waiting lists between October 1987 and June 1990 found that the 7 percent of patients listed in more than one program received kidneys six months faster than others.[5]

Explicit economic barriers notwithstanding, transplant professionals often insist that evenly applied medical factors are used to select patients for their programs. But as Barber's comments show, picking people for transplant is not an objective science. Barber does not want to waste precious kidneys on people too strung out on drugs to take immunosuppressants, or for that matter, too sick to get much use out of them, but there are no rules to help her make that determination. Her recommendations to the transplant surgeon are shaped by her ideas about family, work, and what she called the "drug culture" of inner-city neighborhoods.

Leanne Rockley, Barber's counterpart at Northwestern Memorial Hospital's transplant center, has worked with renal patients for more than two decades. She said that she and her colleagues inevitably exercise a measure of discretion in choosing patients for their programs. "You can't tell me that like or dislike for a patient doesn't sometimes cloud judgment," Rockley said.

Similarly, John Kilner, an ethicist at the Park Ridge Center for the Study of Health, Faith, and Ethics in Chicago, surveyed 453 dialysis and transplant center medical directors and found that their decisions about selecting patients for transplant (or dialysis, if it became a scarce resource) were influenced by everything from patients' ages and psychological stability to how much society benefits if they live. Potential recipients' family support, both emotional and financial, and the scientific knowledge that may be gained by treating them also were considered by about half of the directors surveyed.[6]

Rationing according to socioeconomic criteria has played a powerful role in the history of treatment for kidney disease. When dialysis was introduced in the 1960s as the first treatment for otherwise fatal renal failure, there were not enough machines to meet the demand, so doctors and others decided who would receive the lifesaving treatment. The most infamous example of that process was in Seattle, where a committee comprised of a lawyer, minister, housewife, labor leader, government official, banker, and three physicians decided who would live and who would die. The group, whose deliberations were chronicled in *Life* magazine, was biased toward patients who held good jobs and supported families who otherwise might be on the public dole. Divorce was frowned upon, as was a poor education. "The choices were hard," one member of the committee reflected. "I voted against a young man who had been a ne'er-do-well, a real playboy, until he

learned he had renal failure. He promised he would reform his character, go back to school, and so on, if only he were selected for treatment.
But I felt I'd lived long enough to know that a person like that won't
really do what he was promising."[7]

Commenting on the *Life* article at the time, a lawyer and psychiatrist
observed that it "painted a disturbing picture of the bourgeoisie sparing
the bourgeoisie, of the Seattle committee measuring persons in accordance with its own middle-class, suburban value system: scouts, Sunday
school, Red Cross. This rules out creative nonconformists. . . . The
Pacific Northwest is no place for Henry David Thoreau with bad
kidneys."[8]

Congress's decision to include renal patients in the Medicare program in 1972 was in part a reaction to that unseemly selection process.
No one wanted to take responsibility for the ethical dilemma of choosing one patient over another. Though a parochial God committee no
longer lurks in the background, the same group that received preference for dialysis when it was a scarce, lifesaving resource receives
preference for the new scarce, lifesaving resource: transplant. One
researcher, Dr. Carl Kjellstrand, who studied transplants according to
race, age, and sex among Midwestern kidney patients, summed up the
situation this way: "The most favored recipient of a transplant is similar
to the physicians who make the final decision: a young, white man."[9]

To the extent that racial and economic obstacles block the first gate
to transplant, Robert managed to get around them: he is part of the
University of Illinois transplant program. But because he is black, Robert almost certainly will wait longer for a kidney. In 1988, 63 percent
of the whites on transplant waiting lists in Illinois received kidneys,
compared to 36 percent of the blacks.[10] A report issued in 1990 by
the Office of the Inspector General of the Department of Health and
Human Services found that blacks nationwide waited an average of
13.9 months for a kidney, nearly twice as long as whites.[11]

Transplant professionals often blame the longer waits on the different biological makeups of blacks and whites, combined with the fact
that whites donate more organs than blacks. The two races tend to
have different blood types (more blacks than whites are blood type B,
for example), and blacks supposedly are "highly sensitized" more often
than whites, which means their antibodies repel more donor organs.
In addition, genetic compatibility is weaker between the races than
within them. While some members of the transplant community main-

tain that biology explains whites' advantage, the issue is far from settled. The Inspector General's report, for example, found that even
when blacks and whites had the same blood type and the same level
of sensitization, blacks still waited longer for kidneys than whites.

The transplantation system works like this: the Regional Organ
Bank of Illinois (ROBI) removes kidneys and other organs from donors
within its territory, three-quarters of Illinois and Northwestern Indiana.
The kidneys first are offered nationwide to a pool of close to 20,000
patients listed in the United Network for Organ Sharing (UNOS)
computer bank. The kidneys are flown out of state only if the computer
finds a "perfect match," a close genetic similarity between a donor and
recipient that is quite unusual. Most kidneys stay in Illinois and are
used by one of the seven transplant centers in ROBI's area.

ROBI distributes organs to patients on the local list based on a point
system that takes into account waiting time and genetic compatibility,
measured by what is called "antigen matching." Thought to minimize
the chances of rejection, antigen matching has been part of the UNOS
and ROBI point systems since 1987, but it was given more weight in
1989, a controversial move that seemed likely to push blacks further
back in the transplant line.[12] The change was prompted by a national
study at the University of California at Los Angeles which showed
that after one year patients who received the best matched kidneys
were 13 percent more likely to retain their organs than those who
received the worst matched.[13] Many doctors, however, do not buy the
study's results. No one doubts that the best-matched kidneys last
longer, but anything less than a "perfect match" is irrelevant, say transplant surgeons from Houston to New York City to Chicago. These
doctors, all of whom treat many minorities, report that the drug regi-
mens they use to stave off rejection cancel out the importance of
matching.

Dr. Pollak and other Chicago surgeons who transplant many blacks
were so convinced of matching's insignificance that ROBI obtained a
"variance" from UNOS for the local point system, placing somewhat
less emphasis on matching. Chicago-area blacks still wait longer than
whites, but less so than if ROBI used the UNOS point system, ROBI
officials say.

Even if there were no doubt that matched kidneys invariably lasted
longer, everyone would not be satisfied with the UNOS point system.
It is unfair, critics say, to single out matching when it is only one of

many factors that influence how long a patient keeps a new kidney—and one that discriminates against blacks. "Why shouldn't people get points taken away for having diabetes or lupus or for being retransplant candidates?" ethicist Caplan asked about three medical conditions that are known to hasten rejection. Matching may have earned a special place in the point system because it seemed objective. It's easier to match antigens than to determine, for example, whether patients were too noncompliant during their first transplant (skipping medication or otherwise ignoring doctors' orders) to "deserve" a second chance.

Once they get a spot on a transplant list, blacks' disadvantage in the organ game may have as much to do with the politics of ROBI and the nation's sixty-eight other organ distribution agencies as anything else. Although the agencies increasingly are governed by the dictates of UNOS, they retain significant discretion over divvying up the local supply of organs. That puts transplant surgeons in charge because they dominate procurement agencies.

ROBI's procurement and distribution system has become one of the more evenhanded in the country, even though the organ business in Chicago was once considered an undisciplined free-for-all.[14] Transplant programs elsewhere had to some extent worked together to collect and share organs, but in Chicago, it was every transplant surgeon for himself (or herself—one of the few female transplant surgeons in the country practiced at the University of Illinois). Each transplant program had a separate staff to procure organs from hospitals that they had recruited and considered their own. In one attempt to prevent different programs from claiming the same hospital's organs, Chicago-area surgeons agreed to equally divide donor hospitals, but the informal system devolved into anarchy. Much of the turmoil circled around a particularly aggressive surgeon at Rush–Presbyterian–St. Luke's, Dr. Frederick Merkel. In the late 1970s, he ignored the pact and cut deals to obtain organs from more than half of the state's hospitals.[15] The city's other transplant surgeons, who had incorporated for billing purposes, voted to strip Dr. Merkel of two-thirds of his hospitals in the early 1980s. Soon after, he started his own organ bank.

In 1985, Dr. Merkel gained further notoriety when a Pulitzer Prize–winning series in the *Pittsburgh Press* revealed that he was transplanting kidneys into foreigners who paid exorbitant prices and jumped ahead of Americans languishing on kidney waiting lists. The situation was made more bizarre when Chicago-area hospitals refused to grant Dr.

Merkel surgical privileges to transplant foreign nationals. Ever resourceful, the surgeon flew about the country in search of surgical suites, showing up at hospitals with "a patient in one hand and a kidney in the other," in the words of a Michigan surgeon who received such a visit.[16]

Chicago surgeons were inspired to clean house when they discovered that they might lose control over the local supply of organs, political scientist J. Michael Dennis argued in a University of Chicago dissertation on the politics of organ transplantation.[17] Until the late 1980s, surgeons' hegemony over local organ collection and transplantation had been complete, in Chicago and elsewhere; the federal government did not interfere. That changed in 1987 when the Department of Health and Human Services, responding to Congressional concern that certain groups of patients were not getting an equal chance for a transplant, contracted with UNOS to regulate organ distribution nationwide—to an extent. At about the same time Congress also required Medicare to certify organ procurement agencies and thereby reduce the number of groups jostling for organs. Some experts argued that open organ warfare would sour the public on donation, and one study had suggested that larger agencies would be more effective.[18]

That last reform is what struck fear in the hearts of Chicago transplant surgeons.[19] With the publicity surrounding Dr. Merkel, as well as widely known turf battles that persisted among their own programs, the physicians worried that Medicare would refuse to certify a local procurement agency and would instead transfer responsibility for Chicago to a downstate Illinois group, or to one in Wisconsin.

To head that off, Chicago transplant programs eliminated their own procurement agencies and formed ROBI. They also developed a system for acquiring and distributing kidneys that they hoped was beyond reproach, according to Dennis, who wrote a case history of ROBI and several other procurement agencies.[20] Under the old system, when Chicago transplant surgeons removed two kidneys from a donor, they gave one to the common pool and kept one for their own programs. Such systems were considered necessary to induce transplant surgeons to "carry out the demanding work of procuring organs, often during the middle of the night."[21]

But while "keep one/share one" designs benefit centers by assuring them a somewhat steady flow of organs, they can put some patients at a disadvantage. For instance, hospitals that get many traffic accident victims—who are a major source of organ donors—tend to be located in white, suburban areas close to interstates. If these same hospitals have transplant programs that operate under a "keep one/share one" rule, they will get to transplant more patients than their inner-city counterparts, which have fewer organ donors and thus must depend more heavily on the common pool. More of the suburban hospital's patients are white; more of the city's are minorities.

ROBI has abolished "keep one/share one"—instead, all potential transplant recipients are entered onto a single list, and kidneys are allocated according to matching and waiting time—but just under half of its sister agencies retain it or a similar distribution design, which may account for blacks' longer waiting periods nationwide.

Another deviation from organ procurement practice that happens in Illinois—but over which ROBI has little control—also might skew the waiting period for blacks. Saint Anthony Medical Center in Rockford, 75 miles west of Chicago, reaps a bountiful harvest of organs (an indelicate description typical of the transplantation field). The hospital is technically included in ROBI's region, but hospitals are allowed to give their organs to whatever procurement agency they choose. Saint Anthony sends its kidneys, hearts, and livers to a hospital-based agency in nearby southern Wisconsin. That agency collects organs for only one transplant program, at the University of Wisconsin Hospital and Clinics in Madison, where just 10 percent of the patients are black. The upshot is that if the Wisconsin center gets a disproportionate share of organs relative to Chicago, black Midwesterners may wait longer than whites.

These examples suggest that, to achieve maximum equity nationwide, kidneys should be shared over larger regions. The length of time kidneys can be preserved and the logistics of transporting them put natural limits on region size, but the boundaries are as apt to be gerrymandered by transplant programs reluctant to cede "ownership" over kidneys procured from certain hospitals.

Although the days of unbridled entrepreneurialism have passed, competition for organs—between procurement agencies rather than individual programs—remains keen. No one has ever proved that the Rockford hospital upsets the region's racial balance, but ROBI staffers gripe about how Saint Anthony cheats them out of organs. Meanwhile, the executive director of the Wisconsin agency, Robert Hoffmann, lambasted ROBI for its designs on that hospital's organs. "They deal with 11 million people and a lot of hospitals. Why don't they establish a good relationship with them instead of destroying the one we have?" Hoffmann fumed. "They are the ones at fault." Since the late 1960s, he said his agency had worked diligently to cultivate organ donation at Saint Anthony. "If the goddamned purpose is to get more organs for the whole system, they should leave Saint Anthony's alone."

"Baby, you want to give me a kidney?" Robert asked Jackie, after returning from his appointment with Barber.

Jackie was sitting on the arm of the gold love seat and pulled her head back in surprise. "Will you mess up my kidney?" she said more than asked. "I should spare my kidney for *you?*"

The conversation did not go much further. It made no sense to her to sacrifice her kidney to someone who might neglect it when he took drugs. Robert did not protest; he seemed to expect his wife's response, even her veiled reference to drug use.

He pulled a peanut from a red-and-white striped bag he had bought from a street vendor and popped it into his mouth.

"You shouldn't be eating those," Jackie accused. You can't even follow a proper dialysis diet, her dark eyes reproved.

"I know," Robert replied, another shell cracking open between his fingers.

Because Jackie is not a blood relative, there's a good chance her husband could not use her kidney anyway. But as the demand for cadaver kidneys has grown without a corresponding increase in supply, doctors are looking more toward wives and friends when related donors are not available.

Robert's sister would have a better chance of matching him biologically than Jackie. When he received his first kidney she was under 18, too young to donate. Now she was eligible, but Robert was unwilling to ask her. "Somebody told me she couldn't get pregnant if she gave up her kidney," Robert told Barber, who insisted that was not true but then dropped the subject.

"It's a hell of a thing to ask," Barber acknowledged.

Blacks donate organs of their deceased family members and serve as "living related" kidney donors about half as often as whites. Lack of awareness, fear, superstition, religious beliefs, and distrust of the white medical establishment are the reasons frequently offered by transplant experts.[22] Even Robert, who surely appreciates the benefits of transplant, balked at the idea of donating his organs after his death. "I don't know about letting my heart go out of my body when I die. I might jump back up."

When the subject of racial inequity in kidney distribution is raised, transplant professionals are quick to point out that the simple solution to the problem lies in black hands: they need to donate more organs. "A third of patients waiting for transplant nationwide are black, but only about 10 percent of donors are black," said William LeFor, the chairman of the UNOS committee that changed the organization's rules to emphasize genetic matching. (In Chicago, 42 percent of those on the waiting list are black.)[23] "There is a screeching, screeching need for more black donors."

While increased donation from blacks undoubtedly would be helpful, the comments sometimes sound like accusations. One former Chicago area transplant surgeon said, "People never ask the converse: How many white kidneys go into black people? Blacks disenfranchise themselves by not donating more kidneys. The real issue in my mind is why doesn't the black community get it together and go out and get organs for themselves?"

Though this surgeon blamed the "black community" for its own low donation rates, part of the responsibility has to be assumed by the predominantly white transplant community to which he belonged. The Inspector General's report found that only fourteen of three hundred organ procurement coordinators working nationwide are black.[24] Procurement coordinators approach families about donating their loved ones' organs, a sensitive job, to say the least. The wariness toward the white medical establishment detected in organ donation surveys certainly suggests that blacks might be more open to the idea if asked by other blacks.

Jackie Lynch, a former pharmaceutical salesman who grew up in a Chicago housing project, is ROBI's only black procurement specialist. Beeper on his belt, he takes as many of the agency's black referrals as possible. He does not hesitate to use race to appeal to black families.

"We as a people are often talked to, never spoken with," Lynch told a middle-aged couple reluctant to donate the organs of their brain-dead son. A few hours before, the twenty-two-year-old had been struck by a car as he ran across the street. Now, his parents were talking to Lynch in a small supply room in a South Side hospital.

On the other side of the intensive care unit, their son was attached to a respirator. He had not been removed from life support systems so that Lynch might have a chance to persuade his family to donate organs.

"Do you know why he was running?" the young man's mother asked Lynch.

"Innuendos and rumors, I keep out. I don't think there's any value in that because that won't bring him back," Lynch responded. He already had been informed that the man had been involved in a crime, but discussing that seemed a sure way to discourage organ donation. The man's mother insisted.

"I said I was going to tell you the truth," she continued, her eyes teary. "He was running from the scene, a crime scene. He had a TV."

"Don't worry about that," Lynch consoled.

Over the next few minutes, they went back and forth, with Lynch gradually steering the conversation toward the purpose of his visit.

"His sisters and mother rather keep him together, rather than him being torn apart," the father explained to Lynch.

"If it *were* an issue of being torn apart," Lynch countered. "Those are buzzwords."

"We decided we would not cut him up." The man's tone was firm but not final; it was evident that he and his wife had different opinions on the matter, but he was not going to override her wishes.

"If it was me, and I was his age, and I could help another person," Lynch coaxed.

The boy's mother chimed in. "If they take his organs, I just don't want to know about it."

That did not count as consent for Lynch. "We as a people, so much has been done to us," he said. "We have to be skeptical about how we approach things." Lynch paused. "I want to get back to what you just said about cutting him up and tearing him up. You would not be able to tell."

The couple stared silently at Lynch.

"So you're not consenting," he said.

"I just don't want to know about it," the mother repeated.

"What I'd like is to save other lives of people who are about to die. But that's not your problem."

The father, dressed in a plaid work shirt and jeans, dropped down in a crouch, as if his legs could not support the weight of his sorrow. His eyes were hooded by heavy lids. He muttered something about how only his son's hands and face would be exposed at the funeral.

"It might be the thing that helps you get through," Lynch cajoled. "I can't think of a better gift."

Lynch asked to speak to the boy's father alone. He told him that he could not accept the organs without both parents' consent. "I feel like I'd be back-dooring you otherwise," he said. "I don't want you seeing me on the street and cursing me."

When his wife rejoined them, the man had shifted to Lynch's side. "What do you think, baby?" he said. "We could help another person." She did not answer, but later, Lynch said that, at that point, he had been pretty sure she would agree. Lynch asked the whole family, which included two sisters and an aunt, to join him in a hospital conference room.

"There are five African Americans in this room. Chances are fair each of you know two people on dialysis," Lynch began, surveying the family gathered around the table.

One of the young women agreed, another looked to her mother for confirmation. "That's right," her mother said.

"The kidneys would go into another African American," Lynch said. Although it was likely, Lynch had no way to guarantee the boy's organs would go into another black, but no one challenged him on it.

"Some mother like you, waiting, waiting for that call," he said. "That's the joy, but I can't give it to you." Lynch stopped. He looked steadily at the young man's parents.

"I believe in my heart he would want his organs donated," the mother answered. There it was: Lynch had won, but his face did not betray any satisfaction.

"He was that kind of guy," the young man's mother reminisced. "He was wild, but he was good-hearted." She wiped her face with a washcloth. After more discussion, the couple signed ROBI's consent form, and the boy's father asked to see him one last time.

The young man lay in a bed in the corner of the unit, where the sun shone mockingly through large windows. The father grabbed his son's limp arm, hungrily kissed his face. "I love you, I love you." He backed away from the bed and studied the heart monitor; wavy red, green, and yellow lines ran across it.

"Is he gone, doctor?" the man asked, his eyes expectant, pleading for one last chance. The brain stem was dead, the doctor answered.

It was hard to believe that the man's son was dead, which is one reason families do not easily donate organs. Kept alive by machines, his chest rose and fell underneath a thin blue gown. The way he shuddered when he breathed it was as if he were having a bad dream. Crying, the father touched his son's cheek one last time, and left.

The number of kidneys ROBI obtained from black donors rose from 10 percent of the total in 1988 to 24 percent by 1991.[25] Lynch deserves part of the credit, said Audrey Gordon, a University of Illinois public health professor and hospice expert who has held workshops at ROBI about the ways in which families cope with death. "There is no question that matching cultures helps," Gordon said, drawing on transplant lingo. "This is a time when people are extremely vulnerable because of the shock. When you're in shock, you regress. You want nostalgia. You want the things you absolutely know and don't have to think about."

Public education also may have improved organ donation rates; a ROBI-sponsored task force promotes donations on black radio shows, at church services and community group meetings. Lynch had noted a marked shift in public attitudes during his time at ROBI. "When I first rode in the Bud Billiken parade [an annual black parade held in Chicago] five years ago, I got jeers, people damn near spit on the car. Now people run up to shake your hand."

As important as public education is physician education, or perhaps physician persuasion. Some neurosurgeons are uncomfortable asking families to donate organs, or do not want to take the time or the perceived legal risk of declaring a patient brain dead.[26] They would rather remove patients from life support systems and allow their hearts to stop beating. That precludes organ donation because organs are damaged as the body winds down.

Another problem that depresses organ donation overall is that while some nurses and doctors receive training in organ procurement, others abruptly ask families for consent, instead of waiting for a ROBI specialist. Lynch and his colleagues raise the issue slowly, as soothingly as possible, whereas nurses and doctors may be distracted by the needs of patients who are still alive. They may not have the time to spend with families explaining the touchy concept of brain death, or turning a "no" into a "yes."

In the University of Illinois transplant program, 28 percent of black patients who receive organs reject their kidneys within a year. After four years, another 6 percent reject.[27]

So Robert is one of the more fortunate ones; he kept his kidney for six years and four months before he started feeling fatigued, and before Jackie told him his breath smelled "like something had died inside"—a sign that his kidneys were not filtering wastes. No one knows for sure why the body decides to reject a kidney that it had accepted for so long, but Barber said that what seems to have happened with Robert is common: for whatever reason, patients stop taking the drugs that prevent rejection. "I couldn't take my medication on the job," Robert told Barber, referring to the first time he worked as a security guard. "I would always take my morning medicine. A couple of guys did not like me; I was afraid they might go in my bag."

"Rob, your medicine fits in your pocket."

"If I got stuff jingling in my pocket, that might endanger my life. What if I have to sneak up on someone?"

"You could have taken it all in the morning."

"They always told us not to take it at the same time."

Barber explained that when patients feel good, they may risk not taking their medicine. "Who wants to depend on medication their whole life?"

"I did. I knew it kept me alive," Robert replied.

Sometimes Robert says he took his medication regularly; sometimes he says he did not. Barber had no hard evidence either way because the immunosuppressants Robert took cannot be measured in the blood. If Barber had been aware of his cocaine use, she might not have put him on the transplant waiting list for a second time until he was assessed for addiction and, if necessary, treated. Since organs are a scare resource, it may seem unfair or irresponsible to give a second transplant to someone who did not tend to his first, but those who would want to deny transplants to noncompliant patients face a similar dilemma as those who would want to deny health insurance to smokers: Was the patient willfully noncompliant, or not?

For drug users, some people would answer yes; others would say no, that drug addiction is a disease that reduces or eliminates the addict's culpability for his actions. But drug use, of course, is only one reason transplant patients are labeled as noncompliant. Some stop taking immunosuppressants because they cannot afford to do otherwise.

The most widely used antirejection drug, Cyclosporine, costs $400 to $600 a month, and Medicare picks up 80 percent of the tab for only one year from the date patients are discharged after a transplant. Just how much that policy contributes to noncompliance among the poor is unclear. In a national survey, transplant surgeons reported that half of their patients had trouble paying for their medications. They tallied 143 kidney rejections caused by the high cost of Cyclosporine.[28] On the other hand, an unpublished study of the University of Illinois' transplant population showed that low-income patients were no more likely to stop taking their drugs than wealthier patients, even though the annual cost can be an enormous burden. Some used creative means to pay for their medications; one woman, who supported herself and two children on about $700 a month, borrowed her friend's Medicaid card to cover $200 worth of drugs every three weeks, said researcher Deborah Kiley, who studied compliance for her Ph.D. in psychology at the Illinois Institute of Technology.

Robert said empty pockets never kept him from buying immunosuppressive medication. The drugs that were popular when Robert received his first kidney are much cheaper than Cyclosporine, however, and he managed to come up with the $100 he needed each month. "My grandmother would help me out sometimes," he said.

Barber said that although it increased their risk of rejection, she had taken about twenty-five patients off Cyclosporine because they could not afford it. "I had this Korean grocery store owner. He makes just enough money that he cannot qualify for Public Aid, but he couldn't afford his medication. It would have ruined his business." The grocery store owner and most of the others have handled the change well (some doctors take patients off Cyclosporine after a year anyway, because the drug can be toxic to the kidney). Yet several people have rejected their kidneys after switching medications, Barber said. The University of Illinois has a special Cyclosporine fund, but it is reserved for people who, doctors think, would reject their kidneys were they taken off the drug. In other words, patients can qualify for the program to help them keep their kidneys only when they're in danger of losing them.

Before Robert was officially entered on the transplant waiting list in October, he met with Dr. Pollak. The two probably would not see each other again for at least two years, when Barber had projected that a kidney would become available for Robert. Then, there would be no time for talk, no time for the surgeon to try to ascertain whether Robert was willing to take the precautions necessary to keep a second kidney. Once an organ is identified for a patient, ROBI gives hospital transplant teams an hour to find that person—and to accept or reject the kidney. After that, organs are passed on to the next person on the waiting list.

"I cannot emphasize too much to you that failure to take your medications will result in rejection of your kidney," Dr. Pollak told Robert.

"I know it," Robert replied. The two men were sitting across from each other in Dr. Pollak's office.

"Even skipping for a day is inexcusable as far as God and nature are concerned," Dr. Pollak continued. "See, we won't know about it, but the big man in the sky will know. . . .

"This will be a continuous thing for the rest of your life."

"I know."

12

The Banes family and white doctors

O
H . . . OH . . . OH . . . OH LORD," Mrs. Jackson moaned. She
turned to her side, grabbing one of the low metal bars that kept
her from falling out of the hospital bed. Desperately seeking a
position that would relieve the pain in her remaining leg, she released
the bar and lay back, holding her throbbing thigh underneath the
sheet.

Dr. Mark Angel, the senior resident, accompanied by a fourth year
medical student, Bernadette Cracchiolo, stopped by to check on Mrs.
Jackson. In the summer, Dr. Angel had warned her that her left leg
might also have to be amputated, and that was about to happen.

"Your surgery will be in about two hours," Dr. Angel said. "Hopefully, it will give you some relief from that pain in your leg." Mrs.
Jackson's watery eyes widened in response; she looked scared. The
sore on her foot had never healed, and the infection was beginning to
penetrate the bone. It was a week after Thanksgiving, and Mrs. Jackson
had been in the hospital for nearly a month, during which time doctors
did what they could to save her remaining leg: antibiotics, whirlpool
treatments to stimulate circulation, and surgical cleaning of the foot
ulcer. None of it had worked.

Dr. Angel and Cracchiolo left, and Mrs. Jackson continued to ache
out loud, pausing two times in automatic deference to the hospital
loudspeaker that summoned doctors and nurses. Her breathing was
labored; she wheezed with each intake of air. She had suffered from
mild congestive heart failure for some time, but during this hospitalization, the condition had worsened and fluid was backing up in her
lungs.

Cracchiolo returned to Mrs. Jackson's bedside. In a few months, the
young woman would have her medical degree and begin her intern-

ship. Medical commentators note how doctors tend to occupy a different world than their patients—more than a decade of all-consuming training sets them apart—but so far Cracchiolo seemed at home in both places. Friendly and unusually patient with Mrs. Jackson, she was not wrapped up in medicine's exclusionary white coat.

"Excuse me," she said as she gently pulled aside Mrs. Jackson's gown to check her breathing. "Now take a deep breath."

Mrs. Jackson rattled on with her breathing but did not attempt to do as Cracchiolo had requested.

"Like this," Cracchiolo said, breathing in deeply herself.

Mrs. Jackson responded with a weak rendition. "Good," Cracchiolo told her. "Did your granddaughter come by and see you today?"

"No."

"You think she'll have a chance later on?"

"She might."

The conversation was interrupted by two women who entered Mrs. Jackson's room bearing pamphlets. One had a blue surgical mask over her mouth because Mrs. Jackson had acquired a hard-to-treat infection caused by Methicillin-Resistant Staphylococcus Aureus (MRSA). The bacteria are prevalent in hospitals and tend to take hold in weak, chronically ill patients like Mrs. Jackson. Many patients carry MRSA (and other bacteria) without getting sick, but it can lead to stubborn infections. Thus, hospitals try to prevent its spread. A red, license-plate-size sticker on Mrs. Jackson's door advised visitors to wear a gown and mask and wash their hands before leaving her room.

"We're from pastoral care, and we just want to tell you the Lord loves you," one of the women said. The other smiled and handed Mrs. Jackson a pamphlet that showed a dense forest from which glowed a spiritual light. "The Lord loves you, and he will give you strength; Jesus Christ loves you."

"Ummm," Mrs. Jackson answered, holding the pamphlet listlessly. She was a devout Baptist but at the moment was groggy with pain. The two women stood awkwardly by her bed. "Goodbye, the Lord loves you," one said as she and her partner turned for the door. Mrs. Jackson raised a stiff hand in farewell.

Mercifully, Mrs. Jackson fell asleep a few minutes later, still clutching the religious pamphlet. Her room smelled of an earthy decay, emanating from a withered yellow mum on her bedside table. From the hallway, the two Christian visitors could be heard singing softly.

Mrs. Jackson's peace was short-lived. She awoke with a cry.

"What do you need, Mrs. Jackson?" asked Cracchiolo, who had reentered Mrs. Jackson's room a moment before. She sounded genuinely concerned about her patient. "Did you get a pain shot this morning?"

"No," Mrs. Jackson said clearly.

Cracchiolo left and promptly returned, followed a few minutes later by a nurse. The nurse sauntered slowly into the room. "You do know she's going to surgery," she said, hand on her hip. Nurses often complain, and rightfully so, that doctors treat them like idiots or slaves, but when doctors are very new like Cracchiolo—or women—nurses may take the chance to turn the tables. It is probably in patients' best interest that nurses independently look out for their welfare, but this encounter crackled with a tension that had nothing to do with a mutual desire by doctor and nurse to do right by Mrs. Jackson. It was a power struggle.

Refusing to take the bait, Cracchiolo responded pleasantly that the kind of anesthesia Mrs. Jackson was to receive did not rule out pain killers, but the nurse surveyed her skeptically. She left the room without administering a shot, and a few moments later returned with reinforcement. The other nurse asked Cracchiolo the same questions, and she gave the same answers. The two nurses paused for a moment, then decided to take Cracchiolo's word for it. "Thanks for asking," Cracchiolo said with all the diplomacy she could muster.

Just as the nurse began to give the much disputed shot, the phone rang. It was a preacher from Mrs. Jackson's First Baptist church. "Do you want to talk?" Cracchiolo asked, handing her the phone. Mrs. Jackson put the receiver to her ear.

"Where do you want it, your hip or your arm?" asked the nurse, who, now that she had accepted her mission, was not about to be deterred.

"Hip," Mrs. Jackson said softly into the phone.

The nurse mumbled something.

"She said, 'hip,'" Cracchiolo explained.

"I know," the nurse snapped. "I asked her which one."

Mrs. Jackson got it on the left side.

Distracted by another doctor, Cracchiolo ignored Mrs. Jackson for a few minutes. When she returned to her bedside, Mrs. Jackson was mutely holding the phone at her ear.

"Are you talking to someone?" Cracchiolo asked.

"He hung up," Mrs. Jackson said blankly, still clinging tightly to the phone. Cracchiolo carefully pried it from her fingers.

After Cracchiolo left, Mrs. Jackson rested, her pain vanquished for a while. About an hour later, though, a medical resident who had yet to make an appearance that morning entered Mrs. Jackson's room, heading straight for the end of her bed. She took a quick look at her chart, and without a word, started to unwind the bandages on the old woman's left foot. Mrs. Jackson moaned once again.

Mrs. Jackson did not ask what was going on, but why would the doctor bother putting fresh bandages on her foot, considering that her whole leg was due to be amputated in a few hours?

"She's not having surgery," the resident announced, only after she was asked whether she knew about the scheduled amputation. "The attending [physician] decided her lungs were too congested." So Mrs. Jackson would not be losing her left leg that day, after all.

Compounding an already miserable day, that afternoon Mrs. Jackson and Jackie learned that Cracchiolo was leaving. Medical students spend about a month on each assignment, and Cracchiolo's time on Mrs. Jackson's floor was up. "I hate that," Jackie said when she was informed of the medical student's imminent departure. "When I called her the other day, she called me right back. She was giving me the rundown on Mama better than any of them other doctors they have. Usually, you just sit up there, yeah, uh huh, you just agree, but you don't know what they're talking about. But with her, it was, Wow! This is what it means."

Impoverished black women are not, of course, the only people who complain about being befuddled by doctors. All classes and races of people often perceive doctors as aloof technocrats who confuse patients with scientific jargon rather than engage them in a meaningful give-and-take about their prognoses and treatments. In a 1986 essay in *Newsweek*, columnist Meg Greenfield wrote after a hospital stay that she had "just come back from a foreign place worth reporting on . . . a universe, really, of its own," where she felt like "a tourist in an unfathomable, dangerous land."[1] In *Strangers at the Bedside*, David Rothman, a Columbia University historian and professor of social medicine, attributes the gulf between physicians and patients to a host of structural changes in the practice of medicine: the end of the house call; the extreme specialization of medicine so that doctors follow patients only as long as a particular organ system malfunctions; demographic changes such as those that eliminated the ethnic and religious bonds between Mount Sinai's doctors and patients; technologic advances that make tests better diagnostic instruments than conversations with patients; and, finally, the rigorous, lengthy medical training mentioned earlier.[2]

If medicine is so unfathomable to the Meg Greenfields of the world, imagine the difficulty Robert, Jackie, and her grandmother had getting to the bottom of things. Jackie and Robert had high school educations, but Mrs. Jackson only finished a few years of grade school in Mississippi. Mrs. Jackson and Robert often did not know what was being done to them and did not ask. Or if they did ask and were answered with medical gobbledygook, they did not press for more information. There was Robert on the examining table silently wondering if he had cancer. Then, another time, he came home from the dialysis unit prepared to take a new kind of medication, "stress-tabs," although he had no idea why they had been prescribed. He only found out after Jackie insisted that he call Neomedica to ask. The pills turned out to be vitamins, which relieved Jackie because she thought her husband had been diagnosed with some kind of mental illness arising from stress.

Jackie was more willing to ask questions than the rest of her family, but still her understanding of her grandmother's multiple illnesses was far from complete. The first few times her grandmother was hospitalized, she thought doctors planned to treat her gangrenous foot, but that never happened in the way Jackie expected. She did not know her grandmother had congestive heart failure until Cracchiolo came onto the scene. "Heart failure?" Jackie remembered responding when she was told. "Now you're telling me something different."

Raising the barriers still higher, Jackie did not expect doctors to necessarily level with her. A general distrust of the white establishment inevitably seeped into her dealings with doctors, few of whom are black.[3] A pragmatic woman, she sometimes used me as her intermediary with doctors, figuring that my color and education would give me an edge. "White people are sometimes more official, more legitimate," she told me. "You know many, many words, and how to phrase them. If Mom was going to die, I thought [doctors would] tell you quicker." That did not happen, but Jackie's assumption was not baseless. She had noticed that doctors and nurses tended to treat me differently—that, for instance, they often addressed me before her.

But the cool eyes Jackie and other African Americans cast on medical professionals may have a more specific cause than uneasy racial relations in society at large. A fair number of blacks are convinced, not without reason, that doctors do not always have their best interests at heart. To a degree that confounds many whites, they worry that they could become unwitting subjects in dangerous human experiments.

Tommy, Jackie's father, is one of those leery of doctors' intentions. Tommy told several stories repeatedly, one of them about the harrowing three months he spent in Mount Sinai recovering from his stroke. "When I discovered I couldn't move, boy, that was devastating," he said, slowly shaking his head at the memory. "Buddy, ooh, buddy."

Another subject he regularly injected into casual conversation was how Mount Sinai "experimented" on him after his stroke. "I was afraid to sleep out there. I was a guinea pig," he has said more than once. His evidence for the claim is a purplish vertical scar that runs down the center of his stomach. Hospital records show that Tommy's abdomen was opened up to find the source of persistent abdominal pain that he had developed after his stroke. There is a consent form for the exploratory laparotomy in Tommy's medical record, which he "signed" in an indecipherable scribble. Mrs. Jackson also gave permission for the surgery over the phone. Tommy knows he was in a mental fog during much of his hospitalization and may not remember signing the consent form, but that is not the point. What matters here is how quickly he assumed he was the subject of an experiment.

One of Robert's dialysis buddies, Denny, mentioned similar suspicions about experimentation. He said he was asked to join a clinical trial but refused. The purpose of the experiment, conducted at the Veterans hospital where Denny first received dialysis, was to test a new drug to prevent anemia. "My mom was afraid," said Denny, a retired Navy boiler technician who was in his late twenties when his kidneys failed from uncontrolled high blood pressure. "'Don't let them experiment on you,'" she warned her son. Denny said he became even more adamant about not taking part when, after he declined several times, doctors offered him $500 to participate—a payment he considered tantamount to a bribe.

Dr. Julia Ashenhurst, the chief of clinical hematology/oncology at

Mount Sinai, said she had met many Dennys over the course of her career studying and treating cancer among low-income blacks. "Ever since I can remember, patients have been concerned that they're being experimented on," she said. "It makes it hard to invite people to be part of clinical trials, which is, of course, the only way to really improve cancer treatment."

Tommy's awareness of human experimentation came from direct observation. During his incarceration, he worked as a janitor at the Stateville prison hospital, where from 1945 to the mid-1970s prisoners were infected with malaria to test new drugs. Tommy mopped around the beds of his fellow prisoners who spent weeks in the hospital recovering from malaria, and he also helped breed new batches of mosquitoes—by letting the insects take "blood meals" on his arms. "You could get used to it," he said, referring to the bites that covered his arms. "You can deal with pains. Good God! I've dealt with pains." (By biting already infected prisoners, the mosquitoes Tommy nourished eventually became malaria carriers and spread the disease to new subjects.)[4]

The malaria research began two decades before Tommy entered the maximum security prison, as part of a World War II crash campaign to find alternatives for treating malaria other than quinine. "Many of [the prisoners] suffered from the toxic effects of the experimental drugs," wrote Maurice H. Pappworth, who, as part of a 1967 exposé on human experimentation, examined studies by the Stateville researchers published in the late 1940s, "including abdominal pain which was often severe, loss of appetite, nausea, vomiting, cyanosis (blueness), transient changes in their electrocardiograms, drug fever, skin lesions and marked fall of blood pressure."[5]

Prisoners became crucial cogs in the rapidly expanding pharmaceutical business in the 1950s and 1960s, serving as subjects in the majority of Phase I drug trials, in which healthy people are used to test the toxicity and effectiveness of new compounds. They also participated in other kinds of experiments. *Time* magazine reported in 1963, for example, that prisoners at Cook County Jail in Chicago were injected with blood from leukemia patients to see if the cancer could be transmitted.[6] None of the prisoners developed leukemia, but as Pappworth noted, "*Before* these experiments the possibility that they could have been [infected with leukemia] was quite definite."[7]

For years, prison experimentation was considered harmless. "Prisoners get a valuable feeling of self-respect," *Business Week* proclaimed in a 1964 article.[8] That changed in the late 1960s and early 1970s, when individual rights moved to the forefront of public debate, and a consensus was evolving among the public, lawyers, and ethicists (though not necessarily medical investigators) that prison research was almost inherently coercive. The Nuremberg Code, for instance, which was written after World War II to prevent a repeat of Nazi Germany's horrific concentration camp experiments, said voluntary consent could only be obtained from subjects "so situated as to be able to exercise free power of choice." Unlike the United States, many Western European countries had interpreted that provision to rule out the use of prisoners and other institutionalized populations, such as the mentally ill.

Following a nationwide trend, the Malaria Project at Stateville penitentiary was phased out starting in 1974. Then, four years later, the Department of Health, Education, and Welfare, which funded many of the prison studies, issued regulations that sharply curtailed the use of prisoners in experiments from which they had no hope of benefiting. Today, prisoners' advocates say medical experimentation is not a major concern.

At the time that the malaria project was cancelled, its director, pharmacologist Dr. Paul E. Carson, contended that experiments conducted behind prison walls were no more coercive than those on the outside.[9] But several of Tommy's comments suggest otherwise. To be sure, Tommy favored the medical research, as had most prisoner-subjects interviewed in opinion surveys,[10] and he insisted that his fellow inmates were not forced to participate. Tommy said he did not volunteer to get malaria because he had a job, as a janitor. "I was already getting paid for what I was doing, a dollar a day. That's the only reason any of the others were doing it—for the money."

But as attorney Alvin Bronstein pointed out in 1975, that paltry pay could act as a "coercive force in prison life." Bronstein, who was and is director of the ACLU's prison project in Washington, D.C., used the Stateville research to illustrate his point. An Illinois prisoner could earn from 32 to 55 cents a day for an ordinary prison job, according to 1974 data from the U.S. Justice Department, but such positions were only available to one-third of prisoners. Unemployed prisoners could volunteer for the malaria experiment, however, and earn up to fifty dollars a month.[11]

One California prisoner told a surveyor that he would be "lost" without his medical experiment. "Heh, man, I'm making thirty dollars a month on the DMSO thing [chronic topical application of dimethyl sulfoxide]. I know a couple of guys had to go to the hospital who were on it—and the burns were so bad they had to take *everyone* off for a while. But who gives a shit about that, man? Thirty is a full canteen draw and I wish the thing would go on for years."[12] Journalist Jessica Mitford, who included the California prisoner's quote in her damning account of prison practices, called such bargains the "ultimate exploitation of the prisoner: systematically impoverished by his keepers, denied a decent wage, he is reduced to bartering his body for cigarette and candy money."[13]

Tommy offered one last observation that undercuts the notion that prisoners were "so situated as to be able to exercise free power of choice," as required by the Nuremberg Code. "By working on the [malaria] project," Tommy said, "it increased your chances of getting out." By the 1960s, reduced sentences were not used to entice volunteers to join experiments in U.S. prisons, but inmates almost inevitably held out that hope. Sometimes, researchers did nothing to discourage them. One Iowa doctor instructed his prisoner-subjects that they would not be eligible for early release but at the same time sent a thank-you note to the parole board for each of them. "It is possible," the doctor wrote, "that this letter in the prisoner's file may favorably influence the parole board."[14]

It's tempting to classify prison research as an anomaly, but to blacks it may be viewed as a small piece of a big picture of exploitation by medical investigators. A major source of their suspicion is one of the most unethical (perhaps even criminal, though no charges were ever filed) human experiments ever undertaken: the Tuskegee Syphilis Study. Conducted by the U.S. Public Health Service, the study involved 400 Southern black men who, for forty years, from 1932 to 1972, were not told they had syphilis and were not treated for it so that researchers might discover the "natural history" of the disease. The "end point" of the study, according to its architects, was death, at which point the men were autopsied to see what havoc the disease had wrought on their internal organs. Informed only that they were being treated for "bad blood"—a Southern euphemism for a host of sicknesses—the men were never warned that they could pass the disease to their sex partners or unborn children.[15]

The study started benignly enough. A foundation led by Julius Rosenwald, the longtime president of Sears Roebuck and Co., which was headquartered in North Lawndale until 1973, began in 1929 to fund syphilis testing and treatment projects in several rural, black areas in the South. (In addition to having a strong interest in improving the lives of blacks, Rosenwald was one of the most powerful members of Chicago's Jewish community, embodying the alliance between blacks and Jews that culminated during the Civil Rights movement but disintegrated in the decades after.)

One of the syphilis control efforts began in Macon County, Alabama, where federal epidemiologists discovered that 35 to 40 percent of the population carried the disease. The treatment phase of the project had barely begun when the Depression hit, and Rosenwald's foundation ran short of funds. With their financial support gone, the Public Health Service (PHS) decided that the best way to attract more money for the program was to continue it as a study of untreated syphilis. Poor, uneducated, and isolated in rural Alabama, the men would not have access to treatment, anyway, the government researchers rationalized. If the study showed how devastating the condition was, more money might be forthcoming.

The federal health department hired a trusted black nurse from the community to keep tabs on the men. The PHS also enlisted the cooperation of a nearby black-run teaching hospital located at the Tuskegee Institute, where the men were examined annually to chart the progress of their disease. To entice them to take part, the subjects received free medical care, transportation, and burial stipends.

When the study began, mercury and arsenic were the state-of-the-art therapies to treat syphilis but were so potent that they sometimes killed rather than cured patients. Thus, the government health officials found another rationalization: It wasn't so bad to withhold a treatment that might be as deadly as the disease. Standards about human experimentation and informed consent were much looser during this time, but the experiment lost any veneer of ethical respectability it may have had when penicillin was introduced during World War II. From that point until a PHS whistleblower leaked the story to the media in 1972, the researchers actively prevented the men from receiving penicillin, eventually colluding with local physicians and health departments to keep the drug from the men.

Neither Tommy nor Denny knew directly about Tuskegee, but when Denny was told the basics of the Alabama experiment, he nodded knowingly. "I believe that kind of thing can happen today," he said. "Where do you think AIDS comes from?" Tommy, Jackie, and Robert all hedged when asked whether they believed whites infected blacks with AIDS, but none of them dismissed it outright.

Stephen Thomas, the director of minority health research for the University of Maryland's Department of Health Education, argues that the black community's reluctance to acknowledge AIDS in its midst is perhaps the most tragic result of the mistrust generated by Tuskegee, as well as other abuses of medical authority.[16] For example, many believe that thousands of poor black women were sterilized with federal money during the 1960s and 1970s without their consent—or at least without their informed consent.[17] (The memory of Tuskegee may strangle all kinds of health care initiatives. University of Minnesota ethicist Arthur Caplan, for one, says Tuskegee would doom proposals to provide burial stipends to families as a way of encouraging organ donation.)

One of the few attempts to gauge the extent of blacks' suspicions about AIDS was a 1990 survey of a thousand black church members conducted by the Southern Christian Leadership Conference. More than a third of the respondents believed AIDS was a form of genocide, and another third were unsure. Close to half said that the government was not telling the truth about the disease, and 35 percent were unsure.[18] Thomas suspects that such conspiracy theories are more common among low-income, less-educated blacks, but discussions of the subject have hardly been "ghettoized." Black physicians and scholars have advanced the idea on mainstream black TV programs and in magazines.

To mount a successful AIDS-prevention campaign, health workers must talk candidly about Tuskegee and stop treating the fear of genocide as an irrelevant, fringe belief, Thomas contended. "Given that the conduct of the [Tuskegee] study demonstrated little regard for the lives of the men who participated," Thomas wrote in the *American Journal of Public Health*, "it is no surprise that Blacks today do not readily dismiss assertions that HIV is a manmade virus intentionally allowed to run rampant in their communities."[19]

On one level, a dismissive attitude toward Tuskegee among health educators is understandable. Today, federal regulations explicitly protect human subjects. Institutional Review Boards (IRBs), which are required at all hospitals or universities that conduct federally funded research, decide whether risks to experimental subjects are outweighed by benefits they might receive and potential gains in medical knowledge. IRBs also review procedures for informed consent. With these protections in place, it is hard to imagine that even the most aggressive researcher would seek approval, much less receive it, for anything close to Tuskegee.

But such assurances can ring hollow in a country where racial wounds remain so raw. Harlon Dalton, a Yale Law School professor and member of the National Commission on AIDS, described the difficulties public-health professionals face in educating his race about AIDS in an essay called "AIDS in Blackface." "For most Americans of African descent, our history, especially our trials and tribulations—slavery, discrimination, malign neglect—is a lived thing, something we experience and feel even when we do not know its particulars. We wear Jim Crow like our skin, with precious little choice in the matter. . . . It is, for example, difficult for us to divorce our dealings with white persons as individuals from our dealings with whites who preceded them."[20]

And the truth is, African Americans don't have to search the annals of history (though 1972, the year Tuskegee ended, only barely qualifies as history in the layman's sense of the word) to find instances of medical investigators using them as guinea pigs. In the spring of 1988, the *Chicago Defender*, the city's largest black newspaper, revealed that 240 pregnant women—mostly black or Hispanic—had participated in an experiment at Cook County Hospital without their consent.[21] They were given Dilantin—an anticonvulsant used mainly for epileptics—by an anesthesiologist who wanted to determine whether the drug could increase oxygen flow to children delivered by cesarean section, thereby minimizing fetal distress.

Under the threat of suspension and probation, the anesthesiologist eventually left the hospital, as did his supervisor.[22] Though no physical harm has so far come to the more than 500 mothers and children, the Cook County Board agreed as part of a legal settlement to set aside $1.5 million to compensate the subjects for emotional suffering.

The case suggests several loopholes in Institutional Review Boards' supervision. First, the experiment was not technically governed by federal regulations because it was funded by a private foundation, not by government money. Many large research institutions file "multiple project assurances" with the National Institutes of Health, pledging to follow federal rules for all research, no matter who pays for it. The Hektoen Institute for Medical Research, which is affiliated with Cook County and administers many research projects there, has filed a multiple project assurance with the NIH, but the Dilantin experiment escaped federal regulations because it was not managed by Hektoen. Since Cook County does not have an assurance independent of Hektoen's, technically the hospital did not have to follow NIH standards.[23]

Nonetheless, Cook County Hospital's own rules require that all research involving human subjects be put before its review board. And the protocol for the Dilantin experiment was, indeed, approved by the board. But once an experiment is approved, IRBs typically do not monitor researchers to determine how fully they explain the risks and benefits of clinical trials to potential subjects. In this case, according to one of the attorneys who filed the class-action suit, the doctor tried to obtain consent, but when he wasn't finding enough takers, he decided Dilantin was safe enough to proceed without consent.

Farther from home, but perhaps no less unnerving (or infuriating) to many blacks, were the 1991 revelations that a French scientist had injected eighteen healthy Zairian children with an untested AIDS vaccine. The vaccine was supplied by NIH researchers, who apparently had understood that Frenchman Dr. Daniel Zagury would test the substance on monkeys, not humans. The goings-on in Zaire were bad enough to prompt a general overhaul of the NIH's human subjects' protections in July 1991. A report by a semi-independent watchdog group at the NIH had concluded that no one at the giant health agency had clear responsibility for monitoring research conducted in collaboration with scientists outside the NIH, whether foreign or *domestic*. (The NIH was first alerted to the unethical African experiments by an investigative reporter for the *Chicago Tribune*.) The report went on to note that some government scientists were "unaware" foreign subjects should be afforded the same protections as U.S. subjects.[24]

Poor minorities' heavy use of teaching hospitals is a more mundane but equally powerful reinforcement for their suspicions about experimentation. Not only do more clinical trials take place at teaching hospitals, but, as Mrs. Jackson found out at Mount Sinai, patients are subjected each day to the poking and prodding of as many as a half-dozen different doctors-in-training. When residents receive instruction from senior physicians, they often gather just outside patients' doors, pondering as yet unconsidered causes of illness and new strategies of attack. "It's a different kind of experiment," Caplan, the ethicist, told participants at a 1991 conference on Tuskegee. "You feel like you're being experimented on because the people who are treating you are still in school."

A good argument could be made that such group discussions encourage better care, provided that residents are not dead on their feet from working two days straight, and there may be no other way for new doctors to hone their skills. But a story in the *Chicago Defender* suggests how easily laymen, as well as reporters, may equate untoward experimentation with the everyday care delivered by teaching hospitals. Less than two weeks after the doctor who tested Dilantin on unborn children resigned from Cook County Hospital, an article was published in the newspaper under the headline, "Unauthorized CCH experiments probed."[25] The article cited two cases in which women had died after receiving mismatched blood transfusions. It went on to suggest why the women might have received the wrong blood: "Some County Hospital physicians are routinely conducting unrelated experiments on mostly Black patients which, according to sources, have led to at least two deaths."

The paper's only sources appeared to have been three anonymous letters, parts of which were printed: "'Please look into this problem so it does not happen again. . . . There is no reason why our people should keep dying on the hands of these doctors who are just learnin' their profession.'"

Two women had indeed died at the hospital after they were given mismatched blood. The bad transfusions had nothing to do with a medical experiment—perhaps no less troublesome, negligent medical technicians were to blame—but such stories, true or not, inevitably buttress fears about experimentation.

And finally, in a medical system based on ability to pay, those who have the ability to pay least, the uninsured and Medicaid patients, cannot help but doubt the care they receive. "When you're on the green card, you don't have the big insurance company backing you up," Tommy Markham explained. "The hospital's telling you the green card is only going to cover so much of this and so much of that. They experiment on you [when you have a green card]. They give you different stuffs."

The different stuff may be as potentially harmless as generic drugs, or it may be the more serious difference of an absence of treatment. Medicaid patients, the uninsured, and African Americans—whatever their insurance source—receive fewer coronary diagnostic tests than others, fewer heart bypasses, fewer cesarean sections. They receive less intensive treatment for pneumonia;[26] their sick newborns are discharged earlier than other sick babies.[27] The list goes on.

The perception and the reality of second-class care—including unwanted, experimental care—inescapably stain and strain relationships between medical professionals and poor blacks. And judging from the essay by Yale professor Dalton, doctors and public health workers won't have an easy time convincing blacks that they're on their side. Specifically addressing AIDS, Dalton makes a plea for honest conversations about the deadly disease and attendant fears of genocide. But then he warns: "While we insist that [white public health workers] respectfully come calling, we aren't quite ready to put out the welcome mat. When you predictably bridle at our lack of hospitality, we will peer into your soul to determine whether you are simply one more white person who can't stand to see black folks asserting themselves. But even if we decide that your pique is justified (in the sense that you truly have embraced our concerns and are anxious to work with us), we will expect you to be sympathetic to our predicament while we argue that you cannot expect us to be sympathetic to yours.

"Perhaps that is a lot to ask. But we as a nation must play the hand that slavery has dealt us. We cannot undo history, except through long, hard struggle."[28]

13

Life-sustaining technology

M rs. Jackson's remaining leg was amputated two weeks after the originally scheduled surgery date, and Jackie's hope for her grandmother's recovery had been renewed—but just "for a minute," as she would say. "This lady down the street had the same thing happen to her," Jackie said shortly before the operation. "They nipped and nipped. But once both legs were gone, she was a new person. That extra leg, Mom's not using it. It's just hanging." Though Jackie may sound cold, one of Mrs. Jackson's doctors, resident Dr. Kyu-Jang Oh, made a similar observation some months before. "Unless you condition that one limb, it's more of a burden than anything," he said, explaining that people who've lost one leg often are harder to care for than those who've lost both.

But Mrs. Jackson did not fare as well as the lady down the street. Her body no longer had to fight off the infection that emanated from her foot, but new problems surfaced and other old ones refused to let go. Doctors had given her a diuretic to control the fluid buildup in her lungs, but the medication did not work properly because her kidneys had begun to fail. (Another medication eventually was more successful.) Chronic anemia, prevalent among the sick elderly, sapped Mrs. Jackson's strength and required that she undergo periodic blood transfusions. She came down with pneumonia, another illness that plagues weak patients who are hospitalized for a long time.

Mrs. Jackson also had not been eating well. So, soon after doctors amputated her left leg, they operated on her again, inserting a gastrostomy tube that allowed nutrients to be pumped directly into her stomach. Subsequently, endocrinologists struggled to find a combination of nutrients and insulin that would bring Mrs. Jackson's fluctuating blood sugars under control. Some days she was so lethargic she did not open her eyes when nurses entered her room; other days, she perked up a bit. "I want to go home and be with my children for Christmas," she hopefully told one nurse.

Meanwhile, Jackie worried whether there would be any Christmas to come home to. She sat on the living room couch next to Latrice, whom she had just finished quizzing on her spelling homework. The family was living in the front of the apartment because a rat had been occupying the kitchen and back bedroom for the past couple of days. Until the traps Robert set did their work, Jackie planned to keep the swinging door between the kitchen and living room latched shut. She had even taped a piece of plastic over the door's window, necessary because the landlord had never replaced the glass.

Snapping her book shut, Latrice handed her mother her Christmas list. On it were rap music cassettes, a teen magazine called *Fresh*, and a Precious Cottage doll house.

"Don't you want the mansion?" Jackie asked, studying her daughter's face.

"That costs sixty dollars," Latrice mumbled. Though only eleven, she recognized her mother's financial pressures and did not want to burden her more.

"Sixty dollars is chicken feed," Jackie retorted.

She hated not being able to buy her kids more of what they wanted. Making Christmas merry would be a challenge this year, considering that Robert's drug use had depleted their finances, not to mention their affection. And as usual, Jackie also was concerned about her grandmother.

"Me and my kids might hop the 'L' [elevated train] and see the Christmas tree," Jackie offered, referring to a towering tree that is decorated every year in Daley Plaza. But she hesitated. "But I want the whole family to hop the 'L,' Robert, to go, too." Disgusted with Robert or not, she clung to the ideal of a "whole" family.

Even though Jackie encouraged Latrice to ask for a sixty dollar Christmas present, she was not sure she could afford the much less expensive trip downtown. Train fare would cost only six dollars since the children could ride for reduced rates, but Jackie did not think it would be any fun if they did not at least go to McDonald's for lunch. And what if the kids begged for popcorn or candy apples from street vendors?

Latrice had offered to pay for everyone, with money she had earned from walking her cousin to school, but it embarrassed Jackie to take her daughter's savings. "I won't let her do it," she said. No matter how bad things got, Jackie did not want her children to start feeling as if they had to take care of her. She was the parent; the kids were her responsibility, not the other way around.

Jackie was not as confident about taking charge of her grandmother. "You have to think of Mama like a baby," she said once. "But I can judge Brianna easier than I can judge Mama because Brianna's mine, and I think I know what to do." The responsibility became particularly uncomfortable for Jackie when she had to decide whether to put her grandmother in a nursing home.

The artificial feeding forced the issue. Although Mount Sinai's home health agency assists families with home tube-feeding, Jackie wanted no part of it. "I don't want to be responsible for that. God, I do enough already. Nursing homes are equipped to handle people with tubes." But later in December, after a spartan Christmas for the Baneses and a lonely one for Mrs. Jackson, when one of the hospital social workers began pestering Jackie to choose a home for her grandmother, her resolve slipped.

"I even told the social worker I was immobilized," Jackie said. "Could we do it all over the phone?" she asked her. No, that wouldn't work, the social worker said. "I lied to her and told her I made an appointment [to visit a nursing home]. . . . I don't really want to put her in a nursing home. I feel like the devil doing that."

Jackie sometimes sensed that her grandmother's family—Mrs. Jackson's sister, Eldora, and her only brother lived in Chicago—did not trust her judgment. A few days before Mrs. Jackson's left leg was amputated, her brother went to visit her for the first time since she had been hospitalized. He called Jackie afterward, crying. "He begged me not to have the other one taken off. I told him, 'I am not God.'" Jackie had even detected a hint of accusation in her grandmother's voice after her first amputation. "I didn't know they took my leg off," she told Jackie. "Well, you signed the papers, Mama," Jackie said, sighing.

The pleas of Mrs. Jackson's brother were all the more troubling to Jackie because she doubted her own motivations when she made decisions for her grandmother. Did she want her to go to a nursing home for the wrong reasons, or conversely, did she want her *home* for the wrong reasons? "I don't want to deny her [nursing home care] just so we can have that $600 coming in here; I feel like she need the help the nursing home could give her. I don't want the [Social Security] checks to be the only reason I want her back home."

With that in mind, Jackie went to visit California Gardens nursing home, located a couple of miles away from her apartment and across the street from the Cook County Jail. She thought the place looked clean enough, and she liked the nearby location. "We can visit her whenever we want," Jackie said, pleased that the nursing home, unlike Mount Sinai, allowed children to visit.

But the guilt persisted. Sometimes, when it threatened to get the better of her, Jackie thought back to when she was in high school, when Mrs. Jackson brought her own mother up from Mississippi. The old woman's mind had faltered, but no one was left down South to care for her. After seventy-seven years in rural Mississippi, the urban landscape played tricks on the woman's failing senses. "Down South, she would depend on the screen door for security," Jackie said. But in Chicago: "She would look out the window and think that the chimney stacks were people coming toward her." Jackie remembered entering the kitchen in the middle of the night to find her great-grandmother bent over the stove warming a hot comb to straighten her hair. It was as if the diminutive old woman had become someone else; she had never pressed her hair before. She almost always wore a head scarf, and her long, gray hair was not kinky in the first place.

To try to protect her mother, Mrs. Jackson removed the knobs from the stove. She kept her from wandering by putting her in a recliner and tying a sheet around her lap. "But she managed to wriggle her way out," Jackie said. After several months, Mrs. Jackson decided it was not safe to keep her mother at home and put her in a nursing home. Soon after, she died. "Mama did for her mother what I'm doing for her. She got to know what I'm going through because she went through it. She didn't last as long as I did."

By the beginning of the new year, Jackie was as firm as she could be about sending her grandmother to a nursing home; she had begun to remove the tattered plastic slipcover from her grandmother's couch, which she had not done earlier in deference to Mrs. Jackson's wishes. The decision seemed final.

But Mrs. Jackson would not leave Mount Sinai for quite some time. Her first planned discharge was called off at the last minute when doctors discovered the pneumonia. After that, discharge orders were written for her several times but always rescinded at the eleventh hour. Better one day, she would fall sick the next. Her blood sugars shot up, then plummeted, her fever spiked. "The fever is never really gone," Jackie said. "It just hides for a while." Mrs. Jackson suffered from diarrhea; she developed another bedsore on her thigh. At the beginning of February, she had a few good days and might have been transferred to California Gardens, but the nursing home no longer had a bed.

Another nursing home, Jackson Square, rejected her, too, probably because she carried the MRSA bacteria, explained Dr. Mark Levin, Mount Sinai's chief of infectious diseases. During Mrs. Jackson's hospitalization, Dr. Levin concluded that eradicating the bacteria was hopeless because of her open bed sores. The MRSA was not making Mrs. Jackson sick, but nursing homes did not want her for fear she would transmit it to others, although most homes already had patients who carried the bacteria. MRSA can cause pneumonia or other diseases but in many cases lies dormant, as do countless other harmless bacteria. "We take a lot of protective measures for something that may not cause any problems at all," Dr. Levin explained. "We basically ended up with a group of MRSA lepers."

Rejection of MRSA patients may violate federal law prohibiting discrimination against the handicapped, but public health officials and nursing home advocates have not pressed the case. "There are places that feel comfortable accepting residents with MRSA, so the residents are probably better off going there than some place that doesn't want them," said Dr. John Lumpkin, who at the time supervised nursing home regulation for the Illinois Department of Public Health. Attorneys who represent nursing home clients begrudgingly agreed. They hate letting inadequate nursing homes off the hook—state law requires all homes, with or without MRSA residents, to follow infection control procedures—but they do not know how to pursue the case without endangering their clients.

So Mrs. Jackson's stay in Mount Sinai dragged on. The window of wellness for her transfer to a nursing home was a small one; after California Gardens and Jackson Square refused to take her in early February, her anemia worsened and she could not go anywhere until it improved. Treating her illnesses was like fighting a brush fire; once doctors extinguished one blaze, another burst into flames. Nonetheless, during more than four months of hospitalization, doctors never talked with Mrs. Jackson or Jackie about whether the old woman's quality of life justified taking every measure to prolong it. That meant the artificial feeding was started without discussion of other options, or of the long-term ramifications of that choice. It also meant that if Mrs. Jackson's heart had stopped during her stay at Mount Sinai, a "code blue" would have been called: nurses and doctors would have rushed to her bedside and tried to revive her with cardiopulmonary resuscitation. CPR is routinely performed unless a patient or family, in consultation with doctors, decides that a do-not-resuscitate (DNR) order should be written.

Medical literature is filled with articles that describe doctors' reluctance to discuss forgoing treatment with patients, whatever their class or race.[1] But there is good reason to believe that the poor and poorly educated have perhaps the least say of anybody in decisions about lifesustaining treatment.

To begin with, most doctors relate better to patients whose backgrounds are similar to theirs'. "Affluent people always get more informed consent; physicians respect them more," said Dr. Ronald Cranford, an influential Minneapolis neurologist and the chairman of the American Academy of Neurology's ethics committee.

Another oft-repeated generalization is that the poor are less likely to ask questions that lead to meaningful informed consent. "In our experience, poor families are either in the dark about what's going on, or they have complete trust in doctors," said John Arras, a medical ethicist at Montefiore Medical Center, which serves low-income blacks and Hispanics who live in its New York City neighborhood. The poorer people are, Arras said, the less likely they are to debate quality-of-life issues. "If anything, they are more concerned about getting access to care."

Illinois health care professionals point to the case of Rudy Linares as a tragic example of what can happen when the poor are left out of controversial bioethical decisions. In April 1989, Linares held Rush-Presbyterian hospital staff at gunpoint while he disconnected his permanently comatose son from a respirator. "He was a working-class kind of guy," said Mary Deering, a nurse who helped run Mount Sinai's ethics committee. "If he had had a lot of education and family support, he would have sat down and hashed out the problem with doctors."

In Mrs. Jackson's case, the first decision to initiate long-term lifesustaining treatment came when doctors decided to feed her through the tube surgically implanted in her stomach. The residents who provided most of her day-to-day care were under the leadership of internist Dr. Burton Stone, who had replaced Dr. Gurevich as Mrs. Jackson's attending physician. Dr. Stone said he made an attempt to include Mrs. Jackson in the discussion but determined she was not competent to choose one way or another. "Her clarity was up and down," Dr. Stone said. "We decided [tube feeding] would be in her best interest."

It is easy to criticize that kind of reasoning. As Arras, the New York City ethicist, said, "The fact that someone waxes and wanes is only an argument not to talk to her [about treatment choices] when she's waning. Talk to her when she's lucid." But in the trenches, finding the right time to introduce the subject may seem impossible. Like all attending physicians, Dr. Stone saw his hospitalized patients for only a short time each day, and Mrs. Jackson had many bad days. Proof of that is found in the nurses' notes in her medical record: "Pt. is not responding . . . to verbal stimuli. Is responding to painful stimuli with short moans." Another time, "Opens eyes at intervals to see what is being done to her." Even when she was alert and feeling better, she frequently seemed disoriented.

"I'm going home," Mrs. Jackson announced one day in mid-February, smiling broadly. "I can see it from here." Though her fifth-floor window faced the direction of her apartment, it was about a mile away; the only view she had was of Douglas Park.

"DeMarest and Latrice slept with me last night," she continued.

The children had never spent the night at the hospital, and, sadly, Mrs. Jackson had not had many visitors at all lately. For a couple of weeks she became an "MRSA leper" to her family, too. The hospital had suggested that everyone who enter her room wear a mask and gloves, and Tommy and Mrs. Jackson's sister were scared away. Jackie refused to wear the mask. "I feel like if I wear a mask I might frighten my grandmother. I feel funny approaching her that way." But the MRSA made Jackie squeamish about visiting as often; she did not want to risk transmitting the bacteria to her children or her sick husband. If they were as harmless as doctors said, why all the fuss about masks and gloves?

Jackie's despair about Mrs. Jackson's condition also kept her away from the hospital. Her grandmother's face was so gaunt, her skin peeling, she hardly said a word. Jackie remembered dragging herself to the hospital one day, sure that her grandmother would be uncommunicative, maybe, she feared, even dead. "I walked in and she said, 'Where you been?' I ran into the bathroom and got on my knees and said, 'Thank you, God.'"

Mrs. Jackson had noticed the decline in visitors. She refused to entertain the notion that her family's visits had diminished because they were frustrated at their inability to help her get better. "They can come up here anytime," she said curtly, implying that the company of her family was what she wanted. She did not expect them to cure her.

Unusually talkative that day, Mrs. Jackson volunteered that she had celebrated her birthday the day before (actually, her birthday was that day) and that she was now sixty-nine years old (she had turned seventy). There were no birthday cards in her room, only relics from Christmas. On her bedside table sat a dusty plastic poinsettia. Tied to the artificial flowers was a shiny silver balloon printed with a message in almost unbelievably bad taste: HOPE YOU'RE UP ON YOUR FEET AGAIN SOON.

None of Mrs. Jackson's comments prove that she was incompetent or otherwise—patients who are hospitalized for a long time lose track of time and place but still may be able to participate in treatment decisions—but they shed light on Dr. Stone's hesitation about giving her the chance to refuse artificial feeding. Dr. Stone could have asked residents to raise the subject with her when she seemed lucid, but he chose not to.[2] When it came down to it, Dr. Stone, a devoutly religious man, one who is very cautious about making choices that might accelerate a patient's death, really did not consider the withholding of feeding to be an option.

At this stage of Mrs. Jackson's illness, many doctors would have decided likewise, though not necessarily rightly so, cautioned Stanford University physicians John Ruark and Thomas Raffin in the *New England Journal of Medicine.* "Although few of us may know what it feels like to undergo cardiopulmonary resuscitation or heart transplantation, we all know what it is like to be hungry, thirsty, or short of breath. Health care professionals may provide these basics of care almost as a reflex, without considering whether they are performing a truly caring act. [E]very medical intervention should serve what patients consider to be their best interests as determined in an active dialogue with their families and their physicians."[3]

Jackie did sign a consent form to allow tube feeding, but she was not told enough to make a well-informed choice. She said she approved the artificial nutrition after doctors told her it was the best way to go. They did not say forgoing tube feeding was an option, and she did not ask about it. "They made it sound good, she would never get hungry," Jackie said.

Mary Deering was not surprised at the way the tube-feeding choice was presented. "When I've heard it asked, it's couched in terms of 'Do you want your relative to starve to death, or die of thirst?'" No one told Jackie that there was little hope of her grandmother getting much better, that the tube feeding probably would continue indefinitely, even if her grandmother had a second stroke and fell into a coma, or about any of the other consequences of starting a treatment that is rarely stopped.

That last fact suggests why it may be particularly important for families and patients to make careful, educated decisions about the procedure. While doctors and hospital administrators may be reluctant to with*hold* artificial nutrition or respiration, they are even more reluctant to with*draw* them. Most ethicists say the distinction is meaningless, and Jackie, for one, agreed. "I would want to put any of my family members on a machine to see if they could pull through," she said, adding that she hoped doctors would follow that course were she to become seriously ill: "Throw me on the machine for a while, then cut it off if it doesn't work."

That sounds sensible enough, but of course, things don't work that way. First, some doctors, who have vowed "to do no harm," refuse to take what seems to be an active hand in death. Dr. Stone's religious convictions keep him from pulling the plug, and he has qualms about referring patients to another physician who he knows will do so. "That might be like hiring a hit man," he said.

The long arm of malpractice law also has interfered, pulling the strings at the bedside while doctors and hospitals watch helplessly. Or at least that's the way many health care professionals perceive it, and perception is as powerful as reality.[4] Although very few doctors have been sued for withholding or withdrawing treatment, a deep-seated fear exists in the profession that removing a respirator or feeding tube (rather than just withholding one) increases the chances of getting slapped with a lawsuit. "Concerns about liability overwhelm doctors' ability to think logically," said the Minneapolis neurologist, Dr. Cranford. "They don't ask themselves what's best for the patient, they ask, 'What's legal?'" Such defensive medicine may be more widespread among doctors who treat low-income patients because of another myth: that the poor sue more.[5]

To be sure, in the late 1980s, removing lifesustaining treatment became especially difficult in Illinois for certain categories of patients. The right to refuse treatment is governed by varied state laws and judicial rulings, but the trend in most places had been toward allowing families to make decisions for relatives too incapacitated to do so. Running contrary to that, the Illinois Supreme Court ruled in 1989 that doctors and hospitals must get a court order before removing nutrition and hydration from an "incompetent" patient, a category that may or may not have included Mrs. Jackson.[6] Competent patients were not addressed by the court, but the ruling undoubtedly had a chilling effect on everyone. State senator John D'Arco Jr. noted as much a year later, after the failure of legislation that would have nullified the state Supreme Court opinion, giving families the authority to shut off life support without judicial review. "I think hospitals today are going to . . . be more afraid to exercise their right to pull the plug on patients who are dying because we did not pass this bill," D'Arco said.[7]

While Jackie and her grandmother were at least asked to sign a consent for tube feeding, they were not consulted at all about another key decision to prolong Mrs. Jackson's life. Mrs. Jackson was never asked whether she would want to be artificially resuscitated were her heart to stop. The default position, then, was to administer CPR in all circumstances. CPR commonly involves thirty to sixty minutes of pounding on a patient's chest, giving electric shocks with a defibrillator, inserting a breathing tube into the trachea, and injecting cardiac stimulants. If it works, the procedure literally brings people back to life, although some are left with broken ribs, burns, and brain damage.

Dr. Stone said he did not discuss a do-not-resuscitate (DNR) order with Mrs. Jackson or her family members because he still saw hope for his patient. She seemed comfortable most of the time, he said, and the feeding tube enabled her to receive nutrients and medication without intrusive intravenous lines. "Once you start talking DNR, you're sending out a message. Psychologically, it has an impact on how the staff approach that patient. It's 'Why should I bust my chops for this patient? I've been here sixteen hours; I'm emotionally and physically wiped out,'" Dr. Stone said. "If it's a tie score [between two patients who need care], who gets the call?" The belief that medical staff will abandon patients labeled DNR is reportedly widespread, though many observers discount it.[8]

That Dr. Stone rejected the DNR option without consulting Mrs. Jackson or her family, instead relying on his personal judgment of her best interest, has "tremendous potential for abuse," according to Dr. Stuart Youngner, co-director of Case Western Reserve University's Center for Biomedical Ethics and an expert on DNR orders. "Physicians may use [the concept of best interest or therapeutic privilege] to promote their own values or notions about what constitutes an acceptable quality of life, which may be quite different from those of the patient," Dr. Youngner wrote in a 1987 article on DNR orders. "Physicians can also use it to protect themselves, rather than their patients, from painful discussions about poor prognosis and death. In fact, patients usually sense when things are going badly. They are grateful when a trusted physician is willing to discuss these matters openly."[9]

Dr. Youngner's article mentioned another factor that keeps doctors from initiating discussions about life-sustaining treatment: they get so busy firefighting that they can't see the forest for the trees. He described the phenomenon as one in which doctors get mired in processing each new bit of medical information and forget about a patient's overall condition. "Decision makers may choose to focus on individual organ systems and biological functions," the psychiatrist wrote, "where understanding and control seem more palpable."[10] That mind set seemed to underlie one of Dr. Stone's explanations as to why he had not discussed resuscitation with Mrs. Jackson. "Her sacral decubitus [bedsore] is pink and clean," he said one day in February, enthusiastically noting that the infection had cleared. "I see daylight."

Dr. Stone was aware of the danger of concentrating on individual medical problems rather than the patient as a whole, but he conceded that he was not always successful in attending to the big picture. He had been so wrapped up trying to treat Mrs. Jackson's multiple illnesses, for example, that he neglected to reorder physical and occupational therapy to build back her strength. "You can be following a patient for a long time, and you get locked into certain priorities," he said, adding that there was no good excuse for his lapse. "In medicine, you get what you look for."

As that exchange suggests, Dr. Stone was uncommonly willing to explore the wisdom of his decisions. When asked about the physical and occupational therapy, he did not get defensive or deny responsibility. He said he wished that more of his poor patients had advocates to keep him on his toes. Moreover, though many doctors would deny that their personal beliefs shape life-and-death decisions about patients, Dr. Stone eventually was willing to share his struggle to come to terms with what he considered new, although increasingly mainstream attitudes about lifesustaining treatment.

Dr. Stone is a devoted Orthodox Jew. He has twice taken yearlong leaves-of-absence to study Jewish law in Israel, and from all accounts, he is one of the most widely respected members of Chicago's Orthodox community. Mount Sinai administrator Diane Dubey, herself Orthodox, said, "He's regarded by the most religious people in the community as, I hate to say 'saintly' because it's not a Jewish word, but that may be the best way to describe it." Indeed, he is known among Chicago's Orthodox Jews as one of the rare *lamedvovniks*, Hebrew for the thirty-six righteous men in each generation on whose account God does not destroy the world.

Though Orthodox Judaism has many variants, its leaders generally interpret Jewish law to mean that patients must accept treatment to preserve every possible moment of life, unless death is unequivocally imminent.[11] Defining that point is, of course, difficult; for Dr. Stone, it means "waiting a long time with DNR."

But his approach to life-and-death issues cannot be summed up in a few generalities about his religious faith. Judaism undoubtedly imbues his life, but he continues to explore other ethical concepts: in his personal writings, as a member of Mount Sinai's ethics committee, and as a participant in university-sponsored bioethics workshops. "Explore" is perhaps too mild a word for the way Dr. Stone approaches medical ethics; sometimes he's fairly breathless from the energy he expends wrestling with ethical questions, not to mention the schedule he keeps.

Just before 9 A.M. one Tuesday, Dr. Stone walked quickly into the crowded confines of the Ark, an agency on the North Side of Chicago that he helped found twenty years ago to provide a wide array of medical, social, and legal services for poor Jews. At the time the Ark opened, Dr. Stone and his fellow founders were considered rabble-rousers by the mainstream Jewish community. A rabbi who works at the Chicago Rabbinical Council described the attitude back then: "Poor Jews? There aren't any poor Jews." Today, though, the Ark gets significant financial support from the Jewish Federation.

Head down, Dr. Stone made a beeline for the back of the clinic and slipped into a small medical supply room, where he emptied a plastic grocery bag. It contained a peanut butter jar full of urine and two test tubes of blood, the products of a patient whom Dr. Stone had already visited at home that morning.

He hung his tall black hat on a nail, replacing it with a yarmulke. Dr. Stone has a full brown beard flecked with gray, but the skullcap could not hide the fact that the fifty-five-year-old physician is going bald; only a few wisps of hair fringed it.

Dr. Stone seemed at home at the Ark. The clinic does not charge for any of its services or take insurance because, according to Dr. Stone, billing Medicaid and Medicare was too much trouble. Dr. Stone considers his medical practice an extension of his Jewish obligation to serve others and will not refuse any patient who cannot pay. But with a large family to support, he also has to make a living. He views his life as a balancing act of competing responsibilities, to his family, to the Jewish community, to the broader Chicago community, to the world at large.

"The theme for today is survival," he announced as he walked into a small room to greet the first of twenty-four patients whom he would examine in the next five hours. Some of the patients were quite ill; others were emotionally disturbed; and still others were newly settled Russian-Jews more concerned about making better lives for their children than about their own failing health. What many of them had in common according to Dr. Stone was that they were "survivors." One lady in particular stood out. She was well past eighty and carried only 64 pounds on her 5 foot 4 inch frame. Her eyes bulged in a sunken, wrinkled face; she looked breakable, as if her bones might crack under the pressure of walking.

"How do you feel?" Dr. Stone asked loudly. She was hard of hearing.

"Not good, doctor," she said in a raspy, accented voice. "I feel bad; I feel bad."

"Would you want to move to another place?" Dr. Stone suggested gently. She shook her head sadly, her eyes brimming with tears. She lived on her own, without friends or family for help, but had consistently refused to go to a nursing home. She probably needed to be in an institution, Dr. Stone reckoned, but he was reluctant to initiate guardianship proceedings to have her forcibly removed when she so wanted to stay in her own home. She rested her head in a skeletal hand. Then she pointed to her leg.

"That's a vein," Dr. Stone blared, referring to the thick blue vessel. "Are you taking the medicine?"

"My hearing is gone. Too much upset, too much upset," she croaked.

Dr. Stone wrote his question on a prescription pad and pushed it over to her.

"Sure," she answered softly. At Dr. Stone's request she produced her pill bottles as proof. She had mild hypertension and arthritis, her vision and hearing had deteriorated, but most of all, she was lonely, Dr. Stone said. After promising to see her again in a couple of weeks, he helped her to the door.

To some, this woman might exemplify the dark side of survival— "That's not living; that's just surviving." But to Dr. Stone, survival itself could be a goal, and one woman's darkness was not necessarily another's. He told of a seriously ill stroke patient who was referred to him by another physician. The geriatrician asked Dr. Stone to take the case because he felt uncomfortable acceding to the wishes of the patient's husband, who wanted all measures taken to prolong his wife's life. A stroke had left the woman with severe, seemingly irreversible brain damage, and she could not speak or move. Yet Dr. Stone saw a spark pass between the couple which he felt obliged to keep burning. "The only way she would eat was if he fed her," Dr. Stone remembered, his eyes distant as if conjuring the scene of the elderly man carefully spooning food into his wife's mouth. "There was a special connection between this lady and her husband."

And sometimes survival was rewarded with a light that could not escape anyone's notice. One of Dr. Stone's favorite patients was an elderly Soviet emigré who for some years was confined to bed because of an inoperable brain tumor. The man was barely able to communicate with his wife, who tended to his every need. The situation looked hopeless, especially when he had to be hospitalized at Mount Sinai with septicemia, a life-threatening blood poisoning. At the time, residents asked Dr. Stone whether a DNR order should be issued for him, and the physician suggested that they wait a while. During the next few days, the man's wife complained that her husband could not hear, so doctors had his ears cleaned. And, as is the inevitable climax to the story, the man recovered. His eyes began to move in response to sounds. He spoke for the first time in years. He learned to sit up, then walk. He and his wife eventually embarked on what Dr. Stone called a "second honeymoon," traveling the Midwest by bus. The man had suffered a stroke and was quite ill once again, but he had been gifted with two good years. Dr. Stone pointed to the sky to explain the man's recovery. "I don't want to use spooky terms," Dr. Stone said, "but they got a present."

Yet for all his stories of survival, Dr. Stone acknowledged the perils of basing his medical practice on several successful cases. "The question is, how many people do you torture because one person made it," he said, pushing back his yarmulke and furiously scratching his head. Dr. Stone did not think he was torturing Mrs. Jackson, but he said he felt more comfortable considering termination of treatment for patients whose values he intimately understood, such as the Jews who visited the Ark. "I don't want to manipulate anybody to my way of thinking," he said. "At the same time, I don't want to compromise myself."

At the very least, Dr. Stone said that whatever patients' race or culture, he liked to establish relationships with them before delving into sensitive life-and-death matters. With the Russian-Jewish patient, for example, he said he automatically understood what the man's wife wanted, though he exchanged only a few words with her. "I looked at her, and she looked at me. She says, 'Please,'" Dr. Stone recalled. "It was understood: Do whatever you can." But such intimate relationships are often impossible in North Lawndale. Dr. Stone never laid eyes on Mrs. Jackson until November; he picked her up because he had been on call the afternoon she came through the emergency room. Other times, Dr. Gurevich had been notified when Mrs. Jackson came to the ER, but Jackie had not accompanied her grandmother that day, and evidently her voluminous medical record could not be located.

So worried that he might be imposing his biases on others, Dr. Stone at one point tried to persuade Mount Sinai's ethics committee to hire a "DNR coordinator" to fully discuss termination of life support with patients and families. He raised the possibility at one of the committee's regular meetings, but most of the other members dismissed it. They said it was the physician's job to get the information.

"But I don't have the time and patience to do this," Dr. Stone protested, explaining that many patients assigned to him were complete strangers, without family to give him insight into their beliefs.

"Are you abdicating your responsibility?" a hospital board member asked coolly.

It seemed an unfair question to ask someone whose shoulders almost seemed to sag under the burden of responsibility he felt toward patients, toward humanity even, and Dr. Stone struggled to answer it. "I'm recognizing the areas that I'm weak in," he said, defeated, "the areas that I need help in."

"I don't know about getting an FTE for this," an administrator chimed in.

"What is an FTE?" Dr. Stone asked. The administrator explained that it stood for full-time-equivalent staff position. In other words, no one was sure whether Mount Sinai could come up with the money to pay a DNR coordinator.

Puzzled over FTEs, pulling the plastic from his precooked kosher meal of chicken and green beans while everyone else lunched on deep-dish pizza and Caesar salad, Dr. Stone looked like what he sometimes said he felt like: an anachronism. When he called himself an anachronism, he was referring to his old-fashioned attitudes toward life and death, but other aspects of him fit that description, too. Consider a medical school dean's account of accompanying his doctor/father on housecalls during the 1940s: "I can remember being impressed by the consistently warm welcomes he received. Always he was offered tea, cakes, or cookies by people anxious to hear what he had to say and grateful for his presence. And my father—he seemed to know everyone's friends and relatives. He was full of reminiscences which he and his patients shared. Every visit was an occasion for warm conversation in addition to the medical treatments."[12]

Waiting for Dr. Stone when he arrived at the Ark was a plate of cookies baked by an admirer, which he later wolfed down as a late lunch en route to a house call. And as much as he treated his twenty-four patients that day, he treated them kindly. Instead of seating patients on the examining table, Dr. Stone showed many of them to the chair next to his desk, where they plied him with tales of woe about their bodies, their families, their neighbors, and so on. He counseled a woman who was trying to muster courage to leave an abusive boyfriend; he gave an emotionally disturbed woman referrals for homeless shelters. Some of the encounters were not so grim. A grandmother showed Dr. Stone pictures of her family and a blanket she had crocheted. After another elderly woman whose blood pressure had spiked admitted that she had eaten salty herring and potatoes, Dr. Stone engaged her in a lively discussion of *cholent*, a pot of stew that Orthodox Jews traditionally put on the stove to simmer throughout the Sabbath when they are forbidden to cook.

Dr. Stone, who considers himself a "matchmaker" hooking people to needed services, medical and otherwise, said the chatty appointments were a good way to keep tabs on patients' physical well-being, but sometimes he simply provided a few minutes of companionship. A witty story teller, Dr. Stone reminisced about an eighty-year-old woman who visited him regularly, though she never had a specific complaint. "But one day she came in, drew a deep breath, and I finally thought she was going to tell me her problem. 'Doctor,' she said, 'I'm taking this biology course at Roosevelt University, and I want you to explain miosis.'"

The Ark's volunteer pharmacist, retiree Sam Solomon, praised Dr. Stone—when he was sure the physician would not overhear. Many of Dr. Stone's acquaintances warned that he detested compliments. "He sees what he's doing as nothing out of the ordinary; he's doing what God expects him to do," an Orthodox rabbi said. Another observer explained his modesty this way: "When man stops believing in God, he starts believing in other men." But the pharmacist did not bother comparing Dr. Stone to God; he had Marcus Welby in mind. "You don't see a doctor like this anymore," Solomon said passionately. "People are having problems with their kids, their family, he consoles them."

While Dr. Stone was up-to-date about the goings-on in his patients' lives, they knew personal details about him, too. A half-dozen wished him well on an upcoming two-week vacation to attend a family wedding. "If you need to make more vacation, I'll wait," one elderly woman clucked. "He's very much nice, not just medically but socially; it is very rare," another patient offered. And the pharmacist, while lauding Dr. Stone as a physician, emphasized that he was more than that. Dr. Stone was transformed at jubilant Orthodox weddings, Solomon said. "You should see him jumping up and down dancing."

Watching Dr. Stone care for his Jewish patients was a joy; the sadness was that Mrs. Jackson did not get that from Dr. Stone or any other health care professional. If trusting relationships have not been formed between doctors and patients *outside* of the hospital, they are unlikely ever to happen. "Neither house staff nor attending physicians can linger at the bedside, not because they are uncaring or poorly trained, but because the external pressures to move on to the next case are overwhelming," writes medical historian David Rothman. "On the wards, doctors typically scramble from crisis to crisis. No sooner do they stabilize a patient and get her on the road to recovery, than she is discharged and the next acutely ill patient takes the bed."[13]

That reality inevitably precludes many strong relationships between physicians and poor, inner-city patients, since so many first meet their doctors in that institutional hospital setting. Even for those who have a family physician in the same way that Mrs. Jackson had Dr. Marino, the bonds are tenuous. As happened in her case, doctors in poor neighborhoods often have to abandon their patients when they are hospitalized. And they may not connect well with their patients in the first place. In 1989, approximately eleven doctors had storefront practices in North Lawndale. Physician profiles from the American Medical Association showed that none of them were born in the United States, or went to medical school here. Four were educated in India; two in Korea; the rest in Egypt, Lebanon, the Philippines, China, and Yugoslavia. Though making generalizations about doctors' rapport with patients based on their birthplaces and medical schools is dangerous, it's probably safe to say that few doctors in North Lawndale understood the rhythms of living black, or Hispanic, or poor as well as Dr. Stone understood living Jewish.

As far as the limited issue of artificial life support, the irony is that Dr. Stone's "cultural sensitivity" may well have gotten in the way. Wary of offending, not wanting to overstep his bounds or risk conflict with blacks and others whose beliefs were not second nature to him, he did not engage Jackie in a dialogue about what her grandmother might have wanted concerning further medical treatment. He did not probe Mrs. Jackson or Jackie to learn what they considered a life worth living.

Jackie liked Dr. Stone, at least a lot better than Dr. Gurevich, who had vanished as if he had never existed, even though he had followed Mrs. Jackson for nine months. Jackie thought Dr. Gurevich had been brusque and unwilling to "bring things down to the lowest common denominator." (His thick Russian accent did not help.) As a result, it did not occur to her to ask that he be brought back on her grand-mother's case. Dr. Stone is anything but brusque, and Jackie appreci-ated that. "He seemed a little soft-spoken," Jackie said. "He didn't have a bad word to say."

This is not to say that Jackie would have been eager to talk about terminating treatment for her grandmother, but then again, few fami-lies are. It would have been helpful had Dr. Stone or another physician patiently asked Mrs. Jackson about her wishes before she fell so ill that her competence could be called into question. That way, Jackie would have had some information to go on. "I hate being put on the spot," Jackie brooded. "I wish she could make her own choices." Jackie would not have independently investigated her grandmother's thoughts about prolonging life, or dying. "She already thinks we're neglecting her," she said.

Doctors cannot expect families to take the lead, counseled the Stanford physicians, Dr. Ruark and Dr. Raffin. Attending physicians must assume the delicate task of asking patients and families when they might want to allow death in the door unimpeded, the two doc-tors wrote.[14] As far as Mrs. Jackson was concerned, that meant, of course, that Dr. Stone would have been the man for the job. For numerous reasons, he did not take it. But if he could have overcome his discomfort and found a way to approach the subject, a better man for the job would have been hard to find.

14

Amazing grace

N ancy is already dead," Jackie said one night in mid-April as she awoke from a vivid dream. Robert did not stir, and in the stillness, Jackie pondered the meaning of her dream. Her grandmother had been sitting on the deep freezer in the kitchen chatting with Jackie. She had seemed almost girlish perched on top of the long, white freezer, her legs swinging over the side. That freezer had been Mrs. Jackson's pride and joy; she saved for months to buy it so that she could stock up on meat and fish when they went on sale.

Nancy, Mrs. Jackson told Jackie in her dream, was going to die. Nancy was Mrs. Jackson's daughter and had died in 1981 of liver failure. That's when Jackie awoke, protesting that her Aunt Nancy could not die, she already had.

Jackie eventually fell back asleep, but the next morning she felt uneasy. She called her great-aunt Eldora, Mrs. Jackson's sister down the street. Jackie was sure she would be home; since she had gone blind, the old woman rarely went out. As Jackie had expected, her aunt picked up the phone right away. Jackie related the dream. "That's Cora dying," her aunt said. That clinched it for Jackie; the idea had been in the back of her mind but she had not wanted to acknowledge it. She decided she had to get out to see her grandmother.

In mid-March, Mrs. Jackson finally had been discharged from Mount Sinai. She was transferred to Oak Forest Hospital, a public long-term care facility located in one of Chicago's southwest suburbs, an hour and a half bus ride from Jackie's apartment. Oak Forest's largest unit, a 690-bed chronic disease hospital, houses many patients that other nursing homes refuse to accept. Most are poor, covered by Medicaid. Some had been living in other nursing homes but were transferred to

Oak Forest when they drained their own resources and had to revert to Medicaid. Under state law, nursing homes cannot evict residents for that reason, but if they are subsequently hospitalized, nursing homes can refuse to take them back. Other Oak Forest residents came straight from the hospital. While most nursing homes in Chicago accept some Medicaid patients, they do not want too many like Mrs. Jackson who require heavy care. For the poor with multiple chronic diseases, the only option, then, may be Oak Forest.

That is not to say it is a bad option. Oak Forest is a public hospital, but to look at it, one would never guess that it is run by the same board that presides over the rundown, grimy Cook County Hospital. With sixty buildings spread over broad green lawns shaded by tall, leafy trees, Oak Forest resembles a college campus. The facility is much cleaner than County (though, privately, state nursing home officials rank the quality of its care as no better than mediocre). Far removed from the city, and less expensive to run than County, Oak Forest's appearance is explained in part by its privileged position as a pet of suburban Republican members of the Cook County Board. At one time, rumor has it, board members were so involved with the day-to-day operations of the long-term care facility that they approved admissions.

When Mrs. Jackson was admitted to Oak Forest, her condition, according to medical records, was "poor," her prognosis, "guarded." By the evening of her first day there she already had a fever, and fluid was detected in her lungs, indicating that her chronic congestive heart failure was turning acute again. She was oriented to person only (she knew her name); she didn't know time or place. As Jackie explained it, after visiting her grandmother for the first time at Oak Forest, "She really didn't know it was a hospital. She took a trip; she didn't know where she was. I guess she just thought it was a new apartment or something."

Two weeks into her stay, Mrs. Jackson deteriorated so badly that she had to be transferred to Oak Forest's acute care hospital. Her heart disease had worsened; she had contracted pneumonia again; her glucose level rose precipitously high; her kidneys began to fail in earnest; and she showed signs of septicemia, a life-threatening bacterial blood poisoning that possibly emanated from the large, deep bedsore at the bottom of her spine.

She had been in the acute unit for a week when Jackie had her dream. A few days later, Mrs. Jackson's cousin, B.J., agreed to drive Jackie to Oak Forest. B.J., a retired can factory worker, had taken her on much happier trips in the past. A stand-in father for Jackie and her three cousins when they were young, he took them for hamburgers on Saturdays, or to play on the swing set at the drive-in. "B.J. was an every weekend person," she said. "My father was a once-in-a-blue-moon kind of person."

After winding their way through Oak Forest's sprawling corridors, Jackie and B.J. arrived at the doorway to Mrs. Jackson's room. They hesitated a moment, contemplating the scene. Mrs. Jackson lay in the far left-hand corner of the room by the window. There were three other beds, two of which were occupied. With Jackie in the lead, they proceeded tentatively toward Mrs. Jackson.

Her wiry gray-white hair was brushed back from her face. Her eyes were closed, and her hands rested on top of a neatly arranged sheet, from underneath which emerged the feeding tube, attached to a bag by the bed. An intravenous line grew out of her right arm, and another tube flowed into a small bag that dropped low by the side of the bed, catching urine.

Jackie set flowers and a heart-shaped balloon on her grandmother's bedside table. From a bag, she pulled out a bowl of fruit: strawberries, oranges, bananas, sliced cantaloupe, easy-to-eat treats she hoped her grandmother might soon be able to "pick up and throw in her mouth." As Jackie arranged the flowers in a glass, she glanced sidelong at her grandmother. If Jackie didn't look too hard, she could almost imagine that at any moment the old woman's eyes would flash open and fix on her granddaughter. "Girl, give me a piece of that melon." But as soon as Jackie registered Mrs. Jackson's ashen complexion, her stillness, the fantasy vanished.

In a gesture of respect, B.J. had removed his hat. Well past sixty, he rarely left his apartment without a hat, jacket, and matching trousers. "Miss Mark," he called out. That was his nickname for Mrs. Jackson, whom he continued to address by her first husband's name, Markham. "Mark, you up?"

No response.

B.J. backed away slowly and took a seat by the unoccupied bed facing Mrs. Jackson's. Jackie bent down close to her grandmother, grabbing her limp hand. "Mama, Mama. It's Jackie." Mrs. Jackson's eyelids did not even flutter. Jackie let go of her hand and sat by the window.

"Mama, I brought you some fruit and flowers," Jackie said evenly. "You see B.J. sitting over there." B.J. nodded.

"The kids signed you a card," Jackie went on, searching her grandmother's face for some sign of recognition. "The handwriting you can't read, that's Brianna's."

Dejected, Jackie leaned back in her chair and stared, as if the intensity of her gaze might revive the woman who had taken her for picnic lunches in Douglas Park when she was a girl, who angrily marched into Jackie's high school, coat flying out behind her like a witch, when she discovered the twelfth-grader had cut a month of classes, who never directly acknowledged that her teenage granddaughter had become pregnant but instead bought her a new double bed and warned her about eating too many hot peppers, lest her baby be born blind.

The only way Jackie could tell her grandmother was alive was by the sound of her breathing. Her mouth was held open by a plastic mouthpiece so that she would not get sores on her lips. As a result, each time she exhaled she blew out a poof of air, as if she were making a soap bubble.

Then she made a rumbling sound, probably the result of the pneumonia or fluid in her lungs.

"Looks like she's trying to say something," B.J. said.

"Hopefully so," Jackie responded.

But her grandmother did not speak; her expression remained fixed.

One of the other patients broke the silence, however. "Ya, ya, ya, ya, ya," she shouted. Mrs. Jackson's roommate was sitting up, strapped into a chair next to her bed. The nurse came in. "I think she needs help or something, maybe to get back in bed," Jackie offered.

"She's OK," the nurse assured Jackie. She checked the old woman's restraints and informed her that she was fine, just fine, that she should settle down. She did, and the nurse left.

B.J. and Jackie sat some more.

"Are you ready to go, B.J.?" Jackie asked after a while. "It don't look like she's going to wake up and talk to us."

"Whenever you're ready; I'm in no great hurry."

"OK, then. I know I can't come back tomorrow."

Another few minutes passed quietly, and Jackie rose to leave. She stroked her grandmother's forehead. "Mom, we're fixing to go now,"

Jackie said softly. "When you open your eyes, look over on your table. I doubt if the strawberries will be OK, but the oranges and bananas should keep."

"See you later, Mark," B.J. said from the foot of Mrs. Jackson's bed.

Jackie squeezed her grandmother's hand a last time. "I think I got some pressure here," she said, looking expectantly toward B.J. They turned toward the door.

"Probably so," B.J. answered matter-of-factly, "probably so."

Two days later, on 24 April 1990 at 4:30 A.M., Jackie received a call from Oak Forest. Her grandmother was dead.

Jackie had mixed feelings about the news. "It was heartbreaking, but I had really went through the worst part of it back in November and December, being out there seeing her, and then putting her in isolation," she said pensively. Jackie sat on her grandmother's old, gold couch, which had been completely stripped of its plastic cover. Mrs. Jackson's funeral was a day away. "I had put her shoes away. She had so many shoes. I got tears in my eyes when I was doing it; it was like my grandmother done died."

Jackie paused. The room was quiet. DeMarest and Brianna were napping; Latrice was at school; and Robert was out. "When she died, it hurted. I cried for a long time. But after all that was over with, it's like, 'Thank you, God,' she doesn't have to live like that anymore. I couldn't see nothing else that they could do to help her get any better. She looked very peaceful to me. I'm glad, I guess. To me, she died while sleeping."

According to the medical record, Mrs. Jackson's death was anything but peaceful. After her heart stopped, a medical team tried for a half hour to resuscitate her. They injected her with five separate doses of cardiac stimulants, lay two metal plates on her chest and administered electric shock six times, and, to force air into her lungs, pushed a tube through her nose and down her windpipe.

Their efforts were unsuccessful, as medical literature shows is the case 96 percent to 100 percent of the time when nurses and doctors try to resuscitate hospitalized patients suffering from multiple chronic diseases.[1] Since a DNR order had not been written for Mrs. Jackson, the resuscitation had to be attempted.[2]

Mrs. Jackson's medical record gave no indication that she or Jackie had been consulted regarding their wishes about CPR or other lifesustaining treatments. But Jackie said she briefly discussed the matter with Oak Forest's Dr. Leonard Fisher on the phone, a conversation the former chairman of geriatrics only vaguely recalled.

According to Jackie, Dr. Fisher asked her if she and her grandmother had ever discussed what the elderly woman would want done if her heart failed. Jackie replied that they had not. "He said, 'Would you want your grandmother to be saved if her heart stopped?'" Jackie remembered. "My response was, quite naturally, 'Sure.'"

Family members almost never refuse CPR if asked in that way, said Dr. Youngner. He compared asking Jackie if she wanted her grandmother to be "saved" to another common approach: asking family members whether they want "everything done" for a relative. "It puts the family in the position of executioner," he said.

Dr. Fisher acknowledged that discussing resuscitation over the phone, as he did with Jackie, is far from ideal and can lead to "simplifications so that people understand." But sometimes it is impossible to do otherwise because the relatives of Oak Forest's patients often do not have cars, or are too frail themselves to make it to the hospital. Indeed, Jackie only visited her grandmother once a week during the month she was at Oak Forest.

Even if Jackie had had more regular contact with Oak Forest's doctors, the institution's resuscitation policy discouraged the writing of DNR orders, according to Dr. Fisher and to Dr. Robert Richardson, chairman of the ethics committee. The policy, which was in the process of being rewritten at the time of Mrs. Jackson's death, said that DNR orders could only be issued for patients expected to die within thirty days, a determination that doctors say is impossible to make and inappropriate. "We have people who may hang on for six months to a year, but they don't want to be forced to be resuscitated," Dr. Fisher explained.

The policy also required that DNR orders be renewed once a month, but Dr. Richardson said he and his colleagues did not always remember to comply. The result was that some patients with large, yellow DNR stickers on their charts had been resuscitated because staff didn't want to take any chances when orders had expired, he said. Despite the prevailing fear, no doctor or hospital has ever been successfully sued for allowing a patient to die if requested. Moreover, doctors may be liable for resuscitating patients who want to be allowed to die. In 1990, an elderly Cincinnati, Ohio, man sued a hospital for resuscitating him after he asked not to be.[3] And a New York court decided a man did not have to pay his wife's medical bills after doctors artificially fed her against the couple's wishes, although that decision was later reversed on appeal.[4]

No more than a tenth of Oak Forest's eight hundred (or more) patients were designated DNR at the time Mrs. Jackson died, according to hospital estimates. Such a low number seems foolish, Dr. Richardson said, considering that so many of the hospital's patients are the seriously ill elderly for whom resuscitation rarely works. Of about a hundred CPR attempts reviewed at Oak Forest in 1989, Dr. Richardson said about "99 percent were unsuccessful," either because the patient could not be revived or was revived but lived only a few days.[5]

Concerned about both the human misery and financial burden of CPR among the sick elderly (one day in Oak Forest's intensive care unit costs, on average, $1,089),[6] Dr. Philip Podrid, of the Boston University School of Medicine, suggested in the *Annals of Internal Medicine* that the medical profession consider setting general guidelines for deciding whom to resuscitate. "Is it reasonable and fair to use critical care beds, which are costly and in short supply, to provide intensive care for patients who are unlikely to recover or even survive the hospitalization?"[7]

Dr. Greg Sachs, a fellow in geriatric medicine and clinical ethics at the University of Chicago, was less circumspect: "In a society that claims to have to ration health care and where millions of people are without adequate primary care, it's nonsense to be pouring money into moribund patients."

Cora Jackson might have agreed. Because the irony is that while the health care system gave her everything she needed and perhaps more at the end of her life, she spent most of her earlier years struggling to get decent and dignified care. In the year before she died, there were times Mrs. Jackson couldn't afford transportation to the doctor so Jackie waited until she became sick enough for an ambulance, times when badly needed disposable diapers were beyond her means, times when Jackie scrimped on her grandmother's medication to make it last a few more days. Yet in the last six months of Mrs. Jackson's life, Medicare spent $120,000 for her hospital care. Mount Sinai received $99,300 for the 148 days she spent there from October 1989 to March 1990,[8] and doctors, more than $10,000. In her last month of life,

Medicare paid Oak Forest $8,048. (Hospitalized for such a long time, Mrs. Jackson met her spend-down, so Medicaid kicked in an additional $3,500 for some expenses Medicare did not cover.)[9] Government figures show that Mrs. Jackson's case is not unusual: almost a third of all Medicare dollars go to patients in their last year of life.[10]

That health care may be abundant near the end of life and scarce at the beginning and middle are not unrelated. Although hospitals and doctors certainly could save money with increased efficiency, and Americans could decide to devote more than the current 12.2 percent[11] of the gross national product to health care, there is growing recognition that there will never be enough money for everyone to have all the care they want when they want it.

That has led to debates over rationing, perhaps by limiting care to people over a certain age, or by not providing expensive procedures without proven benefit. But as Mrs. Jackson could have attested, health care has always been rationed, not by procedure or age but by ability to pay and by the nature of government programs, and not at the end of life, but earlier, when debilitating diseases might have been treated or prevented.

For half of the $120,000 that went to Mrs. Jackson in her last six months of life, Mount Sinai could have started a foot clinic to aggressively prevent amputations in diabetics like her. The hospital applied for a $54,000 foundation grant for that purpose in 1984 but was rejected. With that $120,000, the Chicago Department of Health could have hired three new nurses to give immunizations.[12] Drug and alcohol rehabilitation programs could have provided outpatient treatment for roughly 120 of the 757 people waiting for help on the West Side alone.[13] With a mere $2,364, Latrice's school could have replaced its twenty-five-year-old sex education textbooks.[14] The children who attend Paderewski Elementary School live in a community where one of every thirty-two people contracts a sexually transmitted disease each year,[15] where babies die at double the rate of the national average,[16] and where one out of three mothers are teenagers.[17] But sex education has not been taught at Paderewski in a decade.[18]

Such a wish list could go on forever, and it is impossible to determine at what point Mrs. Jackson's "natural death" would have occurred, or if she would have preferred to die sooner. That is not to say that it made sense to try to resuscitate her at Oak Forest. It seems clear that, at least by the time she was transferred to the acute unit, she had reached what Stanford physicians John Ruark and Thomas Raffin call the "critical point beyond which medical interventions may act less to prolong acceptable life than to extend a miserable dying process."[19]

Of course, decisions to shift resources from one area of health care to another cannot be made on a case-by-case basis. And since Mrs. Jackson's care seemed excessive at the end of life, her case does not provide the best example of the difficult trade-offs that the country may need to make. Not much would have been lost—and a modicum of peace and dignity might have been gained—if she had been allowed to die without extraordinary, costly intervention.

Robert's situation is potentially different, however. Kidney failure is the only chronic disease that makes nearly all Americans automatically eligible for Medicare, regardless of age—a situation that strikes many as unfair considering the number of people without access to basic health care. When Congress voted to include dialysis (and kidney transplant) patients in Medicare in 1972, lawmakers figured that the costs of the program would grow slowly, that the treatment would be used only for people who were relatively young and healthy apart from their kidney failure. It quickly became apparent, however, that expenditures would far outstrip projections—not because the price per treatment rose (indeed, the amount Medicare pays for each dialysis session actually has dropped in real dollars since the program began) but because sicker and older patients who never would have been considered for dialysis in earlier years began to receive the treatment as a matter of course. People over 65 comprised 27 percent of the total dialysis population in 1988, compared to 5 percent in 1974.[20] That expansion occurred because Medicare agreed to pay for the new technology, granting doctors and patients control over when it could be used. The standards of the medical profession, economic incentives, and public demand, which both shapes physicians' views and is shaped by them, almost always lead doctors to push the limits of a new treatment's effectiveness. If a terminal cancer patient's kidneys fail and Medicare will pay for dialysis, why not try the treatment if she wants it? Private insurers have not been able to interrupt that momentum any more than Medicare has.

It is not that having Medicare guarantees equal access to care for rich and poor, black and white; Robert's experience (and Mrs. Jackson's) suggests it does not, as do empirical analyses. One recent study that reviewed all of the Medicare-funded heart bypass surgeries performed in 1986 found that white men had four times the number of surgeries as black men, even though both races had similar rates of hospitalization for heart attacks.[21] Still, once Robert got sick enough to qualify, Medicare undoubtedly improved his access to health care. His costly dialysis—$30,000 a year—and, in theory, an unlimited number of kidney transplants were paid for, whereas uninsured women die needlessly from cervical cancer because they cannot afford relatively inexpensive pap smears, and children are born with brain damage because their mothers could not get prenatal care.

Other kinds of organ transplants—liver transplants, for instance—are most often raised in the context of inequitable, even senseless, distribution of resources. The issue here is not that people with liver failure receive special Medicare benefits; they do not. Liver transplants are covered in the usual fashion. Medicare covers the $150,000 operation for people who meet the program's general eligibility requirements of being older than 65 or disabled, and Medicaid and private insurers also pay for it. The question is whether the outcomes of liver transplants justify that large expense. While kidney transplants are in the long run cheaper than dialysis and the vast majority of patients survive for some years following the operation, a third of adult liver-transplant recipients die within one year.[22]

"One of the more fascinating aspects of the policy discussion about transplantation at the federal level has been the virtual absence of discussion about distributive justice," wrote Richard Rettig, one of the leading experts on the politics of organ transplantation. A national task force appointed by Congress in the mid-1980s to study controversial issues in organ transplantation completely ignored "whether resources ought to be spent for other purposes, including [other] health purposes," Rettig continued in a 1989 article.[23]

Left with a federal vacuum, a few states, most notably, Oregon, have begun to try to make explicit decisions about how to best spend a limited amount of state health money. In an effort to extend Medicaid coverage to more of its uninsured residents, the state proposed to ration health care by ranking all services according to their costs and benefits. Everything above a cutoff line, set according to the state's budget, would be covered; everything below would not. Generally, the list favored preventive treatments and those with the most potential to restore health and improve the quality of life. Critics complained the ranking was too crude and did not guarantee a basic package of health care services to Medicaid recipients. They worried that if the state budget got too tight, essential services might be eliminated. Another criticism is perhaps more fundamental. Only Medicaid recipients would be denied the care that fell below the cutoff point. Henry Waxman, a Democratic representative from California, likened the situation to "taking an already small pie and cutting it into more pieces, taking benefits away from the poorest of society."[24] It is hard to see Oregon's rationing plan as a noble attempt to make tough choices when the tough choices would only apply to the poor.[25]

Health care is not a prerogative of the affluent or well-insured in other countries, Canada and Great Britain being the most often cited examples. Their systems are designed differently, but both countries provide health care to all of their citizens, at costs significantly below that of the United States, and with at least equal and often better health outcomes than are achieved here. And though a small percentage of the British have supplementary private health insurance (which is illegal in Canada), by and large, when tough choices need to be made, they apply to all, like a draft without loopholes for the sons of the powerful. As Rettig concluded, "For all the limitations that might be found in the National Health Service, the British have embraced equity as a basic organizing principle, have accepted the reality that not all that can be done technically can be done financially, and have embedded their basic values . . . in institutions that routinely make binding choices that affect the country's citizens."[26]

The salutary effects of that ethic may go beyond enhancing a population's physical well-being. A respected Canadian physician, Dr. Samuel Freedman, said the principle that the same amount and quality of medical care should be available to all had become a transforming national value in his country. "Knowing that everybody gets the same care helps to hold a society together," he said. "It makes everybody feel equally valued."[27]

At the "Homegoing Services for Sister Cora Jackson," Jackie sat in the front pew of the First Baptist Church, between four-year-old DeMarest and Robert's grandmother. Mrs. Jackson had worshipped at this church almost every Sunday since arriving in Chicago from Mississippi, in 1962, and Jackie came here several times a year, for church dinners on Mother's Day, Easter, and other special occasions.

Robert had not come to the funeral. Someone had to watch two-year-old Brianna, and, sadly, it was fitting that he was not there. Jackie felt as if he had never been there for her during her grandmother's illness. When she began to dread going to the hospital in December, scared by her grandmother's labored breathing and unnatural pallor, she mentioned that a companion might give her more courage. "If I could have somebody there, a shoulder to lean on," Jackie lamented. But emotionally estranged from her husband by what she called his "mistress," cocaine, Jackie did not ask Robert to accompany her, and he did not offer. He never once visited his wife's grandmother in the hospital.

Latrice, too, was missing. Before Jackie had married, when she and Latrice lived alone with Mrs. Jackson, the little girl and her great-grandmother had been particularly close. Mrs. Jackson showered Latrice with tokens of affection: puppets, bags of potato chips, little dolls that walked, doughnuts, small plastic balls, gum, peppermint candy. When the girl was a little older, she catered to her great-grandmother in the same way Jackie once had. "Everyday when my grandmother would come in from work, Latrice would have a big cup of water and her house shoes waiting for her," Jackie said. But when Mrs. Jackson had fallen seriously ill, Latrice pulled away. She only shrugged her shoulders when asked what was wrong, but Jackie assumed that she was frightened by her great-grandmother's illness. Perhaps, too, Latrice felt betrayed, abandoned by the woman who had once treated her so specially.

As the guests filled the church, Jackie turned around periodically to see who had come. Wearing a matching skirt and shirt-jacket in navy blue with bold white flowers, Jackie looked quite pretty. Her eyes were clear, and she appeared composed, smiling bright hellos to people she recognized.

All of Mrs. Jackson's closest relatives attended. The first to proceed toward the front of the church were her two out-of-town sisters, one from Cleveland, Ohio, and the other from New York City. All three women liked hats. (Mrs. Jackson's two church hats hung on the corner of her dresser mirror until the day she died.) One sister wore a bright-red felt fedora with a large feather, the other, a beige hat with a fur tail for flourish. Mrs. Jackson's closest sister, Eldora, who had lived nearby ever since the two migrated to Chicago, wore a navy blue hat with a large white brim. She walked tentatively down the church's center aisle, sunglasses hiding her blind eyes. Holding her arm was Mrs. Jackson's only brother, the fifty-one-year-old baby of the family, the one who had been so upset by the prospect of his sister's second amputation. Then came Mrs. Jackson's only son, Tommy, who was just a few years younger than his uncle. Using a cane to support his paralyzed leg, Tommy limped heavily toward the front. He and his girlfriend, Lana, settled in next to DeMarest.

Once the family had been seated, guests shuffled out of their pews, row by row, to pay their respects to Mrs. Jackson. Her gray coffin was located front and center of the church on a cart with wheels. After the last mourner had filed by the coffin, the church ushers pushed it slowly in front of the pew holding the family. Eldora and Mrs. Jackson's sister from Cleveland began to weep. DeMarest whimpered, then sobbed, gulping for air with a little boy's lack of self-consciousness.

Jackie remained dry-eyed; the day before she had gone to the funeral home to say good-bye to her grandmother in private. She was extremely pleased with the way Mrs. Jackson looked. She wore her favorite dress, a long, rose-colored formal, a large gemstone bracelet, and one of her many wigs. "I was expecting to see somebody who looked dead, and to me, she didn't. She looked like a movie star laying up there. You know how I had seen her ailing all the time, and this time she didn't look like she had a problem in the world. Without the machines and all this other junk hooked up on her, in a nice dress and whatnot," Jackie said, trailing off. "She looked real pretty."

A small but enthusiastic choir started the services, swaying and clapping to a hymn that began, "I sing because I'm happy, because I'm free." Mrs. Jackson's pastor, too, celebrated her freedom, her union with God. "I'm happy," he preached, "for Sister Jackson has reached her goal. She made preparations for this a *long* time ago."

Before he spoke, another pastor had warmed up the crowd, directing many of his remarks toward the guests, specifically Tommy. Tommy's boozing and brawling had alienated him from his mother, but after his stroke, he accepted Christ and renounced his past ways. The minister knew Tommy's story well; he was the brother of Lana, Tommy's girlfriend. "Lord, you is a burden-bearer, a heavy-load-carrier," he preached. "Bless Tommy, if he will get his house in order, you will step in where his mother stepped out. Join in with Sister Jackson, who gave her life to the Master." Tommy dabbed his eyes with a large handkerchief.

As the funeral progressed, with rousing gospel songs and tributes to Mrs. Jackson by her fellow parishioners, the central role church had played in her life became increasingly evident. During one particularly bluesy number, an older woman began to murmur and rock slowly. The singer who inspired her had started by accompanying himself on the piano, but as the song gathered momentum, he grabbed a microphone, signaling for the choir director to take over at the keys. As he strode toward Mrs. Jackson's coffin, the woman stretched out her arms and swung them from side to side. Her cries became louder, and trickles of sweat ran down her broad face. "Stop, Mama," her son pleaded, trying to pin down her arms. Only when the song was over did she obey, her cries returning to murmurs and her shoulders relaxing. Her son wiped her brow.

Later, Jackie said the woman was her grandmother's cousin from Michigan. "Mama used to do the same thing. When I was little, she dragged me by the hand to church. I'd say 'Mama, Please don't "shout" today.' She would promise not to, but she couldn't help it. Mom's shouts always ended with fainting."

"She did that?" I asked, surprised.

"Girl, she'd lay out on the floor."

I didn't know about Mrs. Jackson's religious passion, Jackie told me, because I had never met the real woman. "It's the sick mom you learned about," she said.

To Jackie, who was raised by Mrs. Jackson, her grandmother was "like the daddy, the stern one." Because Mrs. Jackson was not a demonstrative woman, not one to tell her family how much they meant to her, Jackie did not find out until the funeral that the old woman had regularly sung her praises. One after another, Mrs. Jackson's friends told Jackie how fond her grandmother had been of her. Jackie was especially pleased to learn that her grandmother had appreciated her cooking. She often had fixed food for Mrs. Jackson to take to church events, peach cobblers and sweet potato pies for dessert, fish and fried chicken for dinner, but she assumed her grandmother claimed the dishes as her own. She was wrong. "Miss Jackson say you're the one who cooked those good cakes and pies," one of the elderly women complimented her.

"Yeah, that's me," Jackie answered, her voice warmed by the evidence of her grandmother's approval. "Thank you."

That Mrs. Jackson revealed more of herself at church than she did at home did not surprise Jackie. She had been gentler with her First Baptist friends than anyone else, Jackie said. Church rejuvenated her after work had beaten her down. "During the week she'd be bending over," Jackie said, "but on Sundays, she stood up like she was in the Army." Her grandmother had often sung at church celebrations and funerals. "She sang grand. Everybody always said she sounded like Mahalia."

Mrs. Jackson probably would have wanted to be remembered that way, the way she was before she became so ill. Wearing her long, rose-colored formal, she stands at the front of the church, preparing to sing her favorite hymn, "Amazing Grace." She insists on singing a cappella, as Jackie says was her way. "Cut the piano," Mrs. Jackson orders. And then, taking a deep breath, she begins.

Epilogue

A year and a day after Mrs. Jackson died, Latrice turned thirteen. At 5 feet 6 inches, she seemed destined to match her mother's height, but in many ways she was still a girl. Sometimes she almost clung to her childhood. Strolling through a suburban mall one afternoon, Latrice and her mother stopped in Montgomery Ward's lingerie department, where Jackie noticed a cotton night shirt that she thought her daughter might like. "That's cute," Jackie said, examining the shirt, which was styled like a baseball jersey, with stripes and a V-neck. Latrice glanced at it sidelong and continued on.

"Too low," she mumbled.

"No one will see you in bed, Latrice," Jackie said, shaking her head, bemused at her daughter's modesty.

The purpose of the trip was to spend the money Latrice had received for her birthday. She chose a pair of black leather high-top gym shoes, turning up her nose at a lavender and pink girls' pair. Latrice shunned most things feminine. She wore her hair in a short curl, hated skirts, and vowed never to wear earrings, despite her mother's love for them. On the way out of the mall, a fake leopard fur stole caught her eye, but she was quick to make sure Jackie knew that she wanted no part of it. "That's too old for me," she said, though no one had suggested otherwise. "Ma, you could wear that."

Jackie laughed. She was, in fact, delighted that Latrice did not seem eager to grow up. "She's thirteen, but she's got a child's mind," Jackie said one time when her daughter was not around. "I *do* not complain." For good reason. In North Lawndale, a third of girls give birth before their twentieth birthdays, and several of Latrice's seventh and eighth grade classmates at Paderewski already had gotten pregnant.

The quality of Latrice's education had not changed much from sixth grade. For the second year in a row, she was in a split class. In the first marking period, Latrice had had three different "permanent" teachers, as well as substitutes; the situation was such a mess that the whole class received all Cs that quarter because no true grades could be determined. One teacher, Sallie Welch, had been there since November. Still, Latrice did not seem challenged in the least, which was probably because Mrs. Welch often gave the sixth and seventh graders the same lessons, explaining that she could not teach two classes at once.

Jackie was not worried about Latrice's schooling, partly because by Paderewski's standards Latrice was doing well. None of her seventh-grade test scores were better than average, but, nonetheless, they put her in the top quarter of her class of 35 pupils, and her grades were solid. After the quarter of meaningless Cs, she received Bs and an A in spelling.

Mrs. Welch described Latrice as "quiet" and "studious." She followed directions well and had a sense of integrity, Mrs. Welch said. On African Market day, a special day where the children dress up and hold a "market" in the halls, Latrice and the other seventh-grade girls sold baubles they had brought from home. They were supposed to keep the money from the sale for a class fund, but instead they pocketed it. When Mrs. Welch confronted them, Latrice was the only one who had not spent her portion of the proceeds. "I knew it was wrong," Latrice told her teacher.

Probably the key factor in Latrice's educational future is which high school she attends. For the most part, the Chicago Public Schools are abysmal. Two-thirds of the sixty-four high schools have a drop-out rate of more than 33 percent; at nineteen schools, more than half of the class drops out.[1] The situation is almost equally bleak for those who graduate: 67 percent test below average in reading, and 70 percent below average in math.[2] Some children are allowed to go outside of their neighborhoods and attend the handful of decent high schools, but Latrice may have trouble qualifying because of her test scores, according to Paderewski's part-time counselor, George McCoy.

As for five-year-old DeMarest, he was attending Head Start preschool, a government-funded program that is widely credited for improving the academic performance of children from poor families.

DeMarest's teachers called him a "little man." When the children were told to get a drink of water or to wash their hands, most raced to the sink. DeMarest hung back, carefully walking to the end of the line. With class projects, he also was slow and deliberate: a perfectionist. His approach to school was epitomized by the way he made his Easter basket. While the other kids grabbed clumps of the bright green grass, DeMarest laid it down in his basket strand by strand.

His reserve had not made him an outcast, however. Rather, he seemed to be a leader; when DeMarest did something, the other children wanted to do it, too. Bored with playing with wooden blocks one day, DeMarest moved over to large foam building blocks. "Hey, I know what," he said, losing his composure and breaking into a little dance, "let's make a stack." He swept his arm toward the sky. By himself, he began pulling the foam slabs out of a cart and stacking them neatly, green, red, yellow, blue. In a few minutes, the other boys hustled over to join him but did not try to take away his job as chief architect.

"Here go one," said his closest friend, Sam, handing him a block.

"Here go one, DeMarest," joined in another little boy.

"Oh, great," DeMarest enthused, thrilled at the prospect of adding a red slab to his growing tower.

DeMarest excelled at his classwork, but his teacher, Joann Reeves, worried that he was *too* well behaved, that he needed to express his feelings more. Once, DeMarest had been made to sit with the girls because the boys' table was too crowded. He had silently complied when Mrs. Reeves asked him to move, but a few minutes later she noticed him shaking with fury. She pulled him aside. "DeMarest, you need to tell me when you want something, when you're mad."

Perhaps DeMarest's reticence was the result of his age. Some of the other children were four, and he was an old five; his birthday was in September, at the beginning of the school year. Then, too, DeMarest may have learned to keep a low profile as a way of coping with the tumult at home.

Even so, teachers of both DeMarest and Latrice said the Baneses were one of the more stable families in the school. That was evident in Jackie's participation in Head Start. In a class of twenty children, she was one of very few parents who regularly attended, though all parents were supposedly required to do so. Some could not come because they had jobs; others just didn't want to, Mrs. Reeves said. Jackie felt she learned a lot from watching the way Mrs. Reeves related to children. The teacher taught her to "accept" her children more, she said, not to expect them to act like miniature adults. She did not snap at them as much, she said, but on the other hand, she tried to be firmer. "I'm trying to make 'No' mean 'No.'"

Jackie's new style of parenting shone forth when she broke up disputes between her children. For example, one afternoon DeMarest had been sitting in a living room chair, when Brianna began trying to push him off. Fed up, DeMarest gave her a shove and, inevitably, Brianna's face crumpled into tears. In the past, DeMarest had often seemed to bear an unfair amount of blame in these situations.

"Come here and talk to me," Jackie said to Brianna from her seat on the couch. Huffing and puffing, Brianna plodded over and stood in front of her mother. Jackie held her small arm and looked her in the eye. "What happened?" she asked.

"DeMarest pushed me."

"What do you say to your sister?" Jackie said, looking over at her son, who was watching the scene intently.

"I'm sorry," he said, keeping his eyes glued to his shoes.

"DeMarest is sitting there now; you can later," she said to Brianna. And that was it. A few minutes later, the two children were swashbuckling through the living room as if nothing had happened, DeMarest brandishing a plastic sword and Brianna an egg beater.

Other mothers with children in Head Start were not able to respond to the program as well as Jackie did. A dentist's visit to Mrs. Reeves' classroom brought out some of these women; to get dental exams, children had to be accompanied by one of their parents.

One little boy cried during his checkup, and when Mrs. Reeves tried to comfort him afterward, offering him a pencil as a reward and telling him that he was "great," his mother snarled, "No, he wasn't."

Another mother, a drug addict, showed up late with her little girl, Shonda. Unkempt and glassy-eyed, the woman stayed in the back of the classroom when Shonda was summoned to the front for her checkup. After a few minutes, however, the dentist called her over. Shonda's teeth were in awful shape, he said. He asked if the child had ever been to the dentist, and the woman said that she had taken her to see someone last year, to a dentist referred by Head Start.

"A dentist in our program? That's hard to believe," he said skeptically.

"They said don't do anything because her teeth are going to fall out," she answered, revealing her own missing teeth. Earlier, the dentist had given a short lecture in which he gave opposite advice. Ignoring cavities in baby teeth could lead to serious problems in the future, he told the class.

Shonda began to wail as the dentist kept probing her infected teeth and gums.

"Oh, shit, girl," her mother said. "Come on now, shut up."

After the checkups ended, the woman and her still weepy daughter headed for the door. She asked Mrs. Reeves if the children had been given lunch. No, the teacher answered, lunch was not served on dentist's day, as a letter home had emphasized. The prospect of making lunch for Shonda seemed to rile the woman, but Mrs. Reeves did not acknowledge her reaction. Instead she asked if Shonda's mother planned to accompany the class to a puppet show on the thirtieth of the month.

"The thirtieth, I have a date," the woman answered, smiling slyly.

"You always have a date," Mrs. Reeves said.

"Do they get puppets?" she asked, edging toward the door.

"No, they just get entertainment."

"Oh," the woman said vacantly.

Jackie tried to go to Head Start every day when she could, but during the winter she wasn't there as often. One of the reasons was that she had a new person to take care of. Tommy, her father, had moved into Mrs. Jackson's old bedroom when his girlfriend put him out in February. "I'm trying to get on my feet," Jackie said, "and I get knocked down again."

It's not that Tommy required nearly as much care as her grandmother. Jackie cooked, laundered, and fetched for him, since he could only walk with great effort, and that was about it. But she did not like to leave him alone in the house for too long. In part, she worried he would need some kind of help, and in part she was not sure she trusted him.

When Tommy was staying with his girlfriend, Lana, Jackie often said she felt sorry for him, but when he actually moved in, she began to see things from Lana's point of view. Tommy could be charming, but he regularly issued abrupt commands to Jackie and the kids. "Jackie, order me a combo," he demanded after she and Latrice had returned home from their birthday shopping. Jackie had picked up hamburgers for dinner, but evidently, Tommy did not like the food they chose. Jackie's response was typical. Tight-lipped, she did what her father requested, phoning in an order for an Italian-beef sandwich to a stand a block away.

Tommy gave half of his $400 Supplemental Security Income checks to Jackie for rent, but he spent a good part of what was left on the lottery. That infuriated Jackie. She felt obligated to replace his threadbare socks and underwear, and he constantly borrowed cigarettes from her. "Go tell your mother to send me a Salem," he liked to say to DeMarest or Latrice. (Jackie had started smoking around the time her grandmother died.) Even with people outside of his family, Tommy showed not the slightest compunction at asking them for one thing or another.

"I need a little pad," he said one day to a social worker who had stopped by the house. She was part of a demonstration project to link chronically ill Medicaid recipients with services that might improve their health and reduce costs. Tommy reached for the pad she had been taking notes on, and looking puzzled, the social worker gave it to him.

"I can't say I didn't get anything from you," he said.

"My time isn't worth anything," she challenged. "This is my second visit and you already are putting me down."

"I'll remember you in my prayers," Tommy said, oozing insincerity.

Tommy's joking with the social worker annoyed Jackie. But then again, almost everything her father did or said these days bothered her. Many of Jackie's complaints about her father centered on money. It was difficult to buy even socks when her family was getting by on $414 in welfare payments, combined with the $368 Robert received from Social Security Disability.

In the end, Jackie did not have much tolerance for her father. When her sick grandmother had barked orders, she drew on a reservoir of gratitude and love to maintain her equanimity. But her father had never nourished Jackie when she was small; he had never cared for her, never lived with her, and in many ways, it was as if a stranger had moved into her apartment.

As for Robert, he still went on periodic binges—trading $50 worth of the family's foodstamps for drugs, for example, part of which had been intended for Latrice's birthday cake. Robert's habit reduced Jackie to hiding everything of value, the family's money (including rolled change), the couple's wedding rings. She got nervous when she left home, wondering what she'd find when she got back.

"I've just got this feeling he's gone," Jackie said the day she and Latrice went to the mall. She had stopped to pick up the hamburgers for dinner, and her eyes darted around the restaurant, as if she half-expected that a glassy-eyed Robert might stumble through the front door. Before she left to go shopping, he had tried to slip away, Jackie thought. He had gone to buy soda for the family, and on his return, rang the buzzer. DeMarest ran downstairs to let him in, but the little boy came back alone, carrying the drinks.

"Where's your daddy?" Jackie asked her son. "Which way did he go?" DeMarest pointed to the back.

Jackie hurried to the rear door and hollered to her husband from the porch: "Robert, where are you going? I told you I'm taking Latrice with me." He turned and headed home, insisting that he had only been going to the corner to buy a bag of peanuts. Jackie knew that would have taken him by a drug house, and she did not want to take any chances.

Jackie was wrong about Robert's leaving that evening, however. When she and Latrice got home, he greeted them at the door. Jackie's face did not register any relief when she saw her husband. She walked impassively past him and set the bag of hamburgers on an end table.

The summer after Latrice finished seventh grade, and DeMarest his first year of preschool, Robert began to look for a job again. He had not worked for almost two years, since he had left his security guard job in the fall of 1989. Good jobs for high school educated black men are limited, and it was even harder for Robert since he had to attend dialysis. Robert's employment opportunities often sounded more like scams than anything else. He checked into selling knockoff perfumes and insurance door-to-door, but both required several hundred dollar investments. He got excited about a bartending course until he learned it would cost nearly $1,000. Finally, near the end of the summer, he landed a job as a cook at a nearby McDonald's.

McDonald's needed Robert during the morning, so he switched to the afternoon dialysis shift at Neomedica. The dialysis clinic had moved to another building a few blocks away, occupying fourth- and fifth-floor suites that looked much cleaner and newer than the old location. The waiting room had padded chairs, in place of the hard cafeteria style variety at the former unit, and each patient could watch a small personal television while their blood filtered through the dialysis machine. The staff/patient ratios had not changed much, however. One day, for example, each staff member supervised at least four patients, although the recommended ratio is 1:3.

While the president and chief executive officer of Neomedica, Dr. Gordon Lang, had complained in 1989 that his company just made ends meet with the low rates Medicare paid, he opened two new dialysis units in 1990, both in the suburbs. That brought Neomedica up to eleven sites.[3]

According to the U.S. Attorney's Office for the Northern District of Illinois, one source of Neomedica's income had been inflated billing. In July 1991, the federal government charged that Neomedica and Associates in Nephrology, the group of physicians who own the corporation in conjunction with Dr. Lang, had "conspired to defraud the United States" out of $1.75 million by using an improper billing code. In addition to supervising dialysis at its own clinics, Neomedica's doctors oversee the treatment for hospitalized patients. The lawsuit alleged that between 1984 and 1986 Neomedica knowingly overcharged Medicare for these patients by using a code that indicated they were "critically ill or multiple injured or comatose" when they were not. While not admitting any wrongdoing, Neomedica settled the lawsuit for $3.5 million, $1.25 million of which was to be made up over five years by providing free dialysis to Medicare patients.

Meanwhile, Robert's worries were not about Neomedica's alleged fraud but about his iron level, which was too low, and about how worn out he felt lately.

At least four of Robert's fellow patients had died since 1989, including Adelle, the Mexican woman. A young man with AIDS, whose funky glasses and tight-knotted hair had earned him the nickname of "Spike Lee," also died. Robert described the last day he saw him, when the two took the elevator together. "He got the shakes real bad, and I ran back up to get the nurse. They took him in an ambulance and he never came back." Ann, the woman who did not work because she feared losing her Social Security Disability payments, looked like she might not be around for long, either, Robert said. "She this big," he said, forming an "O" with his index finger and thumb.

Not all the news was bad, however. The Puerto Rican girl who had found dialysis so painful had received a kidney transplant.

Some of the pressures had been taken from Jackie, too. In September 1991, the preschool teacher at a nearby Catholic school hired her as an assistant. Jackie's attendance at Head Start had paid off. She enrolled Brianna, now three, in her class, which meant she would get two years of preschool instead of one. With Brianna at school, Jackie also did not have to pay for daycare, which would have taken so much from her monthly $1,260 paycheck that she might not have been able to justify working. That was especially true since her job did not provide health benefits. Because Jackie was no longer eligible for welfare, she and the children were not covered by Medicaid anymore.

Some children now qualify for Medicaid even if their families do not get welfare, a result of Congressional reforms enacted in the late 1980s and early 1990s, but Brianna was the only one of the Banes children who could have benefited. There were two main reforms mandated by Congress. One requires states to provide Medicaid to pregnant women and to children under age six whose family incomes are below 133 percent of the poverty level. Overlapping that to an extent, the other reform grants Medicaid to all children born after October 1983 whose family incomes are below 100 percent of the federal poverty level; that group will grow progressively larger each year so that by the year 2002, all children under eighteen in families below the federal poverty level will be covered. These income levels are the minimums mandated by Congress; states were given the option of providing Medicaid to more near-poor families, but Illinois and about half of the other states did not go beyond what was required.

Brianna could qualify for Medicaid under the first reform until she turned five—although Jackie had not been aware of it and had not signed her up—but the second change would not help the family at all. Latrice was born before October 1983, and although DeMarest and Brianna were young enough to qualify, their family was not quite poor enough. Jackie's income put her just $100 over the monthly federal poverty level for a family of four (if she applied for Medicaid, she probably would not report that Robert was a member of the household). If the family needed medical attention, Jackie planned to take them to Lawndale Christian behind the house, which had a sliding scale for the uninsured. Of course, if anything serious happened to Jackie or the children, she would have to consider going back on welfare to get Medicaid.

Working as a preschool teacher may have been risky for Jackie as far as health care coverage, but it was a risk she was willing to take. The job not only gave her extra money, but it provided her with a new sense of self-confidence, of hope for the future—both of which she would need to carry her through the rest of the fall.

A few days before Thanksgiving, Patricia Barber's replacement (Barber had moved to Colorado) called the Baneses' apartment with the news Robert had been waiting for: a kidney was available.

Robert had left the house earlier in the day for dialysis, so Jackie told the nurse to call Neomedica. Time was of the essence; the Regional Organ Bank only gives transplant programs an hour to find their patients before passing kidneys on to the next person on the waiting list. But a few minutes later, the phone rang again. It was the nurse calling back. Robert was not at Neomedica, she said. Did Jackie have any idea where he was? Jackie was stunned. She knew that from time to time Robert skipped dialysis to party. On those days, he came home looking drawn and tired, without the usual bandage over his fistula. But today of all days! She wondered whether she should look for him; she had a pretty good idea of the drug houses he frequented. No, she wasn't going to do that, she told herself. It was too dangerous.

While Jackie was trying to figure out how on earth she was going to find her husband, the phone rang. It was Robert's grandfather. Robert was there, he said, asking for money. Jackie had instructed family members to get in touch with her when Robert came by begging.

"Put him on the phone," Jackie told his grandfather.

"Nah, I don't want him to know I called." He had called Jackie out of earshot of his grandson.

"He's got to know about this," Jackie pleaded. "It's about his kidney."

Jackie gave Robert the news, but moments later the phone rang once more. Robert told Jackie he had called the transplant ward at the hospital, but the clerk knew nothing about his kidney. He accused her of trying to interfere with his fun. Furious, Jackie told him to call the University of Illinois' transplant office, not the hospital itself.

He did, and he reached the nurse in time to be scheduled for a transplant. The next day, in the early morning hours, Dr. Pollak performed the surgery. Robert had been on the waiting list a little over two years, just as Barber had predicted.

As of the winter of 1993, Robert's new kidney was functioning well.

As I write this, it is not clear what changes await the U.S. health care system. Some kind of reform seems imminent, but then again, national health insurance was just around the corner in the early 1970s. My background as a health care reporter does not equip me to lay out a detailed design for change, but after three years spent chronicling the lives of a sick, poor family and the institutions that served or failed to serve them, there are some essential reforms that I think are necessary.

First, a basic level of health care—"basic" being defined by some sort of societal consensus—should be guaranteed to all Americans as a matter of course, as is the case in all industrialized nations other than South Africa. Only in America does it seem vaguely radical to declare that health care is not a luxury item like fancy cars or fur coats. It is inhumane to treat it as if it is. It also can be expensive. In the end, we cannot bear to let the poor die on the streets, so we care for them when they're "damn near death," as Tommy Markham would say, when it costs so much more. It also costs us in other ways; when Jackie and other poor mothers get job opportunities, they must weigh whether they can afford to leave welfare and lose the automatic Medicaid coverage for themselves and their children. Even the expansions in Medicaid leave out many of the children of working poor and near-poor parents, to say nothing of the parents themselves. As things stand now, we say to working poor mothers and fathers: Medicaid may cover your youngest children, as long as your family doesn't creep a dollar over the federal poverty level. You, however, the people who nurture them, you're on your own.

Second, although having Medicaid is marginally better than being uninsured, it should not continue in its present form. It probably would and should be eliminated if the country decided to guarantee some level of basic care to everyone, but if not, its payment rates must be brought in line with those of other health care payors. Otherwise, Medicaid will continue to perpetuate inaccessible, inferior health care for the poor.

Third, any health program that purports to care for the poor must do a better job of figuring out what basic services they need to cope with illness, and how to provide those services in a straightforward way. The poor need more than medical insurance. At least three public programs provide some housekeeping assistance to the homebound elderly, and might have provided Jackie with a much-needed break, but Mrs. Jackson could not take advantage of any of them. For one, the copayment was too high; Jackie did not understand the regulations of another; and she had no idea that the third program even existed. The plethora of programs devised to fill in one gap here, another there, cannot hide the fact that the country has not made a fundamental commitment to meeting the health care needs of those who cannot compete in the marketplace. Navigating the maze of rule-laden programs often defeated Jackie, as it does all but the most savvy and determined.

Bringing adequate health care to all Americans raises the spectre of rising costs, and with the $2-billion-a-day health care tab already eating up 12 percent of the nation's gross national product, and projected to reach an almost unimagineable 37 percent,[4] the American public seems unlikely to support expansions in access that are not accompanied by cost control. Conversely, any form of cost control seems unlikely to work without universal health care access. How can policymakers design plans to contain costs with cost-shifting inexorably pushing up prices for the insured?

To achieve both ends, I am convinced by the arguments of widely published medical ethicist Daniel Callahan that our society needs to rethink its vision of health care and set some kind of global limits on public and private health care spending.[5] He advocates shifting the emphasis of the health care system away from curing and toward "caring" of a kind the Baneses missed most. Caring, as Callahan conceives it, "requires institutions, accommodating social structures, and a society prepared to make room for those it cannot cure or return to 'productive' life. For the dying, the need may be for that of an institutional hospice, for a solid home-care program, for the kind of psychological and social counseling necessary to ease the passage from life to death—which may be true for the family as well as the dying person. . . . For the functioning of the disabled, their families will need technical training and psychological counseling to understand how to do what they must do, and how to live with the enormous pressures that being a caretaker can entail."[6]

Curing, on the other hand, is limitless, he writes. There will always be a "ragged edge," a new disease to conquer, and unless we set explicit restraints, we'll consume all the country's resources chasing immortality, while starving the other institutions that can make life worth living.

That point never was too far from my mind during the past three years. The book sheds a harsh light on how wrong-headed health care policies cheat poor Americans out of an equal chance to lead fulfilling lives, and thereby suggests needed improvements in the medical and health care system. But other problems—drug and alcohol abuse, the risks and everyday strain of living in a violent neighborhood—plagued this family, too, yet such social ills are outside the scope of what a health care program can and should fix. As the use of the word "plague" suggests, drug addiction and alcoholism have no doubt been "medicalized," which is useful inasmuch as it reframes them as conditions that can be treated rather than as immutable character flaws. Violence, too, is increasingly called a public health problem, most recently by the outspoken former Surgeon General, C. Everett Koop, who argued that if violence were considered a public health emergency, lawmakers would encounter less resistance to gun control measures. While casting drugs and violence in terms of public health may have its rhetorical benefits, I believe it misses the essential point: that the virulence of these problems among the urban poor is born out of their lack of opportunity for the future, the joylessness of life in the ghettos. These tears in the social fabric the health care system cannot stitch. Which brings me back to health care reform. Unless we decide that we are going to spend so much on health care and no more—and making this decision stick depends on providing a guarantee of decent health care for all—I fear, as Callahan does, that we will be left with neither the money nor the will to attack the nation's other, equally devastating epidemics.

Appendix

In any project of this kind, reporters face the dilemma of wanting to tell the most accurate story possible, while at the same time wanting to help people they care about. My presence undoubtedly affected the course of the Baneses' care in small ways. As alluded to in chapter 12, Jackie occasionally used me as an advocate because she figured that doctors would pay more attention to me because of my race, class, and education. She was right. Health professionals tended to gravitate toward me—and I could translate some medical jargon—but, in the end, Jackie did not rely on me very much. When she did ask me what a doctor meant, or to get information from one of them, I was glad to help.

I directly influenced the family's care only one time that I can recall. That came in March 1989 when I was interviewing Mrs. Jackson's physician, Dr. Burton Stone. She had been hospitalized since November for a seemingly endless succession of medical problems, and I asked the internist whether she had been receiving physical or occupational therapy to maintain her strength. He realized that she had not, and he subsequently ordered it. But this small change came so late in Mrs. Jackson's illness that I'm certain, sadly, it did little to improve her condition.

The truth is, health care for the poor is such a complicated hodge-podge of programs that I struggled to make sense of it in much the same way the family did. I had covered AIDS and public health for some years, but figuring out the street-level operation of programs as vast and distinct as Medicaid, city clinics, Medicare's kidney program, Medicare coverage for the elderly and disabled, government in-home care programs, and so forth, was a different matter. I was encountering many of these programs for the first time, just as Jackie was, which gave me valuable insight into the confusion and frustration she felt. For example, I was so busy trying to sort out the details of the care given to Mrs. Jackson and Robert that although a childhood measles outbreak hit Chicago while I was working on the book, I did not think to ask Jackie at the time whether Brianna had been fully immunized. She had not been. Jackie missed Brianna's scheduled measles shot for the same reason I neglected to ask her about it. I was overwhelmed translating the Baneses' life; she was infinitely more overwhelmed living it. In one way, I find it appalling that I did not do more to help the family. Mostly, I provided a sympathetic ear.

Before I started working on the book, I had worried about interfering with the family's decisions. It turned out, however, that Jackie never would have let that happen. As much as she sometimes felt burdened by her responsibilities, even resentful of them, she was not about to give them up.

Notes

Introduction

1. *New York Times*/CBS News poll (Storrs, Conn.: The Roper Center), 8 January 1992.

2. Robert J. Blendon, Jennifer N. Edwards, and Andrew L. Hyams, "Making the Critical Choices," *Journal of the American Medical Association* 267, no. 18 (13 May 1992): 2509–20.

3. Some states do provide limited medical coverage for extremely poor single adults, though they receive no federal matching money for it. Illinois had such a program, called General Assistance Medical, until July 1992, when it was eliminated because of a state budget shortfall.

4. Merrill Goozner, "Clout Lets Some Cut Health Bills," *Chicago Tribune*, 9 July 1991, p. 1.

5. American Cancer Society, *Cancer Facts and Figures for Minority Americans*, 1991, pp. 6–7. Sixty-eight percent of white women survive for five years after a diagnosis of cervical cancer, compared to 61.6 percent of black women. This difference suggests that black women are diagnosed with cancer at more advanced stages of disease than are white women, and receive less aggressive treatment. The cervical cancer mortality rate for black women is 8.7 per 100,000; for whites, the rate is 3.2 per 100,000.

Chapter One

1. Chicago and Cook County Health Care Summit, *Chicago and Cook County Health Care Action Plan: System Analysis and Design* (April 1990), ambulatory care chapter, p. 46.

2. Nicholas Lemann, "The Origins of the Underclass," *Atlantic Monthly*, June 1986, p. 36.

3. Chicago Park District and Chicago Public Library, special collections, *A Breath of Fresh Air: Chicago's Neighborhood Parks of the Progressive Reform Era, 1900–1925* (1989), p. 21.

NOTES TO PAGES 16–28

4. The Rev. Michael Doyle's description of depressed South Camden, New Jersey, was included in an article by Wayne King, "Saving an Urban Wasteland," *New York Times*, 16 August 1991, p. B-2.

5. Chicago Department of Planning, *U.S. Census of Chicago: Race and Latino Statistics for Census Tracts Community Areas and City Wards: 1980, 1990* (February 1991), p. 71.

6. *Chicago Tribune* staff, *The American Millstone* (Chicago: Contemporary Books, 1986), p. 96.

7. Personal communication with Marie Bousfield, demographer for the Chicago Department of Planning, 1991. Figure based on calculations from the 1990 U.S. Census.

8. Thomas Bonner, *Medicine in Chicago 1850–1950* (Urbana: University of Illinois Press, 1991), pp. 20–21.

9. *Chicago Tribune* staff, *The American Millstone*, p. 258.

10. Chicago and Cook County Health Care Summit, Chicago and Cook County Health Care Action Plan, draft appendix, communities in need, pp. 1 and 4.

11. Chicago and Cook County Health Care Summit, Chicago and Cook County Health Care Action Plan, draft appendix, pp. 1 and 4.

12. Chicago Department of Health, *Communities Empowered to Prevent Alcohol and Drug Abuse Citywide Needs Assessment Report*, working draft (December 1991), appendix c, p. 71.

13. Colin McCord and Harold P. Freeman, "Excess Mortality in Harlem," *New England Journal of Medicine* 322, no. 3 (18 January 1990): 173–77.

14. Elisabeth Rosenthal, "Health Problems of Inner City Poor Reach Crisis Point," *New York Times*, 24 December 1990, p. 9.

15. Personal communication with Thomas Dunn, National Center for Health Statistics, vital statistics branch, January 1993.

16. Ibid.

17. Personal communication with Robert Armstrong, actuarial advisor, Division of Vital Statistics, National Center for Health Statistics, March 1993.

Chapter Two

1. Chicago Transit Authority, on-time performance of CTA Special Services transportation companies 1989–1991, obtained through a Freedom of Information Act request, December 1991.

2. Renal Network of Illinois, "Chicago Dialysis Population: Race within Age," special data run obtained through a Freedom of Information Act request, July 1989.

3. Committee for the Study of the Medicare ESRD Program, Institute of

Medicine, prepublication copy, *Kidney Failure and the Federal Government* (Washington, D.C.: National Academy Press, 1991), p. 122.

4. National Center for Health Statistics, "Advanced Report of Final Mortality Statistics, 1989," in *Monthly Vital Statistics* 40, no. 8, suppl. 2 (Hyattsville, Md.: Public Health Service, 1992). The 1989 age-adjusted stroke rate for whites was 25.9 per 100,000 population, for blacks, 49.0 per 100,000.

5. Elijah Saunders, "Epidemiologic Factors in the Management of Hypertension," *Journal of the National Medical Association* 81, suppl. (April 1989): 9. The excess death rate is the number of deaths minorities would not have suffered had they died at the same rate as whites.

6. Renal Network of Illinois, "Chicago Dialysis Population: Race within Age within Zip Code, Diagnosis Hypertension," special data run obtained through Freedom of Information Act request, July 1989.

7. Committee for the Study of the Medicare ESRD Program, *Kidney Failure and the Federal Government*, p. 126.

8. D.R. Levy, "White Doctors and Black Patients: Influence of Race on the Doctor-Patient Relationship," *Pediatrics* 75, no. 4 (April 1985): 639–43.

9. Robert J. Blendon et al., "Access to Medical Care for Black and White Americans," *Journal of the American Medical Association* 261, no. 2 (13 January 1989): 278–81.

10. In 1991, 35,445,000 people were uninsured. Personal communication with Shirley Smith, Income Branch, Housing, Household, and Economic Statistics, U.S. Bureau of Census, 1993.

11. Larry R. Churchill, *Rationing Health Care in America* (Notre Dame, Ind.: University of Notre Dame Press, 1987), p. 14.

12. Medicare reimburses the average dialysis facility at a rate of $125 per treatment, but Neomedica gets a little more because of Chicago's relatively high wage-scale. Medicare only pays 80 percent of that rate; the secondary insurers—Medicaid, private insurance companies, and the special state plan—make up the difference.

13. Matthew Purdy, "Dialysis: The Profit Machine," *Philadelphia Inquirer*, reprint of series, 1988, p. 2. Bernadette Shoemaker, a federal official who oversees Medicare's End Stage Renal Disease Program, told Purdy: "We don't ask questions about how [dialysis clinics] parcel out that amount of money. We pay the [money]. It's up to the [clinics] to divvy up the amount."

14. Dr. Lang's financial interest in Neomedica was included in the Medicare cost reports Neomedica filed with Blue Cross and Blue Shield of Illinois for fiscal 1990. Judging from cost reports filed in 1988 and 1989, his percentage of the business seems to change slightly from year to year, as medical directors at other units are brought into the company.

15. Dun & Bradstreet, Inc., credit report for Neomedica, 30 June 1990.

16. Neomedica's Medicare cost reports, filed with Blue Cross and Blue Shield of Illinois for fiscal 1989.

17. In a 1992 interview, Dr. Lang told me he received the monthly Medicare payment for forty-five to fifty dialysis patients.

18. To arrive at the $100,000 estimate of Dr. Lang's payments from Medicare for outpatient dialysis at Neomedica, I multiplied the number of patients for which he said he received the monthly Medicare fee—45 to 50—by the average monthly payment per patient, $173, according to *Kidney Failure and the Federal Government*. For 45 patients, at $173 per patient per month, Dr. Lang would earn $93,420 annually from Medicare. For 50 patients at the same rate, he would earn $103,800.

19. Gordon R. Lang and Angelika Lang v. Commissioner of Internal Revenue, filed 20 August 1991.

20. Another reason Congress easily voted to extend Medicare to kidney patients was that, at the time, many lawmakers believed national health insurance was imminent, and so providing government coverage to a new group of people simply seemed the first step along this path.

21. Purdy, "Dialysis: The Profit Machine," *Philadelphia Inquirer*, p. 2.

22. End Stage Renal Disease Network Coordinating Council No. 15 (now the Renal Network of Illinois), *Rehabilitation Status of ESRD Patients in Network 15*, November 1985, p. 9.

23. In fiscal 1989, the Illinois Department of Rehabilitation Services found jobs for only thirteen of twenty-three clients on dialysis. In contrast, the agency rehabilitated 84 percent of 652 deaf clients that year and 77 percent of 709 blind clients. Personal communication with Lisa Wolfe, public information officer, Illinois Department of Rehabilitation Services, 1989.

24. A drug called erythropoietin was introduced in mid-1989 to treat dialysis-induced anemia. Neomedica did not start using it until the end of that year, when payment from Medicare for the drug was assured. Robert did not feel the drug increased his energy level much, although other patients reportedly have been helped quite a bit by EPO.

25. End Stage Renal Disease Network, *Rehabilitation Status of ESRD Patients in Network 15*, p. 9.

26. Clinics located in suburban Cook and DuPage counties have slightly more patients on home-dialysis than those in Chicago. Overall, 9 percent of Chicago blacks versus 14 percent of whites dialyze at home. Renal Network of Illinois, "Chicago Dialysis Population: Race within Age, Setting Home," special data run obtained through Freedom of Information Act request, July 1989.

27. U.S. Department of Labor, Bureau of Labor Statistics, *Geographic Profiles of Employment and Unemployment, 1991* (Washington, D.C.: U.S. Government Printing Office, 1992), table 23.

28. Personal communication with Cheryl Anderson, quality assurance co-ordinator, Renal Network of Illinois, 1991.

29. Dr. Alan Kanter, president of North Central Dialysis Centers, which has four units in Chicago, blamed declining Medicare rates for transforming social workers into glorified insurance clerks. Social workers "increasingly are responsible for obtaining and maintaining insurance information. This latter activity, so necessary for NCDC's fiscal health, is a sad waste of their professional skills." Committee for the Study of the Medicare ESRD Program, *Kidney Failure and the Federal Government*, p. 258.

30. Renal Network of Illinois, "Staffing Patterns among Dialysis Social Workers in Network 10," 1991, p. 8.

31. The more generous payments of private insurers may not entirely explain why patients at Highland Park get more one-on-one medical attention, not to mention soup and crackers. Unlike Neomedica, Highland Park is a nonprofit operation, meaning that any money left over after the bills are paid is pumped back into the clinic. Most dialysis units are for-profit businesses owned by physicians and others who expect returns on their investments.

Chapter Three

1. Martin Ruther and Charles Helbing, "Health Care Financing Trends: Use and Cost of Home Health Agency Services under Medicare," *Health Care Financing Review* 10, no. 1 (Fall 1988): 105.

2. Committee on Ways and Means, U.S. House of Representatives, *1991 Green Book* (Washington, D.C.: U.S. Government Printing Office, 1991), p. 133.

3. Personal communication with public information office, U.S. Department of Agriculture. The federal poverty level for a family of one in 1991 was $6,620; in 1989, it was $5,980.

4. Philip J. Hilts, "Millions of Elderly Poor Paying Too Much for Medicare Coverage," *New York Times*, 18 June 1991, p. 1.

5. Committee on a National Agenda for the Prevention of Disabilities, Institute of Medicine, *Disability in America: Toward a National Agenda for Prevention* (Washington, D.C.: National Academy Press, 1991), p. 227.

6. The medically needy level in 1989 was set by the Illinois Department of Public Aid at $3,204 a year for a single person. The department does not count $25 of each client's monthly income, so that brings the amount of income an individual can earn before going into the spend-down program up to $3,504 a year, or $292 a month. The 1992 medically needy

level was raised slightly to $308 a month, which includes the $25 disregard.

7. Personal communication with Dean Schott, public information officer for the Illinois Department of Public Aid, 1990. Number of spend-down clients was for January 1990.

8. I reviewed Mrs. Jackson's Illinois Department of Public Aid file at the agency's Western field office, 3910 W. Ogden Avenue.

9. Committee for the Study of the Future of Public Health, Institute of Medicine, *The Future of Public Health* (Washington, D.C.: National Academy Press, 1988), p. 10.

10. Though all U.S. citizens age 65 and older are eligible for Medicare, those who do not qualify for Social Security retirement benefits can only get it if they pay special premiums, $156 a month in 1989.

11. Steffie Woolhandler and David U. Himmelstein, "The Deteriorating Administrative Efficiency of the U.S. Health Care System," *New England Journal of Medicine* 324, no. 18 (2 May 1991): 1253–58.

12. As of October 1990, the federal government required all states to provide AFDC for one year to two-parent families in which the main breadwinner is unemployed. The families also receive Medicaid coverage for six of the twelve months that they are eligible for the program, called AFDC-Unemployed Parent. The program rules are quite tight, however, and AFDC-UP recipients comprise only a small portion of total AFDC enrollment. In Illinois, the 10,619 families receiving AFDC-UP in fiscal 1991 made up 4.6 percent of the total AFDC families in the state.

Some states sponsor their own medical programs for absolutely destitute single adults. Illinois had such a program, called General Assistance, but it was eliminated in July 1992.

13. Peter Ries, "Characteristics of Persons with and without Health Care Coverage: United States, 1989," *Advance Data*, no. 201 (18 June 1991), p. 7.

14. The Robert Wood Johnson Foundation, *Special Report, Access to Health Care in the United States: Results of a 1986 Survey* (Princeton, N.J.: The Robert Wood Johnson Foundation, 1987), pp. 3–10; Joel S. Weissman et al., "Delayed Access to Health Care: Risk Factors, Reasons and Consequences," *Annals of Internal Medicine* 114, no. 4 (15 February 1991): 325–30; Mark B. Wenneker, Joel S. Weissman, and Arnold M. Epstein, "The Association of Payer with Utilization of Cardiac Procedures in Massachusetts," *Journal of the American Medical Association* 264, no. 10 (12 September 1990): 1255–60; Paula A. Braveman et al., "Differences in Hospital Resource Allocation among Sick Newborns According to Insurance Coverage," *Journal of the American Medical Association* 266, no. 23 (18 December 1991): 3300–08; E.R. Greenberg et al., "Social and Economic Factors in the Choice of Lung Cancer Treatment," *New England Journal of Medicine* (10 March 1988): 612–17.

Chapter Four

1. Randi S. Most and Pomeroy Sinnock, "The Epidemiology of Lower Extremity Amputations in Diabetic Individuals," *Diabetes Care* 6, no. 1 (January/February 1983): 87.

2. National Center for Health Statistics, *Health, United States, 1990* (Hyattsville: Public Health Service, 1991), p. 139. In 1964, 42 percent of blacks but only 32 percent of whites had not seen a doctor in the past year. In 1989, the comparable figures were 23 percent and 22 percent. In 1964, 41 percent of people in families with incomes under $14,000 had not seen a doctor in the past year, compared to 26 percent of people in families with incomes greater than $50,000. In 1989, the comparable figures were 24 percent and 18 percent.

3. The Robert Wood Johnson Foundation, *Special Report 1986.*

4. National Center for Health Statistics, *Health, United States, 1990,* p. 137.

5. Emily J. Goodwin et al., "Access to Health Care: Medicare and the Poor Elderly," in *Poverty and Health in the United States,* ed. Melvin I. Krasner (New York: United Hospital Fund, 1989), p. 124.

6. I reviewed all available inpatient and outpatient medical records for Mrs. Jackson kept at Mount Sinai Hospital. The chronology of her experience on Coumadin is based on those records, as well as interviews with several physicians who participated in her care.

7. Mount Sinai home health nurses write progress notes each time they visit a patient; I reviewed Mrs. Jackson's notes.

8. Sandy Lutz, "Home Care's Growth Hinges on Winning over Physicians," *Modern Healthcare,* 29 September 1989, pp. 20–22.

9. William H. Herman et al., "Diabetes Mellitus," in *Closing the Gap: The Burden of Unnecessary Illness,* ed. Robert W. Amler and H. Bruce Dull (New York: Oxford University Press, 1987), p. 72.

10. Maureen I. Harris, "Non-Insulin Dependent Diabetes Mellitus in Black and White Americans," *Diabetes/Metabolism Reviews* 6, no. 2 (1990): 71–90.

11. Ibid.

12. Goodwin, "Access to Health Care: Medicare and the Poor Elderly," pp. 111–12.

13. Letter to Hector Marino, M.D., from Mabel Patterson, manager, Health Care Standards Section, Bureau of Medical Quality Assurance, Illinois Department of Public Aid, 11 December 1991. Letter included findings of peer review and informed Dr. Marino that he would be placed on "continuous monitoring status."

NOTES TO PAGES 72–94

14. Physician peer review data obtained through Freedom of Information Act request to Illinois Department of Public Aid, 24 March 1992.

15. Physician financial data obtained through Freedom of Information Act request, 24 March 1992.

16. James W. Fossett et al., *Medicaid Patients' Access to Office-Based Obstetricians* (Chicago: The Institute of Government and Public Affairs, 1989), p. 5.

Chapter Five

1. As of July 1992, Mount Sinai and Schwab stopped sharing board members and staff, although they remain affiliates.

2. Mount Sinai Hospital Medical Centers, Minutes of Meeting of Board of Trustees, 2 November 1988, pp. 9–10.

3. Medicare rules, for example, do not require rehab facilities to provide psychological services, though most do.

4. Judith R. Lave and Howard H. Goldman, "Medicare Financing for Mental Health Care," *Health Affairs* 9, no. 1 (Spring 1990): 19–30.

5. *Physicians' Desk Reference* 46 (Montvale, N.J.: Medical Economics Data, 1992), pp. 1404–5.

6. Emily Mumford et al., "A New Look at Evidence about Reduced Cost of Medical Utilization Following Mental Health Treatment," *American Journal of Psychiatry* 141, no. 10 (October 1984): 1145–58. The study used a technique called meta-analysis to summarize fifty-eight reports on how the use of outpatient mental health services affects the use of medical services.

7. Committee on Health Promotion and Disability Prevention, *The Second Fifty Years: Promoting Health and Preventing Disability* (Washington, D.C.: National Academy Press, 1990), p. 206.

8. Cash grants were eliminated as an option from the Circuit Breaker program in spring 1992. In addition, pharmaceutical cards must now be purchased; the cost is $40 to people below the poverty level, $80 to people above it, such as Mrs. Jackson. In addition, the program now has an $800 cap, after which the state will pay for only 80 percent of medication costs.

9. Older Women's League, *Failing America's Caregivers* (Washington, D.C.: Older Women's League, 1989), p. 3.

Chapter Six

1. Mount Sinai Hospital, *Mount Sinai Hospital Medical Center and the State of Illinois: Safeguarding the Future of the Community*, 1991, p. 13. The hospital's daily census in fiscal 1991 was more than 81 percent.

2. Personal communication with Dr. Karen O'Mara, Mount Sinai's director of emergency medicine.

3. Various studies peg the average loss for Chicago Level One trauma patients as between $3,389 and $6,000. Chicago and Cook County Health Care Summit, *Chicago and Cook County Health Care Action Plan: System Analysis and Design,* trauma section, p. 5.

4. Personal communication with Charles Weis, Mount Sinai's chief financial officer.

5. Chicago and Cook County Health Care Summit, *Chicago and Cook County Health Care Action Plan: System Analysis and Design,* ambulatory care chapter, p. 45.

6. See, for example, Gregg A. Pane, "Health Care Access Problems of Medically Indigent Emergency Department Walk-in Patients," *Annals of Emergency Medicine* 20, no. 7 (July 1991): 730–33.

7. Robert J. Rydman and Ross H. Mullner, *Medicaid Reimbursed Hospital Ambulatory Health Care,* unpublished report for the Illinois Department of Public Aid, 1988, pp. 3–12.

8. Illinois Department of Public Aid, "Waiver Application to the Health Care Financing Administration for Medicaid Partnerships," submitted July 1990, p. 11.

9. At least 15 percent of the population in North Lawndale and four contiguous West Side communities is uninsured. That group receives less than half the primary care of the average American. *Chicago and Cook County Health Care Action Plan: System Analysis and Design,* ambulatory care chapter, p. 46.

10. *Emergency Department Overcrowding Project* (Chicago: Roosevelt University Institute for Metropolitan Affairs, 1992), pp. 7–22.

11. One of the closed community health centers, Mile Square Health Center, reopened one of its three sites in late 1990, but as of 1991, the clinic was underutilized, struggling to attract back patients.

12. Arsenio Oloroso, "Traumatic Tale: ER Costs," *Crain's Chicago Business,* 19 February 1990, p. 1.

13. Personal communication with Charles Weis. In 1992, the nursing shortage at Mount Sinai diminished as the hospital successfully recruited nurses, many from the Philippines.

14. *Emergency Room Hospital Survey, Midnight, Tuesday, 10 January 1989* (New York: New York State Department of Health, Office of Health Systems Management, 1989).

15. Personal communication with Melvin I. Krasner, senior director of research for the United Hospital Fund of New York, March 1993.

16. Emergency Medical Services Commission of Metropolitan Chicago and the Illinois Department of Public Health, "Survey on ED Overcrowding and Supplement for Trauma Centers," January 1992.

17. Ronda Kotelchuck, "Down and Out in the 'New Calcutta': New

York City's Health Care Crisis," *Health/PAC Bulletin* 19, no. 2 (Summer 1989): 8.

18. Kotelchuck, "Down and Out in the 'New Calcutta'," p. 10.

19. William Recktenwald, "City's Top Crime Rates Still Haunt Poor Areas," *Chicago Tribune,* 15 April 1991, p. 1.

20. *Chicago Tribune* staff, *The American Millstone,* p. 53.

21. U.S. General Accounting Office, *Trauma Care: Lifesaving System Threatened by Unreimbursed Costs and Other Factors* (Washington, D.C.: U.S. General Accounting Office, 1991), p. 27.

22. Nancy Gibbs, "Do You Want to Die?" *Time,* 28 May 1990, p. 65.

23. As part of the state's budget-tightening, General Assistance recipients, single adults who receive small monthly cash grants, lost hospital coverage in July 1991. (They still got Medicaid cards to cover outpatient care.) The Illinois Department of Public Aid instead agreed to pay hospitals a lump sum based on the amount of uncompensated care they delivered annually, with the tacit understanding that hospitals would not turn away patients formerly covered under the GA medical program. The budget got still tighter in July 1992, and the state eliminated the General Assistance program altogether, which ended both cash grants and the remaining medical coverage.

24. Oloroso, "Traumatic Tale," p. 1.

Chapter Seven

1. Oloroso, "Traumatic Tale," p. 1.

2. Rosemary Stevens, *In Sickness and in Wealth: American Hospitals in the Twentieth Century* (New York: Basic Books, 1989), p. 314.

3. Sarah Gordon, *All Our Lives: A Centennial History of Michael Reese Hospital and Medical Center* (Chicago: Michael Reese Hospital and Medical Center, 1981), p. 9.

4. Stevens, *In Sickness and in Wealth,* p. 24.

5. National Conference of Jewish Charities, "Chicago Survey of Jewish Charities," 1919.

6. Letter from Morris Kurtzon, president of the board of Mount Sinai Hospital, to Samuel A. Goldsmith, executive director of the Jewish Charities of Chicago, 5 June 1939.

7. Memo from Samuel A. Goldsmith to members of the Jewish Charities of Chicago's Medical Care Sub-Committee, 25 July 1940.

8. Letter from Samuel A. Goldsmith to Frank L. Sulzberger, 23 July 1940.

9. Minutes from 30 March 1939, Medical Care Subcommittee meeting,

Jewish Charities, citing service and pay days for both hospitals from 1 January 1938 through 28 February 1939.

10. Stevens, *In Sickness and in Wealth*, p. 112.

11. The Charities resisted the building of the Nurses' Home as strenuously as the five-story expansion. See "Report of the Medical Care Committee to the Board of Directors," 29 November 1943.

12. Stephen Manheimer, "Mount Sinai Hospital Then and Now: 1919–1949," *Today* (Chicago: Mount Sinai Hospital, January 1950), p. 4.

13. Stevens, *In Sickness and in Wealth*, pp. 6 and 7.

14. Letter from Edward Katzinger to Lewis H. Cahn, 15 June 1922.

15. A graph of Jewish admissions to Mount Sinai and Michael Reese, 1935 to 1963, was prepared for the Jewish Federation by the consulting firm, Booz, Allen & Hamilton in 1963 or 1964.

16. "Negro" admissions were tabulated by Mount Sinai for the Federation until 1963, according to a memo from Federation staffer Saul Kaplan to Federation executive director James P. Rice, 13 June 1974. The practice may have ceased because of worry about appearances of overt racial discrimination. Nonetheless, Kaplan's memo, other documents, and interviews with Federation officials and board members indicate that concern about the large number of black patients versus an increasingly small number of Jews continued until at least the mid-1970s.

17. "Committee of Racial Equality Action Pamphlet," testimony of Pauline Mathewson, 1947.

18. "Committee of Racial Equality Action Pamphlet," testimony of Margaret I. Alton, 1947.

19. Louise Stephens, "Hospital Plan Fails for 50,000 Negroes," *Chicago Defender*, 14 November 1948, p. 1.

20. Ibid.

21. Chicago Commission on Human Relations, "Mount Sinai Admissions and Segregation," 24 September 1957, pp. 1–5.

22. Ibid.

23. Patricia Anstett, "Is Presbyterian-St. Luke's Doing Poorly by the Poor?" *Chicago Sun-Times*, 11 June 1973, pullout section two, p. 1.

24. Nicholas Lemann, *The Promised Land: The Great Black Migration and How It Changed America* (New York: Alfred A. Knopf, Inc., 1991), p. 81.

25. Lemann, *The Promised Land*, p. 82.

26. E.D. Rosenfeld, *Survey and Report: An Outline of a Master Program of Expansion, Modernization and Renovation for the Mount Sinai Hospital of Chicago* (New York: E.D. Rosenfeld, M.D. & Associates, 1961), p. 14.

27. In an interview, Abram Davis, president of the Jewish Federation from 1965 to 1967, said that the eventual secondary role of Mount Sinai was well understood by everyone involved in the failed merger.

28. David K. Fremon, *Chicago Politics Ward by Ward* (Bloomington, Ind.: Indiana University Press, 1988), p. 158.

29. See, for example, Mount Sinai's application for the Foster G. McGaw Prize Program, 10 December 1987.

30. Mount Sinai Hospital Medical Center of Chicago, Minutes of Meeting of Board of Directors, 2 May 1973, p. 2.

31. Personal communication with DePaul University geography professor Donald Dewey, author of *Where the Doctors Have Gone*, a 1973 report on physician supply for the Chicago Regional Hospital Study.

32. "Chicago Hospital Bets on Group Practices to Win Doctors, Cash and Community," *Modern Hospital*, August 1972, 22–24.

33. Judy Nicol, "Mt. Sinai Closing Outpatient Clinic," *Chicago Sun Times*, 27 June 1972, p. 10.

34. Ibid.

35. Robert L. Schiff et al., "Transfers to a Public Hospital," *New England Journal of Medicine* 314, no. 9 (27 February 1986): 552–57. The authors prospectively reviewed 467 medical and surgical patients transferred to Cook County Hospital from emergency rooms at other Chicago hospitals. Eighty-seven percent were transferred because they lacked adequate insurance coverage, and 89 percent were black or Hispanic.

36. Alan P. Henry, "Hospitals Dumping Poor Here: County," *Chicago Sun Times*, 20 September 1981, p. 8.

37. Rush-Presbyterian-St. Luke's Medical Center, *A Report of Stewardship*, annual report, 1977, pp. 2, 7, and 9.

38. Fifty-three percent of Rush's patients were commercially insured in 1988; 30 percent were covered by Medicare and 15 percent by Medicaid. Chicago and Cook County Health Summit, Chicago and Cook County Health Care Action Plan, draft appendix, hospital utilization profiles, p. 31.

39. Mount Sinai, Minutes of Meeting of Board of Directors, 3 October 1973, p. 5.

40. "Mt. Sinai Halts Medicaid," *Chicago Defender*, 9 March 1976, p. 3.

41. Mount Sinai, Minutes of Meeting of Board of Directors, 3 March 1976, p. 4.

42. Ronald Kotulak, "Thirteen City Hospitals Face Fiscal Crisis, 8 May Close Doors," *Chicago Tribune*, 30 January 1977, p. 1.

43. Mount Sinai, Minutes of Meeting of Board of Trustees (formerly Board of Directors), 7 September 1977, p. 4.

44. Mount Sinai, Minutes of Meeting of Board of Trustees, 3 September 1980, p. 3.

45. Mount Sinai, Minutes of Meeting of Board of Trustees, 6 January 1982.

46. Mount Sinai, Minutes of Meeting of Board of Trustees, 5 May 1982, p. 3.

47. Mount Sinai, Minutes of Meeting of Board of Trustees, 6 February 1985, p. 4. Only 62 percent of the beds Mount Sinai still had in service were filled during a six-month period ending 31 December 1984. In addition to Mount Sinai's unique problems, the hospital's patient census was affected by large, nationwide trends, such as the vastly increased use of outpatient surgery.

48. Mount Sinai Hospital Medical Center, *Novel Exposures*, annual report, 1986, p. 1.

49. Lisbeth B. Schorr, *Within Our Reach: Breaking the Cycle of Disadvantage* (New York: Anchor Press Doubleday, 1988), p. 117.

50. Personal communication with Jackie Beverly, executive director of the clinics, called Sinai Family Health Centers, 1992.

51. Sixteen hospitals have closed in Chicago since 1985, according to the Illinois Department of Public Health. Nationwide, 247 urban hospitals closed between 1985 and 1990, according to the American Hospital Association Data Center.

52. John Grezenbach and Associates, Inc., *Development Study for Mount Sinai Medical Center*, 1976, pp. 10 and 13.

53. Ibid.

54. "Mount Sinai's Sad Decision," *Chicago Sun Times*, 1 July 1972, p. 29.

Chapter Eight

1. Fiscal 1992 marked the first significant federal funding hike for community health centers, a $65 million increase over the previous year. The National Association of Community Health Centers estimates that the increase will allow fifty community health centers to either open or expand their operations. Still, that is far short of the need, according to the association. In a plan called "Access 2000," the association figured that 3,000 centers (up from 540 today) would be needed by the turn of the century to reach the 30 million Americans with the least access to care.

2. Paul Starr, *The Social Transformation of American Medicine* (New York: Basic Books, 1982), p. 372.

3. Daniel R. Hawkins and Sara Rosenbaum, *Lives in the Balance* (Washington, D.C.: National Association of Community Health Centers, March 1992), pp. 1–42.

4. Louis W. Sullivan, speech before National Medical Association, Internal Medicine Section, Las Vegas, Nevada, 1 August 1990.

5. Louis W. Sullivan, speech before National Medical Association, House of Delegates, Las Vegas, Nevada, 1 August 1990.

6. U.S. Department of Health and Human Services, *Report of the Secretary's Task Force on Black and Minority Health* (Washington, D.C.: U.S. Government Printing Office, 1985), pp. 9–45. I found this observation in an article by Leith Mullings, "Inequality and African-American Health Status: Policies and Prospects," in *Race: Twentieth Century Dilemmas—Twenty-First Century Prognoses*, ed. W. Van Horne (Madison: University of Wisconsin Institute on Race and Ethnicity), p. 170.

7. U.S. General Accounting Office, *Health Insurance Coverage: A Profile of the Uninsured in Selected States* (Washington, D.C.: U.S. General Accounting Office, 1991), p. 41.

8. Daniel Wikler, "Who Should Be Blamed for Being Sick?" *Health Education Quarterly* 14, no. 1 (Spring 1987): 11.

9. Associated Press, "Americans' Diet Still Unhealthy, Survey Finds," *Chicago Tribune*, 4 June 1992, p. 3.

10. Reinhard Priester, "Overview of Individual Responsibility for Health," in *Individual Responsibility for Health*, ed. Reinhard Priester (Minneapolis, Minn.: Center for Biomedical Ethics, 1991), p. 3.

11. Robert M. Veatch, "Voluntary Risks to Health," *Journal of the American Medical Association* 243, no. 1 (4 January 1980): 50–55.

12. S. Heurtin-Roberts and E. Reisin, "Health Beliefs and Compliance with Prescribed Medication for Hypertension among Black Women—New Orleans, 1985–86," *Morbidity and Mortality Weekly Report* 39, no. 40 (12 October 1990): 701–4.

13. Ibid., p. 702.

14. Eric J. Bailey, "An Ethnomedical Analysis of Hypertension among Detroit Afro-Americans," *Journal of the National Medical Association* 80, no. 10 (October 1988): 1110.

15. Loudell F. Snow, "Traditional Health Benefits and Practices among Lower Class Black Americans," *Western Journal of Medicine* 139, no. 6 (December 1983): 820–28.

16. Loudell F. Snow, "Sorcerers, Saints, and Charlatans: Black Folk Healers in Urban America," *Culture, Medicine and Psychiatry* 2 (March 1978): 60–106.

17. Hypertension Detection and Follow-up Program Cooperative Group, "Educational Level and Five-Year All-Cause Mortality in the Hypertension Detection and Follow-up Program," *Hypertension* 9, no. 6 (June 1987): 641–46.

18. Personal communication with Rose Stamler, professor of community medicine, Northwestern University Medical School, 1989. Stamler is one of the Chicago members of the Hypertension Detection and Follow-up Program Cooperative Group.

19. Hypertension Group, "Educational Level and Five-Year All-Cause Mortality in the Hypertension Detection and Follow-up Program," p. 641.

Chapter Nine

1. U.S. General Accounting Office, *Medicare: Increased Denials of Home Health Claims During 1986 and 1987* (Washington, D.C.: U.S. General Accounting Office, 1990), p. 2.

2. Ibid., p. 43.

3. Duggan v. Bowen, 691 F. Supp. (D.D.C. 1988), p. 1487. Case in U.S. District Court of the District of Columbia. Decision handed down by U.S. District Court Judge Stanley Sporkin on 1 August 1988.

4. "Mount Sinai Hospital Medical Center Home Health Agency: Report for Board of Trustees," 25 April 1990. The agency made 1,207 Medicare-funded visits in July 1989 and 1,644 in March 1990.

5. "Mount Sinai Home Health Agency Summary," February 1989, p. 2.

6. Tish Sommers and Laurie Shields, *Women Take Care: The Consequences of Caregiving in Today's Society* (Gainesville, Fla.: Triad Publishing Company, 1987), pp. 117–18.

7. In Illinois, blacks represented 21 percent of the elderly poor in fiscal 1990 but received only 15 percent of the care provided by the state's Medicaid program (Legal Assistance Foundation of Chicago, "Racial Disparities: Medicaid Coverage for Nursing Home Care," 1992). A similar pattern has been documented in many states, including Florida, Pennsylvania, Texas, and Mississippi. "If nursing home coverage reflected medical need," the Legal Assistance Foundation document said, "blacks would receive a disproportionately higher—not lower—share of total care because blacks' health status is worse than whites."

8. Katharine R. Levit et al., "National Health Expenditures, 1990," *Health Care Financing Review* 13, no. 1 (Fall 1991): 53.

9. Many states have some version of the Community Care Program, but Illinois' is one of the largest.

10. Four months after Jackie cancelled her grandmother's homemaker, the monthly income cutoff for a single person to qualify for a homemaker without a copayment was raised to $498, the federal poverty level for one person. But Mrs. Jackson still would have had to share the homemaker's cost because her income was $100 over that amount.

11. Illinois Department on Aging, *Older Women in Illinois: A Test of Courage* (Springfield, Ill.: Illinois Department on Aging, 1990), p. 5.

12. Sadelle T. Greenblatt and C. Jean Rogers, "Impact of a Fee upon

Utilization of In-Home Services," unpublished paper, 1987, pp. 7, 91, and 92.

13. Nursing home and Community Care Program expenditures were for fiscal 1991, compiled by Illinois Department of Public Aid, Bureau of Management and Budget, 20 August 1991.

14. Carol Kleiman, "Lack of Health-Care Benefits Keeps Low-wage Workers on Welfare's Edge," *Chicago Tribune*, 6 April 1992, section 4, p. 5.

15. Office of the Inspector General, *Home Health Aide Services for Medicare Patients* (Washington, D.C.: Department of Health and Human Services, 1987), pp. 15-17.

16. Middle-class Americans might compare the phenomenon to one that has hit their ranks: "job-lock," where chronically ill workers remain with dead-end jobs because they cannot get health insurance from a new employer. Note that the middle-class problem is not called "dead-end job dependency." Perhaps poor women would get more attention to their plight if they called it "welfare-lock."

17. David T. Ellwood, *Poor Support: Poverty in the American Family* (New York: Basic Books, Inc., 1988), p. 20.

18. Ibid., p. 142.

19. Robin Palley, "Street Beats: Missing the Story," *IRE Journal* (September-October 1991): 9. Quote from Carol Tracy, the former executive director of the Mayor's Commission for Women in Philadelphia.

20. Mount Sinai Home Health Agency Summary, p. 1.

21. Sommers and Shields, *Women Take Care*, p. 45.

22. Dr. Noel List, a geriatrician who practiced at Mount Sinai, pointed out to me that several of the patients on the hospital's geriatric floor were illegally restrained. He subsequently asked the staff to free patients who had been restrained without doctors' orders.

23. Mary S. Harper, "Behavioral, Social and Mental Health Aspects of Home Care for Older Americans," *Home Health Care Services Quarterly* 9, no. 4 (1988): 77.

Chapter Ten

1. Three-quarters of the 1989 cases occurred in children under the age of five, more than 80 percent of whom were overdue for immunizations. Letter from Dr. Walter A. Orenstein, director of the Centers for Disease Control's Division of Immunization Services, to Richard Krieg, then acting commissioner of the Chicago Department of Health, 4 June 1990, p. 2.

2. Chicago Department of Health, *Clinics in Crisis*, September 1989, p. 13. More recent figure, for 1991, is from personal communication with

Steve Ochoa, administrative director for CDOH Bureau of Community Health.

3. Chicago Department of Health, *Clinics in Crisis*, pp. 23–26.

4. Letter from Walter Orenstein, p. 6.

5. Personal communication with Virginia Parker, Chicago Department of Health deputy commissioner, administration.

6. Chicago Department of Health, "Immunization Program Operational Reviews," for seven Neighborhood Health Centers, conducted from September 1990 through January 1991.

7. Letter from Walter Orenstein, p. 6.

8. Chicago Department of Health, "Immunization Program Operational Reviews," West Town Neighborhood Health Center, 16 October 1990; Lakeview Neighborhood Health Center, 26 September 1990; Uptown Neighborhood Health Centers, 18 September 1990.

9. I called each of the clinics in the winter of 1991, asking if I could get a child immunized that day.

10. Alan R. Hinman, "What Will It Take to Fully Protect All American Children with Vaccines?" *American Journal of Diseases of Children* 145, no. 5 (May 1991): 559–62.

11. Letter from Walter Orenstein, p. 4.

12. Hinman, "What Will It Take to Fully Protect All American Children with Vaccines?" pp. 559–60.

13. Physician Payment Review Commission, *Annual Report to Congress* (Washington, D.C.: Physician Payment Review Commission, 1991), p. 290.

14. Personal communication with Candy Masten, supervisor of the Illinois Department of Public Aid's Assistance Support Unit, 1992.

15. Children's Defense Fund, "Analysis of 1989 Legislation," January 1990, table 1.

16. National Vaccine Advisory Committee, *The Measles Epidemic: The Problems, Barriers and Recommendations*, 8 January 1991, p. 8.

17. Personal communication with Diane Hayes, Illinois Department of Public Aid, Medicaid provider services coordinator, winter 1992. She said the card program started sometime in the mid-1980s and did not stop until November 1991.

18. Public Aid stopped sending the useless cards in November 1991, replacing them with another notification program. Mothers now are sent a letter informing them when their children are due for doctors' appointments. Jackie received such a letter in June 1991, advising her that Brianna needed a well-child exam. PLEASE ACT NOW! the letter said. "Please take Brianna Banes to the doctor or dentist for a Healthy Kids medical or dental screening." For the record, Jackie was confused about the letter. She thought

NOTES TO PAGES 174-178

there might be some special Public Aid medical clinic where she had to take Brianna, or that the letter meant she had to take the little girl to the eligibility office on Ogden. She is accustomed to receiving letters from Public Aid that command her to appear at the office; not showing up could mean the loss of her grant and medical card.

19. Health Care Financing Administration, Region V, "Illinois Early and Periodic Screening, Diagnosis and Treatment (EPSDT) Review," June 1986, p. 4. The review stated: "When cards are returned requesting assistance they are batched and entered into the automated system which produces notices to the local offices requiring contact with the recipients requesting the services. All notices to Cook County offices are being suppressed. . . ."

20. Illinois Department of Public Aid, "Healthy Kids Program, Fiscal Year '92 Conditions for the Application."

21. Personal communication with Ben Behrent, an EPSDT supervisor for the Illinois Department of Public Aid, July 1991.

22. Personal communication with Ben Behrent, July 1991.

23. Joseph Tiang-Yau Liu, *Increasing the Proportion of Children Receiving EPSDT Benefits: A South Carolina Case Study* (Washington, D.C.: Children's Defense Fund, 1990), p. 6.

24. Paul Starr, "Health Care for the Poor: The Past Twenty Years," in *Fighting Poverty: What Works and What Doesn't*, ed. Sheldon Danzinger and Daniel H. Weinberg (Cambridge, Mass.: Harvard University Press, 1986), p. 108.

25. House Select Committee on Children, Youth, and Families, *Opportunities for Success: Cost Effective Programs for Children*, 1985, pp. 5–8.

26. American Academy of Pediatrics, "Medicaid State Reports, Fiscal Year 1990," March 1992.

27. U.S. General Accounting Office, *Medicaid Expansions: Coverage Improves but State Fiscal Problems Jeopardize Continued Progress* (Washington, D.C.: General Accounting Office, 1991), p. 4. Data for 1989.

28. Harris Meyer, "Seniors Find Loopholes for Medicaid Nursing Home Coverage," *American Medical News*, 2 December 1991, p. 10.

29. I get a half-dozen notices a year from my veterinarian reminding me about shots and so forth for my cat, Emily.

30. Felicia Lee, "Immunization of Children Is Said to Lag: Third World Rate Seen in the New York Area," *New York Times*, 16 October 1991, p. B1.

31. Chicago Department of Health, "Kindergarten Retrospective Survey," 1990, p. 10. The survey showed that in the ten poor black and Hispanic neighborhoods where the 1989 measles epidemic took its biggest toll, 49 percent of children had been immunized by their second birthdays.

In comparison, 78 percent of the children that age in four white communities had been immunized, and very few got measles.

Chapter Eleven

1. Roger W. Evans, *Executive Summary: The National Cooperative Transplantation Study* (Seattle, Wash.: Battelle-Seattle Research Center, June 1991), pp. C-4 and E-2.

2. See Office of Inspector General, *The Distribution of Organs for Transplantation: Expectations and Practices* (Washington, D.C.: Department of Health and Human Services, August 1990); Philip J. Held et al., "Access to Kidney Transplantation: Has the United States Eliminated Income and Racial Differences?" *Archives of Internal Medicine* 148, no. 12 (December 1988): 2594–600.

3. Based on my analysis of data from the Renal Network of Illinois and the Regional Organ Bank of Illinois. "Blacks Hold Low Card in High Stakes Transplant Game," *Chicago Reporter*, October 1989, p. 5.

4. V.E. Pollack and A. Pesce, "Analysis of Data Related to the 1976–1989 Patient Population: Treatment Characteristics and Patient Outcomes," prepared for the Institute of Medicine (Cincinnati, Ohio: Dialysis Clinic, Inc., 1990).

5. Fred P. Sanfilippo et al., "Factors Affecting the Waiting Time of Cadaveric Kidney Transplant Candidates in the United States," *Journal of the American Medical Association* 267, no. 2 (8 January 1992): 247–52.

6. John F. Kilner, "Selecting Patients When Resources Are Limited: A Study of U.S. Medical Directors," *American Journal of Public Health* 78, no. 2 (February 1988): 144–47.

7. Renee C. Fox and Judith P. Swazey, *The Courage to Fail* (Chicago: The University of Chicago Press, 1974), p. 246.

8. David Sanders and Jesse Dukeminier, Jr., "Medical Advance and Legal Lag," unpublished paper, 1968, pp. 377–78.

9. Carl M. Kjellstrand, "Age, Sex, and Race Inequality in Renal Transplantation," *Archives of Internal Medicine* 148, no. 6 (June 1988): 1309.

10. Abraham, "Blacks Hold Low Card in High Stakes Transplant Game," p. 3.

11. Office of Inspector General, *The Distribution of Organs for Transplantation*, p. 8.

12. Fred P. Sanfilippo, "Factors Affecting the Waiting Time of Cadaveric Kidney Transplant Candidates in the United States," pp. 250–52. This study, conducted after the 1989 change in the UNOS point system, suggested that the shift in emphasis had not been as dramatic as supposed;

blacks continued to wait longer than whites for kidneys, but not much longer than they had before.

13. Paul I. Terasaki et al., "Overview," in *Clinical Transplants*, ed. Paul I. Terasaki (Los Angeles: UCLA Tissue Typing Laboratory, 1988), pp. 409–11.

14. J. Michael Dennis, "The Politics of Kidney Transplantation" (Ph.D. diss., University of Chicago, Department of Political Science, 1992), pp. 159–81.

15. Dennis, "The Politics of Kidney Transplantation," pp. 163–65.

16. Mary Pat Flaherty and Andrew Schneider, "Selling the Gift: Floating Transplant Service," *Pittsburgh Press*, 5 November 1985, p. 6.

17. Dennis, "The Politics of Kidney Transplantation," pp. 169–71.

18. Jeffrey Prottas, "The Structure and Effectiveness of the U.S. Organ Procurement System," *Inquiry* 22, no. 4 (Winter 1985): 365–76.

19. Dennis, "The Politics of Kidney Transplantation," pp. 169–71.

20. Ibid., p. 170.

21. Office of the Inspector General, *The Distribution of Organs for Transplantation*, p. 15.

22. Clive O. Callender et al., "Attitudes among Blacks toward Donating Kidneys for Transplantation: A Pilot Project," *Journal of the National Medical Association* 74, no. 8 (August 1982): 807–9.

23. Personal communication with Dr. Velta Lazda, laboratory medical director, Regional Organ Bank of Illinois, 1992. Data as of the winter of 1992.

24. Office of the Inspector General, *The Distribution of Organs for Transplantation*, p. 11.

25. Personal communication with Lorraine Willmont, public information officer, Regional Organ Bank of Illinois, 1992.

26. Jeffrey Prottas and Helen Levine Batten, "Neurosurgeons and the Supply of Human Organs," *Health Affairs* 8, no. 1 (Spring 1989): 119–31.

27. Personal communication with Dr. Raymond Pollack, chief of the University of Illinois transplant program, 1992. Data for May 1989 to September 1991.

28. American Society of Transplant Surgeons, "Survey on Present Status of Reimbursement for Immunosuppressive Drugs," unpublished paper, 1990.

Chapter Twelve

1. Meg Greenfield, "The Land of the Hospital," *Newsweek*, 30 June 1986, p. 74. Greenfield's comment was noted in this context by David Rothman, *Strangers at the Bedside: A History of How Law and Bioethics Transformed Medical Decision Making* (New York: Basic Books, 1991), p. 127.

2. Rothman, *Strangers at the Bedside,* pp. 127–34.

3. In 1989, blacks represented 13.6 percent of the population between the ages of 20 and 29 but received only 5.3 percent of medical degrees awarded that year. Robert G. Petersdorf et al., "Minorities in Medicine: Past, Present, and Future," *Academic Medicine* 65, no. 11 (November 1990): 663–70.

4. Dr. Robin Powell, an internist who was clinical director of the malaria research during Tommy's incarceration at Stateville, told me in a 1992 phone interview that, indeed, some prisoners in the experiment fed mosquitoes. He, not Tommy, used the phrase "blood meal."

5. Maurice Henry Pappworth, *Human Guinea Pigs: Experimentation on Man* (Boston: Beacon Press, 1967), p. 62.

6. "Volunteers behind Bars," *Time,* 12 July 1963, p. 72.

7. Pappworth, *Human Guinea Pigs,* p. 65.

8. "Drug Tests behind Bars," *Business Week,* 27 June 1964, pp. 58–62.

9. Paul E. Carson, "Prison Project Being Closed: A Lethal Blow to Malaria Research," *Chicago Tribune,* 24 August 1974, p. 10.

10. National Commission for the Protection of Human Subjects of Biomedical and Behavioral Research, *Research Involving Prisoners: Appendix to Report and Recommendations* (Washington, D.C.: Department of Health, Education, and Welfare, 1976), chapter 10, pp. 1–87. A survey of prisoner/subjects' attitudes toward research showed a "near consensus" in favor of it. Close to 200 prisoner/subjects were interviewed at four prisons. Eighty-seven percent said they would be "very willing" to participate in medical research again, and 11 percent said they would be "somewhat willing." Other surveys, the report said, had similar results.

11. National Academy of Sciences, *Experiments and Research with Humans: Values in Conflict* (Washington, D.C.: National Academy of Sciences, 1975), p. 133.

12. Jessica Mitford, *Kind and Usual Punishment* (New York: Alfred A. Knopf, 1973), pp. 144–45.

13. Ibid., p. 163.

14. Robert Hodges and William Bean, "The Use of Prisoners for Medical Research," *Journal of the American Medical Association* 202, no. 6 (6 November 1967): 513–15.

15. History of the experiment based on an account by James Jones, *Bad Blood: The Tuskegee Syphilis Experiment—A Tragedy of Race and Medicine* (New York: The Free Press, 1981).

16. Stephen B. Thomas and Sandra Crouse Quinn, "The Tuskegee Syphilis Study, 1932 to 1972: Implications for HIV Education and AIDS Risk Education Programs in the Black Community," *American Journal of Public Health,* 81, no. 11 (November 1991): 1499.

17. Annette Dula, "Toward an African-American Perspective on Bioethics," *Journal of Health Care for the Poor and Underserved* 2, no. 2 (Fall 1991): 259-69.

18. Thomas, "The Tuskegee Syphilis Study," p. 1499.

19. Ibid., pp. 1502-3.

20. Harlon Dalton, "AIDS in Blackface," *Daedalus* 118, no. 2 (Summer 1989): 223.

21. Henry Locke, "Dead Infants Trigger Probe," *Chicago Defender*, 28 May 1988, p. 1.

22. Sonya Rose, "Doctor in Dilantin Probe Quits," *Chicago Defender*, 6 February 1989, p. 3.

23. Pursuant to a Freedom of Information Act request, I received a letter, dated 16 April 1992, from Ann DuLaney, of the NIH's Office for Protection of Research Risks, that confirmed that Hektoen had a Multiple Project Assurance, but Cook County Hospital, independent of that, did not.

24. Office for Protection from Research Risks, Division of Human Subject Protections, "Findings and Required Actions Regarding Investigation of Noncompliance with HHS Regulations for the Protection of Human Research Subjects Involving the National Institutes of Health Intramural Research Program," 3 July 1991, pp. 6-16.

25. Sonya Rose, "Unauthorized CCH experiments probed," *Chicago Defender*, 18 February 1989, p. 1.

26. See, for example, Council on Ethical and Judicial Affairs, "Black-White Disparities in Health Care," *Journal of the American Medical Association* 263, no. 17 (2 May 1990): 2344-46.

27. Paula Braveman et al., "Differences in Hospital Resource Allocation among Sick Newborns According to Insurance Coverage," *Journal of the American Medical Association* 266, no. 23 (18 December 1991): 3300-8.

28. Dalton, "AIDS in Blackface," p. 223.

Chapter Thirteen

1. See, for example, Susanna E. Bedel and Thomas L. Delbanco, "Choices about Cardiopulmonary Resuscitation in the Hospital: When Do Physicians Talk with Patients?" *New England Journal of Medicine* 310, no. 310 (26 April 1984): 1089-93; Cynthia J. Stolman et al., "Evaluation of Patient, Physician, Nurse, and Family Attitudes toward Do Not Resuscitate Orders," *Archives of Internal Medicine* 150, no. 3 (March 1990): 653-58.

2. Palmi Jonsson, Michael McNamee, and Edward W. Campion, "The 'Do Not Resuscitate' Order: A Profile of Its Changing Use," *Archives of Inter-*

nal Medicine 148, no. 11 (November 1988): 2372–75. The study found that of 100 patients who died with DNR orders, only 14 percent had been consulted about the orders, although 77 percent of their families took part in the decision. "This is partially explained by the fact that the DNR decision appears to be made close to the time of death, when many patients have clouded mental status or are unconscious," the authors wrote.

3. John Edward Ruark and Thomas Alfred Raffin, "Initiating and Withdrawing Life Support," *New England Journal of Medicine* 318, no. 1 (7 January 1988): 27.

4. Alan Meisel, "Legal Myths About Terminating Life Support," *Archives of Internal Medicine* 151, no. 8 (August 1991): 1497–1501. Meisel cites seven such myths that permeate the medical profession and "can lead to tragic results for physicians, health care institutions, patients and families."

5. Mary G. Mussman et al., "Medical Malpractice Claims Filed by Medicaid and Non-Medicaid Recipients in Maryland," *Journal of the American Medical Association* 265, no. 22 (12 June 1991): 2992–94.

6. Cook County State's Attorney's Task Force on the Foregoing of Life-Sustaining Treatment, *Report of the Cook County State's Attorney's Task Force on the Foregoing of Life-Sustaining Treatment*, March 1990, p. 18. The report notes that despite its restrictive ruling in *In Re Dorothy M. Longeway*, the Illinois Supreme Court invited the state legislature to "'streamline, tailor, or overrule the procedures outlined in this opinion.'" The legislature was the best place to resolve right-to-die issues, the court said.

7. Lynn Sweet and Greg Tasker, "House Committee Rejects 'Pull-the-Plug' Proposal," *Chicago Sun-Times*, 7 June 1990, p. 32. Legislation similar to that which was rejected in 1990 was passed a year later. Overturning the earlier decision by the state's high court, the law allows family members, or "surrogate decision makers," to decide to shut off life support without judicial review. It also provides immunity from legal action for doctors and hospitals who follow its provisions.

8. Some of the worry about abandonment undoubtedly stems from physicians' differing interpretations of DNR orders, a situation that has prompted calls for more specificity in the orders. Instead of simply writing "DNR," doctors should specify what, if any, other lifesaving treatments should be withheld, some experts believe. See Richard F. Uhlmann, Christine K. Cassel, and Walter J. McDonald, "Some Treatment-Withholding Implications of No-Code Orders in an Academic Hospital," *Journal of the American Medical Association* 253, no. 1 (4 January 1985): 54–57. This study documented doctors' divergent views about the meaning of the same DNR orders and concluded that the potential for misinterpretation was greatest at large teaching hospitals, such as Mount Sinai, where many doctors and nurses participate in each case.

9. Stuart Youngner, "Do-Not-Resuscitate Orders: No Longer Secret, But Still a Problem," *Hastings Center Report*, February 1987, pp. 28–29.

On the other hand, some doctors and ethicists blame the proliferation of CPR on hospital policies that require *too much* patient and family involvement. They argue that doctors should not have to perform CPR on patients when it is medically futile, even if patients have requested it or the issue has not been discussed. Until about a decade ago, doctors made such decisions on their own. See Elisabeth Rosenthal, "Rules on Reviving the Dying Bring Undue Suffering, Doctors Contend," *New York Times*, 4 October 1990, p. 1.

10. Youngner, "Do-Not-Resuscitate Orders: No Longer Secret," p. 27.

11. *Report of the Cook County State's Attorney's Task Force on the Foregoing of Life Sustaining Treatment*, p. 28.

12. Lane Gerber, *Married to Their Careers* (New York: Tavistock Publications, 1983), p. xiv.

13. Rothman, *Strangers at the Bedside*, p. 131.

14. Ruark and Raffin, "Initiating and Withdrawing Life Support," p. 27.

Chapter Fourteen

1. Donald J. Murphy, "Do-Not-Resuscitate Orders: Time for Reappraisal in Long-term-Care Institutions," *Journal of the American Medical Association* 260, no. 14 (14 October 1988): 2098–2101. A "successful resuscitation" is defined as one in which the patient survives to hospital discharge.

2. Because of the poor outcomes, some doctors believe that the presumption for resuscitation in the chronically ill elderly should be reconsidered. William G. Bartholome, "'Do Not Resuscitate' Orders: Accepting Responsibility," *Archives of Internal Medicine* 148, no. 11 (November 1988): 2345–46. "Increasingly, I have become convinced that we need to think of sick patients in hospitals or nursing homes as being 'at risk' of becoming the unwitting patients (victims?) of 'code blue teams,'" Dr. Bartholome wrote. "Perhaps if we could come to understand that in most tertiary medical centers and nursing homes the only predictably 'good candidates' for the use of CPR techniques are staff and visitors."

3. David Margolick, "Patient's Lawsuit Says Saving Life Ruined It," *New York Times*, 18 March 1990, p. 1. The Cincinnati, Ohio, man lost in the state trial and appeals courts. The case was appealed to the Ohio Supreme Court in December 1992.

4. Lisa Belkin, "In Right-to-Die Fight, Court Finds Family Liable for Care," *New York Times*, 24 September 1992, p. B6.

5. In the two years following Mrs. Jackson's death, new laws gave dying patients more freedom to steer the course of their care, but she may or

may not have benefited from the changes. In its first ruling on the subject, the U.S. Supreme Court in June 1990 affirmed patients' right to refuse life-sustaining treatment. For incompetent patients, however, the court said states could require "clear and convincing evidence" of their prior wishes before life support systems could be refused or removed—a standard that might only be met with a living will or other written proof, documents Mrs. Jackson did not have.

But the Supreme Court opinion only *allowed* states to ask for "clear and convincing" evidence of prior wishes; it did not compel them to adopt that rule. In Illinois and a few other states, legislatures decided to explicitly grant families decision-making power in cases where patients' wishes were not clearly known. Congress also passed the Patient Self-Determination Act, which, starting in December 1991, required hospitals and long-term-care facilities to inform newly admitted patients about their right to refuse life-sustaining treatment. Some observers say that changes such as the Patient Self-Determination Act will not make much difference to the poor. Deborah Pinkney, "Law May Encourage Talk about End-of-Life Care," *American Medical News*, 25 November 1991, p. 1. In this article, Dr. Greg Sachs, of the University of Chicago's Center for Clinical Ethics, called the new law an "upper-middle-class construct." "People who don't have regular access to health care are not going to understand where you're coming from when you start talking about the right to refuse treatment and they don't have the right to access health care," he said.

6. Personal communication with Paul Scaletta, associate administrator for finance at Oak Forest, 1992. Data for 1991.

7. Philip Podrid, "Resuscitation in the Elderly: A Blessing or a Curse?" *Annals of Internal Medicine* 111, no. 3 (1 August 1989): 194. In earlier years, setting such guidelines would have been anathema to the medical profession, which has traditionally resisted what it considered "cookbook medicine." But pressured by insurers to justify their decisions, and embarrassed by large studies that suggest some medical procedures are used inappropriately, doctors' groups, even the conservative American Medical Association, are accepting the idea of guidelines.

8. Personal communication with Charles Weis, chief financial officer, Mount Sinai Hospital, 1990.

9. Personal communication with Lisa O'Toole, public information officer, Oak Forest Hospital, 1992.

10. Personal communication with James Lubitz, chief of the analytical studies branch, Office of Research and Demonstrations, Health Care Financing Administration. The exact figure is 28 percent. This analysis was done with 1978 data, but Lubitz said that preliminary results of a new study indicate that the percentage has not changed appreciably since then. Although

this figure suggests a misallocation of resources, no one knows what the "right" percentage should be. After all, one of the reasons that such a large portion of Medicare money goes to people in their last year of life is that that tends to be when they are sickest. For some patients, that "last year" could have been the year in which they recovered.

11. Personal communication, Office of the Actuary, Health Care Financing Administration, 1992. U.S. health care expenditures totaled $666.2 billion in 1990, the latest year for which figures were available.

12. The starting salary and benefits for a Chicago Department of Health clinic nurse are approximately $37,600. Personal communication with Tim Hadac, public affairs, Chicago Department of Health, March 1993.

13. Chicago Department of Health, *Communities Empowered to Prevent Alcohol and Drug Abuse: Citywide Needs Assessment Report,* December 1991, p. 42. The figures reported were from the 1990 waiting list for outpatient drug treatment kept by the Illinois Department of Alcohol and Substance Abuse (DASA). Citywide, there were 5,871 slots in outpatient drug programs in 1990 and close to 2,000 people waiting for treatment. The cost of outpatient treatment averages $30 an hour, with a minimum of 25 hours needed, according to Tom Green, public affairs, DASA, March 1993.

14. Personal communication with Beverly Biehr, facilitator, Family Life/ AIDS Education, Chicago Public Schools, 1992.

15. Lisa Capitanini, "City Losing Battle Against Epidemic in Black Communities," *Chicago Reporter,* November 1991, p. 1. The report, based on 1990 Chicago Department of Health statistics, found that North Lawndale and twelve other black communities had the highest rates of gonorrhea, syphilis, and chlamydia. In more affluent white areas, only one out of every 2,371 residents contracted an STD in 1990.

16. Personal communication with Ben Squires, program administrator, Families with a Future, Illinois Department of Public Health, 1992. Forty babies died in North Lawndale before reaching their first birthdays in 1990, for an infant mortality rate of 21.6 deaths per 1,000 births. The national infant mortality rate for 1989, the latest year in which figures were available, was 9.8 for all races, 8.1 for whites, and 18.6 for blacks. National Center for Health Statistics, "Advanced Report of Final Mortality Statistics, 1989," *Monthly Vital Statistics Report* 40, no. 8, supp. 2 (Hyattsville, Md.: Public Health Service, 1992).

17. Personal communication with James Long, program coordinator, Illinois Department of Public Health, 1988 data, 1991.

18. Personal communication with Beverly Biehr, facilitator, Family Life/ AIDS Education, Chicago Public Schools, 1992.

19. Ruark and Raffin, "Initiating and Withdrawing Life Support," p. 28.

20. Committee for the Study of the Medicare ESRD Program, *Kidney*

Failure and the Federal Government, pp. 108–12. A fraction of that 27 percent are elderly transplant recipients, not dialysis patients.

21. Kenneth C. Goldberg et al., "Racial and Community Factors Influencing Coronary Artery Bypass Graft Surgery Rates for All 1986 Medicare Patients," *Journal of the American Medical Association* 267, no. 11 (18 March 1992): 1473–77.

22. United Network for Organ Sharing, *Annual U.S. Scientific Registry for Organ Transplantation and the Organ Procurement and Transplantation Network* (Richmond, Va.: United Network for Organ Sharing, 1990), appendix, p. E-V. Thirty-five percent of liver transplant recipients, aged nineteen to forty-four, die within one year after receiving a transplant; the comparable figure for older recipients, aged forty-five to sixty-four, is 35.7 percent.

23. Richard Rettig, "The Politics of Organ Transplantation: A Parable of Our Time," *Journal of Health Politics, Policy and Law* 14, no 1 (Spring 1989): 218.

24. Timothy Egan, "For Oregon's Health Care System, Triage by a Lawmaker with an M.D.," *New York Times,* 9 June 1991, p. 18.

25. The Department of Health and Human Services granted Oregon a waiver to try its plan in March 1993.

26. Rettig, "The Politics of Organ Transplantation," p. 221.

27. *The New Yorker,* "Notes and Comments," 20 April 1992, pp. 29–30.

Chapter Fifteen

1. The Chicago Panel on Public School Policy and Finance, *Chicago Public Schools Databook: School Year 1988–1989,* February 1990, p. 237. The dropout statistics are for 1986.

2. Ibid., pp. 25–27.

3. By 1993, Neomedica had opened two more units in suburban Chicago, bringing the chain up to thirteen sites.

4. Robert Pear, "Darman Forecasts Dire Health Costs," *New York Times,* 17 April 1991, p. 14. President Bush's budget director had projected that health care could reach 37 percent of GNP by 2030.

5. Daniel Callahan, *What Kind of Life* (New York: Simon and Schuster, 1990).

6. Callahan, *What Kind of Life,* p. 148.